Readings in Insect-Plant Disease Relationships

Edited by
J. W. Brewer
M. D. Harrison
Colorado State University

MSS Information Corporation
655 Madison Avenue, New York, N. Y. 10021

This is a custom-made book of readings prepared for the courses taught by the editors, as well as for related courses and for college and university libraries. For information about our program, please write to:

MSS INFORMATION CORPORATION
655 Madison Avenue
New York, New York 10021

MSS wishes to express its appreciation to the authors of the articles in this collection for their cooperation in making their work available in this format.

Library of Congress Cataloging in Publication Data

Brewer, Jesse Wayne, 1940-
    Readings in: insect-plant disease relationships.

    1. Insects as carriers of plant diseases--
Addresses, essays, lectures. I. Harrison, Monty
DeVerl, 1934-   joint comp. II. Title.
III. Title: Insect-plant disease relationships.
SB931.B684   632'.7'08   72-10029
ISBN 0-8422-5071-9
ISBN 0-8422-0264-1 (pbk)

CONTENTS

INTRODUCTION TO SECTION I:
THE INTERRELATIONSHIPS OF INSECTS AND PLANTS

This collection of papers is concerned primarily
with insect-plant disease relationships. We feel, however, that it is first necessary to consider some of the
general associations between insects and plants. Leach,
in his book on Insect Transmission of Plant Diseases,
classified these numerous associations into the following
six basic groups:

1. Insects that feed upon plants (phytophagous
    insects)

2. Plants that feed upon insects (entomophagous
    plants)

3. Plants that cause diseases of insects (ento-
    mophthorous plants)

4. Plants that are pollinated by insects (ento-
    mophilous plants)

5. Insects and plants that live in symbiosis

6. Insects that disseminate plant pathogens or aid
    in the development of plant diseases.

Phytophagous insects feed on plants in various ways,
ranging from direct removal of plant tissue by chewing
insects to removal of plant liquids as occurs with

sap-sucking feeders. Although many phytophagous insects have a general association with plants, some form very intimate relationships with their host. The paper on the needle gall midge by Houseweart and Brewer (1972) describes the latter situation.

A few plants have turned the table on insects (in both figurative and literal sense) and have developed the ability to use insects as a food source. These entomophagous plants vary considerably in their approach to capturing insects but one of the most interesting is the Venus fly trap. Jones (1923) presents an excellent discussion of this fascinating plant.

Entomophthorous plants provide one means of natural control for certain insects. The types of plants that cause insect diseases are many and varied but perhaps the fungi are the most interesting. MacLeod's paper (1934) on the genus Empusa describes one of these specialized plant groups.

There are many highly specialized relationships that exist between entomophilous plants and their insect pollinators. One such association is well-illustrated in the paper on pollination of alfalfa and red clover by Bohart (1957).

Perhaps the most highly evolved insect-plant relationship exists when both insect and plant are completely dependent on each other for survival. Such a mutualistic symbiotic relationship exists between insects and several plant groups but one of the most interesting involves the ants that raise fungi as a food source. This relationship is well-presented by Weber (1967) in his discussion of the "Fungus-growing ants".

The various associations that exist between insects and plant pathogens will be covered in the following sections of this collection.

Biology of a Pinyon Spindle Gall Midge
(Diptera: Cecidomyiidae)[1]

MARK W. HOUSEWEART[2] AND J. W. BREWER[3]

Pinyonia edulicola Gagné caused spindle-shaped galls to form at the bases of the needles of *Pinus edulis* (Fig. 1), a popular landscape tree in urban areas of Colorado. After the emergence of this cecidomyiid midge the galls turned brown and dropped off prematurely, thus causing serious defoliation under heavy infestations. Although the spindle-shaped gall has been found in native pinyon stands, it does not occur at the high population levels found in landscape plantings. Perhaps the increased water and nutrients, along with the lack of native predators and parasites in the urban environment, have allowed the midges to become more abundant than was possible in native pinyon stands.

Felt (1940) reported only 1 needle gall on *P. edulis*. However, his description and sketches were quite different from the spindle-shaped gall discussed here. Little (1943) noted a spindle-shaped needle gall on *P. edulis* but gave no further information. Gagné (1970) described the midge that causes this spindle-shaped gall as a new genus and species.

Although *P. edulicola* has been recognized as causing a serious problem on landscape pinyons for several years, its life cycle has not been previously studied. The objective of the research reported here was to learn more about its life history, habits, and ecological relationships.

MATERIALS AND METHODS

The primary study sites were landscape plantings in Fort Collins and a native pinyon stand near Salida, Colo. Other pinyon stands in Colorado were visited to determine the distribution of the gall.

[1] Journal paper no. 1665 of the Colorado State University Experiment Station.
[2] Graduate Research Assistant. Portion of a thesis presented in partial fulfillment of the requirements of the M.S. degree Present address: Texas Forest Service, Pest Control Section, P.O. Box 310, Lutkin 75901.
[3] Assistant Professor.

ANNALS OF THE ENTOMOLOGICAL SOCIETY OF AMERICA, 1972, Vol. 65, pp. 331-336.

Collections were made at the Fort Collins location every 3 days from July 14, 1969, until June 23, 1970, except during emergence periods when collections and observations were made daily.

Emerging adult midges and parasites (*Platygaster* sp.) were collected by placing 8×4×2-in. plastic bags over infested branches. The bags were changed daily and the insects were taken to the laboratory for examination. The midges were sexed and preserved in 70% ethyl alcohol. Parasitic wasps were treated in the same manner except that they were not sexed.

In the laboratory, infested branches were placed in rearing cages made from 3¼×7×2-in. plastic boxes. The period of emergence of both midge sexes as well as that of the wasp parasite was recorded. Parasite oviposition was also observed in the laboratory. Infestation levels were determined by counting the number of galled needles in the current year's growth and computing the percent of needles attacked. Needles on about 125 branches were examined in this manner.

The duration of the egg stage and the number of eggs laid were determined by observation in both the field and laboratory. Maximum egg production was determined by dissecting 100 gravid females. Larval development was studied by making microscope slide preparations of larvae from 10 galls every 3 days throughout the year. The number of larvae per gall and the size of the galls were recorded and used to determine if gall size was related to larval numbers. The gall collections also made it possible to determine the onset and duration of the various life stages of the insect.

Changes in plant tissues caused by gall formation were investigated by studying tissue sections of deformed and normal needles. Microtome sections 10 μ thick were prepared, using standard embedding techniques. The number and size of cells in various tissues were recorded.

An artificial midge infestation was established on pinyon seedlings by releasing midges into an insectary measuring 10×30×10 ft. *Pinus ponderosa* (Laws.) and *Pinus contorta* (Dougl.) seedlings were placed in the insectary to determine if the midge would infest these species as well as *P. edulis*. Ponderosa and lodgepole pine seedlings were also placed in an area of naturally infested pinyons during midge emergence.

The ability of the wasp *Platygaster* sp. to parasitize the midge was studied by collecting adult wasps and caging them over midge-infested needles.

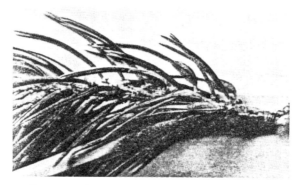

FIG. 1.—Galls on pinyon caused by *P. edulicola.*

The resulting galls were later opened and the number of parasitized and normal midges counted.

RESULTS AND DISCUSSION

Life Stages.—The duration and occurrence of life stages of *P. edulicola* are shown in Fig. 2.

Egg.—The eggs averaged 0.383 long and 0.096 mm wide immediately after being deposited. They were light orange, torpedo-shaped, and had an adhesive substance which stuck them to the outside of the new needles. They were laid longitudinally parallel to the length of the 2 needles in groups of 6 to 12 across the split (Fig. 3). The groups averaged 10.8 eggs (±4.67). Usually only 1 egg group was found on a needle although as many as 3 groups were observed.

The 1st eggs were observed on June 25, 1970, in Fort Collins. Egg laying extended over a period of about 2 weeks. The midges on the lower ⅓ of the tree emerged first and those higher up emerged later. The egg stage lasted 5–9 days.

Larva.—The orange, oblong larvae (Fig. 4 a) had a smooth cuticle and did not appear to possess a spatula. First-stage larvae were observed on June 30, 1970, mid-way down between the 2 needles of a fascicle. Once the larvae reached the base of the needles they started to feed. This feeding seemed to be associated with gall formation since there was no evidence of tissue deformation until the larvae reached the base of the needle. The larvae remained inside the gall throughout the fall and winter.

The changes in larval length throughout the year are shown in Fig. 5. Larval length increased rapidly at first but then decreased over the winter months. Although this may not be an unusual occurrence for

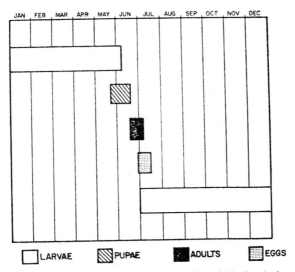

JAN | FEB | MAR | APR | MAY | JUN | JUL | AUG | SEP | OCT | NOV | DEC

▢ LARVAE   ◩ PUPAE   ■ ADULTS   ▨ EGGS

Fig. 2.—Seasonal life history of *P. edulicola* during 1969 and 1970 in Colorado.

overwintering larvae, it is possible that the decrease in length might have been caused in part by unseasonably low temperatures in October. By February and March, larval length began to increase again and during April, May, and early June it increased very rapidly.

Prepupa.—The prepupae were orange with white "heads" (Fig. 4 b). The prepupal stage began when the last larval instar became quiescent and started to form a definite head capsule. At this time the prepupae started to spin or exude a silken, frothy communal pupal case inside the gall (Fig. 4 c).

Pupa.—The onset of the pupal stage varied considerably. In 1969 the 1st pupae were observed in late May, and by mid-June all midges were in this stage. In 1970 this stage occurred about 2 weeks later than in 1969. The pupal stage lasted 2–3 weeks. Early pupae were light orange while the later ones were dark orange to a dull red with black eyes and black wing pads (Fig. 4 d). Just prior to the end of the pupal period the pupae wiggled up between the needles of a fascicle by means of abdominal movements. When they reached the tip of the gall, the dorsal side of the pupal exoskeleton split open and the adult midges crawled free, leaving the pupal cases at the tips of the galls. The adults moved up to the tip of the needles and remained for a few minutes before flight.

Adult.—Emergence of adults started on June 18,

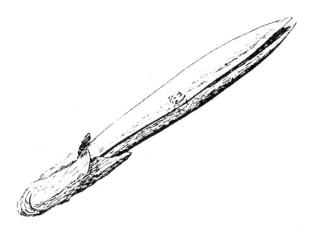

Fig. 3.—Egg group of *P. edulicola* laid across split of *Pinus edulis* needles.

1969, and reached a peak June 23–27. Nearly all midges had emerged by July 10 in all study areas in Fort Collins.

The newly-emerged female midge was larger than the male and had a large dark-orange abdomen filled with eggs (Fig. 6 a). Over the 2-year study, 100 ♀ were dissected. An average of 85.8 eggs/midge was found (±14.51). The female laid eggs parallel to one another in small groups. The groups were then covered with a gluelike substance.

The smaller male had 2 claspers on the tip of the light orange abdomen (Fig. 6 b) making sex identification easy.

Mating was never observed but it was believed to have occurred in flight while the midges swarmed about the trees. Adults were never observed feeding. The sex ratio was about 1:1. Of 3611 midges collected, 1853 were males and 1758 were females. A χ^2 test indicated that these numbers were not significantly different.

Parasites.—The midges were parasitized by a small black wasp of the genus *Platygaster* (Platygasteridae[4]) (Fig. 7 a). The wasp emergence followed that of the midge. The duration of the wasp-emergence period was about 15 days both in 1969 and 1970. Soon after emergence, the wasps oviposited on the midge eggs. The parasites were not visible inside the midge larvae until the midges were well into the pupal stage the following spring. At that time 2 white structures appeared inside the midge exo-

[4] Identified by Lubomir Masner, Entomology Research Institute, Central Experiment Farm, Ottawa, Canada.

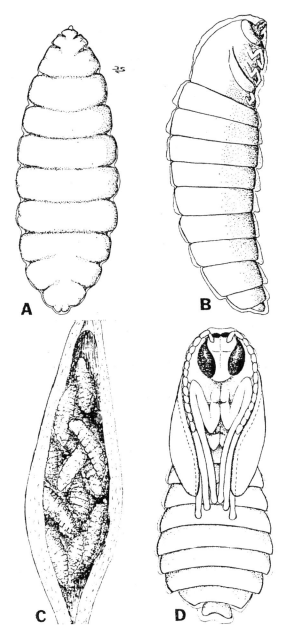

Fig. 4.—*P. edulicola:* (A) Larva; (B) Prepupa; (C) Communal Pupal Case; (D) Pupa.

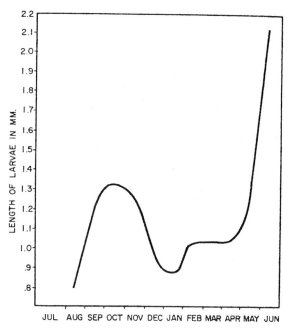

F<small>IG</small>. 5.—Changes in larval length of *P. edulicola* throughout the year.

skeletons. These became black shortly before wasp emergence. The wasps emerged by chewing out the end of the midge exoskeletons. Most frequently there were 2 wasps (headed in opposite directions) per midge exoskeleton, occasionally only 1, but never more than 2. Peak parasite oviposition was observed in the field in 1969 from July 3 to July 9. Wasp oviposition observations in the laboratory and field showed that female wasps searched for and found eggs using their antennae. Beginning at 1 end of an egg group, the wasps, in a straddling position, backed up and inserted their ovipositors into each egg (Fig. 7 b). After the complete group of eggs had been parasitized in this manner, the wasps moved on, apparently searching for another group of eggs. On occasion a wasp was observed to oviposit more than once on the same egg group; however she first left the immediate area in search of other eggs. Likewise, several different wasps repeatedly parasitized a single group of eggs. It appeared that the parasites could not determine whether an egg group had been previously attacked.

In 1969 parasites were introduced into plastic bags and placed on midge-infested needles in the

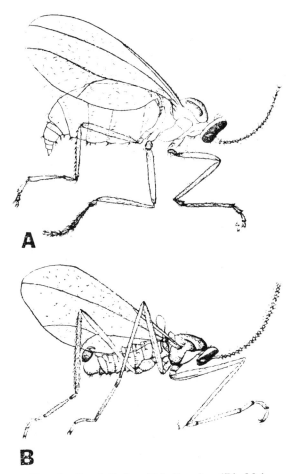

Fig. 6.—*P. edulicola:* (A) Female; (B) Male.

field. The ability of the wasp to parasitize the midge was determined in 1970 by opening the galls which had formed and calculating the percent of parasitized midges. All the midges in these galls had been parasitized; therefore, the wasp was considered to be 100% effective in controlling midges under experimental conditions. Since the wasp did not kill the midges until the gall had already formed, we have some reservations about the true potential of the parasite as a short-term control agent. Nevertheless, a long-term biological control program with these wasps may keep the midge populations reduced.

Emergence Patterns.—Midge emergence started on June 18 and lasted until July 11, while parasite emergence occurred from July 1 to July 14 (Fig. 8).

Peak wasp emergence did not occur until after the midges had oviposited.

Laboratory emergence tests (Fig. 9) showed that on the 1st day of midge emergence there were more female midges than males. More females than males continued to emerge each day until June 19, when the number of emerging males surpassed that of the females. The peak of male emergence occurred after the peak of female.

Host Damage.—During 1969, 1 study site in Fort Collins had 10.5% of the current year's needles attacked. Two trees at another location in Fort Collins had an average of 33.6% of the current year's needles infested in 1969. However, several individual branches had infestation rates ranging from 60 to 79%. The infestation rates were much lower

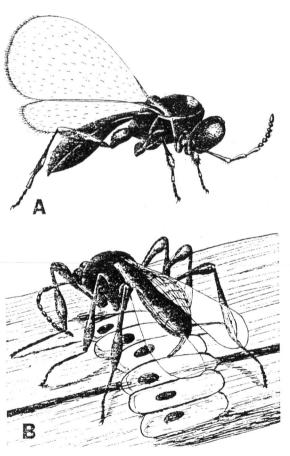

FIG. 7.—*Platygaster* sp. (A) Male; (B) Female ovipositing in eggs of *P. edulicola.*

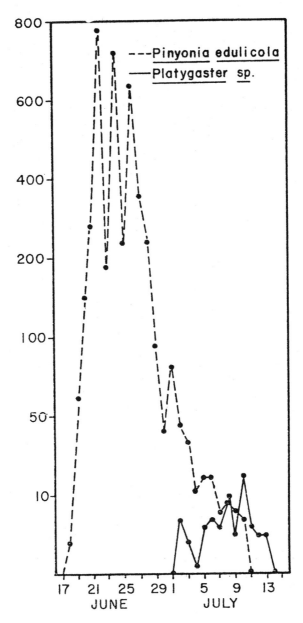

FIG. 8.—Field emergence of *P. edulicola* and *Platygaster* sp. during 1970 in Colorado.

in the native stands near Salida, where there were seldom more than 10–30 galls/tree. Since infested needles dropped shortly after adult emergence, serious defoliation resulted from infestations as high as those found on some trees in Fort Collins. Complete defoliation of a pinyon by this gall midge may be possible.

Host Selection and Distribution.—No galls developed on the *P. ponderosa* or *P. contorta* seedlings in the host-distribution tests. The midges flew around and landed on these trees, but no eggs were observed. A total of 84 galls was found on 11 pinyon seedlings in this test. Therefore, it appears that this midge does not attack these other species, or at least it prefers pinyon. Attempts to establish artificial infestations on pinyon seedlings in small cone cages in the greenhouse were not successful with laboratory-reared midges but were successful with those collected in the field. Collections from several locations in the state have revealed that the spindle gall is present on pinyons near the following cities: Montrose, Salida, Breen, Durango, Mancos, Bayfield, Cortez, Manitou Springs, Denver, and Fort Collins.

Gall Characteristics.—The midges apparently induced gall formation by stimulation of the developing needles. Although the exact source of the stimulus was not found, observations indicated that this was a feeding rather than an oviposition stimulus because the eggs were placed on the needle rather than being inserted into them. Also, the area of needle deformation was generally located some distance from where oviposition occurred.

The considerable variation observed in gall size was thought to be caused by the varying number of larvae found inside the gall. A correlation coefficient (r value) of 0.786 was found between the gall length and number of larvae. A coefficient of 0.511 was found when the gall width was computed against the number of larvae. However, when both variables, length and width, were used together in a stepwise regression the correlation was 0.798. The r^2 value indicated that almost 64% of the variability in gall size could be accounted for by the number of larvae found inside.

When 1050 galls were dissected, the mean length, width, and number of larvae found inside with respective standard deviations were 13.06±2.80, 4.31± 0.75 mm, and 11.78±5.69. In most cases larvae from only 1 egg group apparently caused a particular gall. However, it appeared that very large galls containing 40 or more larvae may have been caused by lar-

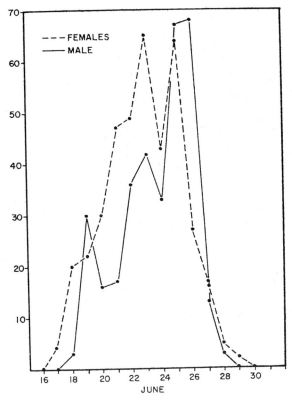

F$_{IG}$. 9.—Laboratory emergence of *P. edulicola* males and females during 1970 in Colorado.

Table 1.—Number of cells from various tissues of normal and deformed (galled) pinyon needles per unit area.

	Needle	Average	S$_D$
Epidermal (10× 0.2 mm)	Normal	11.2	1.35
	Infested	6.2	.42
Parenchyma (10× 0.2 mm)	Normal	4.7	.45
	Infested	3.3	.90
Xylem (45× 0.045 mm)	Normal	5.3	.23
	Infested	4.4	.71

vae from several egg groups acting together to form 1 gall.

Normal and galled needles were sectioned for microscopic examination. The results (Table 1) show that for each type of tissue examined the normal needles had more cells per unit area than the galled needles. This seems to indicate that the cells from the galled tissue were larger, thereby suggesting that the gall was the result of an increase in the cell size (hypertrophy) in the area of deformation.

REFERENCES CITED

Felt, E. P. 1940. Plant Galls and Gall Makers. Hafner Pub. Co., New York. 364 p.

Gagné, R. J. 1970. A new genus and species of Cecidomyiidae on pinyon pine (Diptera). Entomol. News 81: 153–6.

Little, E. L. 1943. Common insects on pinyon (*Pinus edulis*). J. N. Y. Entomol. Soc. 51(4): 239–53.

"The Most Wonderful Plant in the World"

WITH SOME UNPUBLISHED CORRESPONDENCE OF CHARLES DARWIN

By FRANK MORTON JONES

IN 1867 Charles Darwin received a letter from his American correspondent, Asa Gray, enclosing one which Doctor Gray, in turn, had received from William M. Canby, of Wilmington, Delaware. The subject of the Canby letter was the American insectivorous plant, *Dionæa*, Venus's-fly-trap; and Darwin's reply says,[1] "This letter fires me up to complete and publish on *Drosera*, *Dionæa*, etc., but

when I shall get time I know not." Though he had also written,[2] "I care more about *Drosera* than the origin of all the species in the world," five years elapsed before Darwin was able to resume in earnest his work on insectivorous plants; then, recalling the American botanist as a source of information in regard to *Dionæa*, and admittedly confusing Mr. Canby's home, Wilmington, Delaware, with the habitat of the

[1] *Letters of Asa Gray.* Edited by Jane Loring Gray. Published by Houghton, Mifflin & Co., 1893.

[2] *The Life and Letters of Charles Darwin.* Edited by Francis Darwin. Published by D. Appleton & Co., 1899.

on the Dionea, which I look at as the most wonderful plant in the world.

If you do visit the proper district I shd be very much obliged if you wd open a dozen oldish leaves to see what sized insects they capture.

I am aware that a very minute insect wd start the leaf, but I suspect that they wd generally escape through the apertures at the bases of the spikes

before they are completely interlocked.

With my best thanks,

believe me dear Sir

yours faithfully

Ch. Darwin

Dated from Down, Beckenham, Kent, February 19, 1873, this letter from Charles Darwin to the American botanist, William M. Canby, begins with the admission, "I find that I erred in supposing that the leaves never opened a second time. I did suppose that you resided near the habitation of the Dionea [Dionæa], which I look at as the most wonderful plant in the world"

NATURAL HISTORY, 1923, Vol. 23, pp. 589-596.

plant, Wilmington, North Carolina, he wrote requesting further information, and especially that field observations should be made on the insect-catching habits of the plant in its native home.

Within the last few months, in a half-forgotten chest in the attic of Mr. Canby's home, this Darwin-Canby correspondence of fifty years ago, relating to Dionæa ("which I look at as the most wonderful plant in the world"), has been found. These letters, with the published letters of Darwin and Gray of the same period and regarding the same subject, typically illustrate Darwin's intuitive, almost uncanny, facility in seizing upon apparently minor characters of structure or behavior and in finding there significances hidden from the observers upon

whose evidence he builds his edifice of inference and deduction; and they most forcibly call to our attention the paucity in our literature of direct and detailed field observations on Dionæa,— if not "the most wonderful plant in the world" yet undeniably among the most remarkable of all our native flora.

Dionæa muscipula, Venus's-flytrap, belongs to the same plant family as the more familiar Drosera, the sundews; but while some species of Drosera are almost world-wide in their distribution, Dionæa, represented by its single species muscipula, is confined, if one excepts hothouse specimens, to a narrow strip of about fifty miles along the coast of North and South Carolina: and even within these limits its dis-

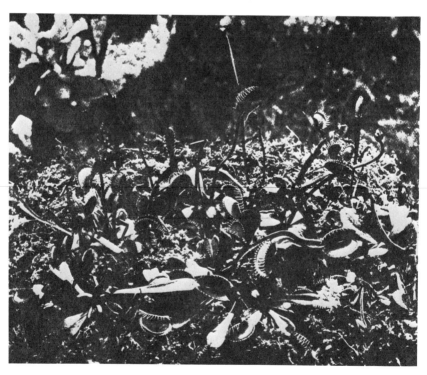

Dionæa is not a conspicuous plant, for its leaves rise, at most, only a few inches above the sand, where they are often half-hidden by other herbage

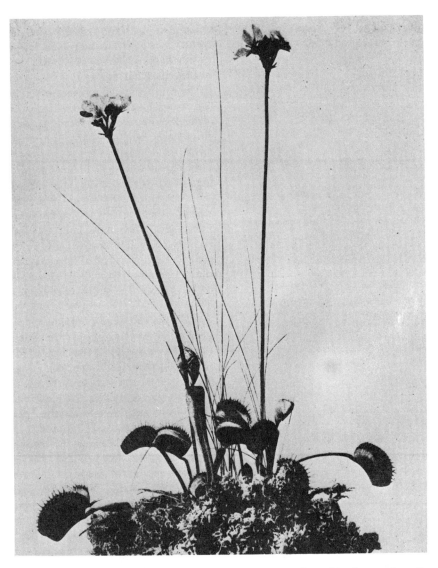

Only when the slender flower stalk raises its cluster of modest white flowers above the level of the leaves, is the discovery of *Dionæa* always possible without prolonged search

tribution is strictly localized, for it seems to be very particular in the selection of its growing place.

To the non-botanical observer, untroubled by problems of comparative morphology, the "leaf" of *Dionæa* is borne on a flattened or winged petiole; the broadly rounded halves of the leaf are set at an upward angle to the mid-rib, and the outer edge of each half bears more than a dozen evenly spaced finger-like spikes; the slightly concave disk of each leaf-half bears three (sometimes more), fine, short, tapering bristles, which are the "triggers" to set off the trap; for the whole structure is a trap for the capture of insects. Touch one of the trigger hairs twice, or any two of them in close succession (gently, even with a hair) and like a closing hand the halves of the leaf clap to, the marginal fingers interlace, and if the capture be of nutrient material (an insect), or if it continues its struggles (for the leaf responds both to chemical and mechanical stimulation), the leaf-halves press more and more closely together, the innumerable glands which stud their upper surface pour out an abundant ropy secretion, which bathes the captive in a digestive juice, and when days later the leaf reopens, the insect has been reduced to a mere chitinous shell from which all the softer parts have been dissolved out and absorbed for the nourishment of the plant.

This is the usual (and apparently justified) interpretation of the activities of *Dionæa*. The mechanism of the closing of the leaf; the conditions under which the digestive liquid is poured out and nutritive material absorbed; even the minute electrical disturbances set up in the leaf in closing,—all these have been made the subject of extended research; but it was in reference to none of these that Darwin wrote Canby. In the closing movement of the leaf one detail had puzzled him. When the trigger hairs are touched and the leaf claps to, it does not at first close tightly; the fingers interlace but do not close to their bases, and a row of crevices remains through which for a time a small insect might squeeze out. Darwin's son actually observed a small ant make its escape in this manner. But after the first quick closing movement, if a capture is actually made, the marginal fingers soon tighten their grip, the leaf edges are pressed into closer contact, and eventually even the form of the imprisoned insect, under the pressure

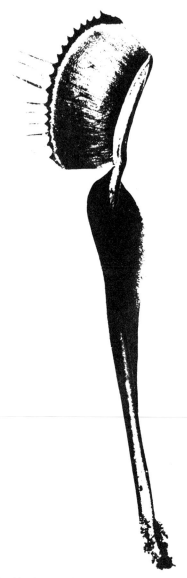

In this photograph one half of the leaf has been removed, to show distinctly the marginal spikes, the three trigger hairs, and the slightly concave and densely glandular area forming the digesting and absorbing surface of the leaf

24

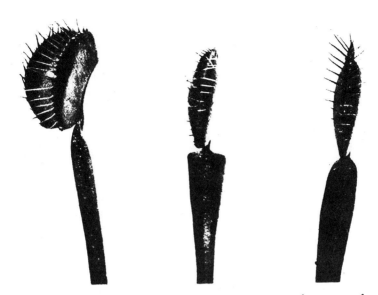

Why does the leaf of *Dionæa*, in its first quick closing movement, leave a row of crevices between the "fingers," through which a small insect may make its escape, and then very gradually close these orifices? It looks as though the small insects were given an opportunity to escape; but why?

exerted, becomes visible as it bulges out the thin walls. In explanation of these peculiarities of the closing movements of the leaf Darwin had a theory; but his sickly greenhouse plants ("I cannot make the little creature grow well," he wrote[1] Hooker) did not furnish conclusive evidence of its correctness; so his queries to his American correspondent were, "How many times, successively, does a single leaf capture and digest prey? What sized insects do they capture?" Canby replied, writing from memory, six years after his observations had been made: "As to the specific point about the plant capturing large or small insects, the answer is that so far as I am aware it catches everything it can, large or small. . . . As far as I can remember, any insect from the size of a small fly, say a line or two in length, to

a beetle or other insect of *nearly* the length of the leaf would be closed upon and . . . devoured. As to the proportion of 'large' or 'small,' I cannot distinctly remember; but after what I have written it would be fair to suppose that within the limits mentioned above it would probably be almost the proportion of insects in the neighborhood of the leaves, except that insects which habitually fly, as a class, would probably be less liable to capture than those which crawl. . . Now about the leaves becoming callous and unexcitable after 'catching' an insect, I have several times known leaves to devour insects *three* successive times, never more than that, and then they were the most vigorous. Ordinarily twice, and quite often once, was enough to render them unserviceable."

This reply was not conclusive, and on February 17, 1873, Darwin wrote Canby: "I find that I erred in sup-

[1]*More Letters of Charles Darwin.* Edited by Francis Darwin. Published by D. Appleton & Co., 1903.

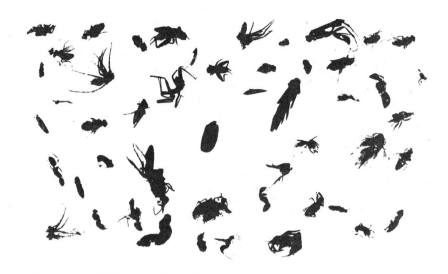

The captures of fifty mature leaves of *Dionæa* consisted of Hymenoptera (wasps and large ants), 10; Diptera (flies), 9; arachnids (spiders), 9 (one with an egg sack); Coleoptera (beetles), 9 (each distinct as to species); Orthoptera (grasshoppers, locusts, roaches), 7; Hemiptera (predacious bugs and leaf hoppers), 4; Lepidoptera (caterpillars), 2. The average length of the fifty victims was 8.6 mm., or about one third of an inch

posing that the leaves never opened a second time. . . If you do visit the proper district I shd be very much obliged if you wd open a dozen oldish leaves to see what sized insects they capture. I am aware that a very minute insect wd start the leaf, but I suspect that they wd generally escape through the apertures at the bases of the spikes before they completely interlocked."

And again on May 7 of the same year Darwin wrote: "I thank you very sincerely for the leaves, of which I have examined the [captures] with great interest. The results support my anticipation that the leaves are adapted to allow of the smaller fry escaping. Eight of the fourteen leaves had caught beetles of relative considerable size. There were also a good-sized spider & a scolopendra. Three of the leaves had caught ants. I wish the leaves had been of full size, but I think my results may be trusted."

The examination of the captures of fourteen small leaves, then, is the principal basis upon which Darwin builds his theory of the significance of the initial partial closing of the leaf of *Dionæa*. In *Insectivorous Plants* he reviews this evidence, concluding, "It would manifestly be a disadvantage to the plant to waste many days in remaining clasped over a minute insect, and several additional days or weeks in afterwards recovering its sensibility; inasmuch as a minute insect would afford but little nutriment. It would be far better for the plant to wait for a time until a moderately large insect was captured, and to allow all the little ones to escape; and this advantage is secured by the slowly intercrossing marginal spikes, which act like the large meshes of a fishing net, allowing the small and useless fry to escape."

Before the appearance of *Insectivorous Plants* Gray wrote to Canby thus:[1]

[1] *Letters of Asa Gray*. Edited by Jane Loring Gray Published by Houghton, Mifflin & Co., 1893.

"Conundrum? Why does the Dionæa trap close only part way, so as to cross the bristles of edge only, at first, and afterwards close fully? Darwin has hit it. I wonder you or I never thought of it. . . Think what a waste if the leaf had to go through all the process of secretion, etc., taking so much time, all for a little gnat. It would not pay. Yet it would have to do it except for this arrangement to let the little flies escape. But when a bigger one is caught he is sure for a good dinner. That is real Darwin! I just wonder you and I never thought of it. But *he* did." Gray was right, and "That is real Darwin!" But is it true? Darwin, after examining the captures of fourteen leaves gathered in the field, writes, "I think my results may be trusted." Perhaps by these methods his theory of this significance of the leaf behavior is not susceptible of absolute proof; but it seemed worth while, by further direct observation upon the plants in their native home, and by the examination of a large number of leaves which had made captures, to determine whether an actual sorting out of visiting insects by size does take place.

On May 31, 1921, Dionæa was found in full bloom, in abundance, and in fine condition, within a few miles of Wilmington, North Carolina. It was an easy task to gather fifty well-developed leaves with captures; these were opened carefully, and their captures were dropped into alcohol, for measurement and approximate identification at leisure. Of the fifty, only one was less than 5 mm. in length, and only seven, less than 6 mm.; ten were 10 mm. or more in length, with a maximum of 30 mm. We may then safely conclude that the habitual captures of mature leaves range from the largest insect the leaf is able to close upon and hold, down to those approximately one quarter of an inch in length; and that insects materially smaller than this, if they spring the trap, usually take advantage of the opportunity afforded by the partially closed leaf and make their escape.

One capture not tabulated deserves special mention. When one leaf was opened, its contents were found to be a single wing cover of a large beetle (shown in the center of the plate of captures) and an ant much smaller than any of those captured by the other leaves examined. It is not diffi-

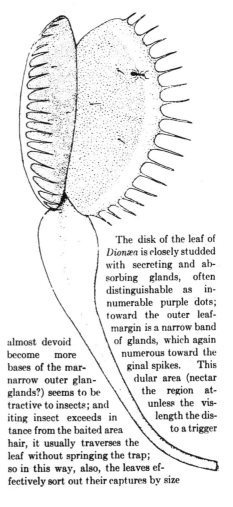

The disk of the leaf of Dionæa is closely studded with secreting and absorbing glands, often distinguishable as innumerable purple dots; toward the outer leaf-margin is a narrow band of glands, which again become more numerous toward the bases of the marginal spikes. This narrow outer glandular area (nectar glands?) seems to be the region attractive to insects; and unless the visiting insect exceeds in length the distance from the baited area to a trigger hair, it usually traverses the leaf without springing the trap; so in this way, also, the leaves effectively sort out their captures by size

cult to picture the minute ant, desperately tugging the wing cover across the leaf, bumping into the trigger hairs, and refusing to desert its booty until the time for possible escape had passed.

With this evidence of the size of the actual captures of the leaves, it was desirable to determine what insects could be observed upon the leaves, subject to capture; and parts of two days were devoted to this, with some unanticipated results. Ants were the only insects frequently noticed upon the leaves. Nearly all of these ants belonged to small species, 3 mm. or less in length, and consequently smaller than any of those captured by the fifty leaves. None was actually observed to set off the trigger hairs, but we repeatedly sprung the leaf traps with slender grass stems without disturbing the ants, each leaf closing upon its visiting ant, which crept out after the expiration of a few seconds, either between the crossed fingers, as Darwin had surmised and recorded, or at the end of the leaf, where also a slight crevice remains after the first closing movement; and none failed thus to make its escape in time to elude the slow tightening and closing of these apertures.

The plants *were* sorting out their captures by size; but to accomplish this not one method, but two, were employed; and the second and unrecorded method with respect to these small ants was the more effective. Most of these little ants (sometimes two of them on a single leaf) were observed to occupy a uniform position on its upper surface, their heads close to the bases of the marginal spikes. As they moved slowly across this belt of the leaf, they made frequent and prolonged pauses, during which, their mouth parts were observed under the lens, to be in motion against the surface of the leaf. A larger and winged hymenopteron was observed to be engaged in the same performance Obviously, they were feeding upon some attractive exudation of the leaf. The behavior of visiting insects is entirely convincing to the observer that a baited area extends across the leaf on its upper surface just within the bases of the marginal spines. This baited marginal band is so situated upon the leaf surface that a visiting insect *in length too small to extend from the bait to the trigger hairs*, usually does not spring the trap. Whether or not these conditions are to be interpreted as adjustments to that end, the effect of this arrangement, in conjunction with the peculiarities of the closing movement by which small insects are given an opportunity to escape, is to limit the usual captures of the leaves to insects approximating one quarter of an inch or more in length.

Living plants of *Dionæa* were exhibited in England more than 150 years ago, even prior to the first published description by Ellis (1775). The voluminous literature of research upon this plant has increased rather than decreased our recognition of its almost unique interest, and is at least proof that *Dionæa* still withholds answer to some of its more fascinating problems. As a hothouse plant it continues to be fairly familiar both here and abroad, but its survival in its restricted native habitat should not be left to chance. Let us hope that means for its preservation may be found, and that for all the future we may have opportunity to "look on *Dionæa* as the most wonderful plant in the world."

NOTES ON THE GENUS EMPUSA COHN

By D. M. MacLeod

Introduction

The following account deals with preliminary observations on a number of *Empusa* species isolated from naturally infected insect material obtained either from collections sent directly to the Laboratory of Insect Pathology or from routine collections of the Forest Insect Survey of the Division of Forest Biology.

The Genus *Empusa*

No general monograph of the numerous *Empusa* species (including 134 epithets), described and named in various parts of the world, has yet been prepared. According to Fitzpatrick (6) the genus *Empusa* was founded by Cohn (2) on *E. muscae*, parasitic in the housefly. The name *Empusa*, however, had already been applied to a genus of orchids and Fresenius (7), recognizing this fact, proposed *Entomophthora* to replace it. The two names have subsequently been used indiscriminately until separated as two distinct genera by Brefeld (1) and Nowakowski (11), who by so doing recognized the validity of the name *Empusa*.

In Nowakowski's arrangement, *Entomophthora* is largely characterized by branched conidiophores (Fig. 3) and *Empusa* by unbranched or simple conidiophores (Fig. 2). Thaxter (22), who prepared the first really critical account of the group, stated that these characters are inconstant and that borderline species make the maintenance of this separation impossible. He therefore united all the species under *Empusa*. Thaxter further pointed out that the orchidaceous genus *Empusa* is now placed as a synonym and hence seems unlikely to cause confusion.

More recently, cytological investigations tend to show that the branching habit of the conidiophore (*Entomophthora*) is correlated with a uninucleate condition of the conidia, whereas in forms with simple conidiophores (*Empusa*), the conidia are multinucleate (12). These observations indicate (6) that the earlier usage of Nowakowski, in applying the names *Empusa* and *Entomoph-thora* to species with unbranched and branched conidiophores, respectively, was probably in the main phylogenetically sound and in all probability later students will return to it. However, owing to the considerable variation found in the general appearance of conidiophores of individual species under varying environmental conditions, the writer prefers to follow Thaxter's treatment of this group, by incorporating all the species under *Empusa*, until a clearer understanding of the nomenclature of this genus is available.

Two other related genera are *Tarichium* named by Cohn (3) in 1875, and *Lamia*, erected by Nowakowski (11) in 1884. The identity of the former was based on the resting spore condition of an unknown species of *Empusa*; the latter is a group intermediate between *Empusa* and *Entomophthora*. Neither *Tarichium* nor *Lamia* has found general acceptance (6 and 22).

In infected insects, *Empusa* isolates do not generally develop profusely branching mycelium; instead they form short thick segments, called hyphal bodies, that undergo a process of division and budding. These, in the final stages of infection, give rise to conidiophores that penetrate the outer covering of the host and form conidia in the air (Figs. 4, 5, 6, and 7).

Besides the type of "air spore" or conidium just described, some species under certain conditions may produce another type, generally formed internally and known as resting spores, with walls approximately three microns thick. These spores may be either sexual (zygospores) or asexual (azygospores). The zygospores result from a true sexual conjugation between a pair of hyphal bodies or hyphal cells with the young spore budding out from the point of union. At maturity the spores are usually large and spherical, and generally smooth-walled (Fig. 8); although a few are characteristically rough-walled (Fig. 14). In azygospore formation, a bud is put out from a hyphal body or cell and enlarges to form a spore similar to the zygospore. A modification of this process sometimes occurs in the chlamydospores* (with walls approximately 0.5μ thick (Fig. 9) which may be transformed directly into azygospores by the deposition of a third inner wall.

Very little is known concerning the formation and germination of resting spores. Schweizer (20) reported in 1945 that in *E. muscae* they form after the substratum has been used up, or earlier if unfavorable growth conditions develop. In general they are believed to afford the fungus a means of hibernation or a way of withstanding adverse conditions. A single season is thought to be the normal period of this resting state, although it has been suggested that it may extend over more than one season.

Conidia are germinable for several days after discharge, resting spores are not. The latter are believed (20) to require a special biocatalytic stimulus, which may be simulated in the laboratory by means of pure cultures of chitin-splitting bacteria.

---

* *Under unfavorable environmental conditions hyphal bodies may develop heavier walls and enter a period of rest as chlamydospores, which, on the return of favorable conditions, germinate readily and eventually form conidiophores.*

Members of *Empusa* are all entomogenous and were long thought to be obligate in their parasitism. Some degree of success (20, 21, and 24), however, has attended attempts to culture these forms and it now seems probable that many of them will be found to develop saprophytically on favorable media. A number of *Empusa* forms isolated in this study were successfully established on Sabouraud maltose agar when infected larvae (freshly dead or with hyphal bodies still viable internally and free from contamination) surface-sterilized in a 2–5% "Javex" (sodium hypochlorite) solution were transferred to sterile medium. Under these conditions the fungus soon appeared on the surface of the insect, and later spread to the medium, where it developed a colony with a very irregular and convoluted surface (Fig. 16).

TABLE I

INSECT SPECIES WITH WHICH *Empusa* SPECIES ARE ASSOCIATED IN CANADA
(SEE TEXT-FIG. 1, FOR DISTRIBUTION)

No.	Host	Family	Order	*Empusa* species
1	*Anisota rubicunda* Fabr.	Citheroniidae	Lepidop.	*Empusa grylli* type
2	" *virginiensis* Dru.	"	"	" species
3	*Anthelia hyperborea* Hlst.	Geometridae	"	" "
4	*Archips cerasivorana* Fitch	Tortricidae	"	" *grylli* type
5	*Arge pectoralis* (Leach)	Argidae	Hymenop.	" species
6	*Calliphora* sp.	Metopiidae	Diptera	" *bullata*
7	*Camnula pellucida** Scudd.	Acrididae	Orthop.	" *grylli*
8	*Caripeta divisata* Wlk.	Geometridae	Lepidop.	" species
9	*Choristoneura fumiferana* Clem.	Tortricidae	"	" *grylli* type and *sphaerosperma*
10	*Dioryctria reniculella* Grt.	Pyralidae	"	" species
11	*Dissosteira carolina* (Linn.)	Locustidae	Orthop.	" *grylli*
12	*Ectropis crepuscularia* Schiff.	Geometridae	Lepidop.	" *grylli* type
13	*Estigmene acrea* Dru.	Arctiidae	"	" " "
14	*Haploa lecontei* Guer.	"	"	" species
15	*Hesperumia sulphuraria* Pack.	Geometridae	"	" "
16	*Hypera punctata* F.	Curculionidae	Coleop.	" "
17	*Lambdina fiscellaria fiscellaria* Gn.	Geometridae	Lepidop.	" *grylli* type and *sphaerosperma*
18	" " *lugubrosa* Hlst.	"	"	" species
19	*Lygus communis* var. *novascotiensis* Knight	Miridae	Hemip.	" *erupta*
20	*Macrosiphum albifrons*† Esseq.	Aphiidae	Homop.	" *aphidis*
21	" *pisi* (Klth.)	"	"	" "
22	" *solanifolii* (Ashm.)	"	"	" "
23	*Malacosoma americanum* F.	Lasiocampidae	Lepidop.	" *megasperma*
24	" *disstria* Hbn.	"	"	" *grylli* and *megasperma*
25	" *pluviale* Dyar	"	"	" *megasperma*
26	*Melanolophia imitata* Wlk.	Geometridae	"	" *grylli* type
27	*Melanoplus bivittatus** Say	Locustidae	Orthop.	" *grylli*
28	*Monoctenus juniperinus* MacG.	Diprionidae	Hymenop.	" " type
29	*Musca domestica* Linn.	Muscidae	Diptera	" *muscae*
30	*Nematocampa filamentaria* Gn.	Geometridae	Lepidop.	" *grylli* type
31	*Neodiprion abietis* (Harr.)	Diprionidae	Hymenop.	" species
32	" *lecontei* (Fitch)	"	"	" "
33	" *tsugae* Midd.	"	"	" *sphaerosperma*
34	*Nepytia canosaria* Wlk.	Geometridae	Lepidop.	" *grylli* type
35	*Orgyia* sp.‡	Arctiidae	Lepidop.	" *grylli*
36	*Pristiphora erichsonii*§ (Htg.)	Tenthredinidae	Hymenop.	" " type
37	*Psyllia mali* Schmidb.	Chermidae	Homop.	" *sphaerosperma*
38	*Sarcophaga aldrichi* Park.	Metopiidae	Diptera	" species
39	*Sciaphila duplex* Wlshm.	Olethreutidae	Lepidop.	" *grylli* type
40	*Semiothisa granitata* Gn.	Geometridae	"	" " "
41	*Stenoporpia albescens* Hlst.	"	"	" " " "
42	*Typhlocyba pomaria* Mca.	Cicadellidae	Homop.	" species
43	Unidentified sp.	Arctiidae	Lepidop.	" *grylli* type
44	" "	Phalaenidae	"	" " "

* *Infected material received from Dr. G. E. Bucher, Belleville, Ontario.*
† *Material received from Conn. Agr. Expt. Station, New Haven, Connecticut, U.S.A.*
‡ *Collected in Newfoundland (22, p. 161).*
§ *Material also received from Forest Insect Laboratory, Milwaukee, Wisconsin, U.S.A.*

Identity of *Empusa* Species Isolated from Insects in Canada

In all named species known to form resting spores, the mature zygospores as well as the azygospores are spherical in shape, except in *E. fresenii*, and *E. coleopterorum*. The spores in the former are elliptical or ovoid, and in the latter globose, or broadly oval, or sometimes pyriform. In an estimated three-fourths of these species the resting spores are smooth-walled (Fig. 8) and indistinguishable in the different species except for slight variations in size, while in the remaining one-fourth the resting spores are rough-walled (Table III, Figs. 10, 11, and 14). On this basis the forms studied in the present survey are divided into two groups: *A*, forms with smooth-walled resting spores and *B*, forms with rough-walled resting spores. Several isolates included under "*A*" did not develop resting spores but are included here, because they appear to be closely allied to *E. grylli*.

Empusa species were found on 44 different species of insects (Table I) representing 20 different familes from the following orders: Lepidoptera, Hymenoptera, Diptera, Orthoptera, Coleoptera, Hemiptera, and Homoptera. Although the forms in 12 insect species had not sporulated they, nevertheless, could be readily recognized as an *Empusa* by the presence of coenocytic hyphae *ca.* 13μ in diameter (Fig. 1) and hyphal bodies of various sizes and shapes.

A. Forms with Smooth-walled Resting Spores

The isolates from the 20 different insect species listed in Table II contained spores characteristic of *E. grylli* Fres. Those from insect species 1 to 7 also

TABLE II

VARIATION IN SIZE AMONG SPORES OF THE "*E. grylli*" TYPE

No.	Source of *Empusa* isolates	*Empusa* sp.	Dimensions	
			Range	Average
1	*P. erichsonii*	*E. thaxteriana**	$28.5 - 48.5\mu \times 23.0 - 37.5\mu$	$34.0 \times 29.0\mu$
2	*C. fumiferana*	" "	$23.0 - 42.0\mu \times 17.5 - 30.0\mu$	$32.0 \times 22.5\mu$
3	*M. juniperinus*	" "	$25.5 - 39.5\mu \times 24.0 - 27.5\mu$	$33.5 \times 26.0\mu$
4	*A. cerasivorana*	" "	$22.0 - 32.0\mu \times 18.5 - 25.5\mu$	$28.0 \times 22.0\mu$
5	*M. disstria*	" "	$26.5 - 35.0\mu \times 18.5 - 27.5\mu$	$30.0 \times 23.0\mu$
6	*S. albescens*	" "	$25.5 - 32.0\mu \times 18.5 - 28.5\mu$	$28.5 \times 23.0\mu$
7	*N. filamentaria*	" "	$21.0 - 36.5\mu \times 13.0 - 29.5\mu$	$31.5 \times 24.0\mu$
8	*C. pellucida*	*E. grylli†*		
9	*D. carolina*	" "	$27.5 - 40.0\mu \times 21.0 - 36.0\mu$	$33.5 \times 25.5\mu$
10	*M. bivittatus*	" "		
11	*L. f. fiscellaria*	" "	$27.5 - 32.0\mu \times 17.5 - 21.0\mu$	$29.0 \times 19.0\mu$
12	*M. imitata*	" "	$27.5 - 33.0\mu \times 17.5 - 22.0\mu$	$28.5 \times 21.5\mu$
13	*S. duplex*	" "	$23.0 - 39.5\mu \times 18.5 - 33.0\mu$	$33.5 \times 26.0\mu$
14	Arctiidae	" "	$28.5 - 39.5\mu \times 25.5 - 33.0\mu$	$34.0 \times 26.0\mu$
15	Phalaenidae	" "	$36.5 - 43.0\mu \times 27.5 - 33.0\mu$	$40.0 \times 30.0\mu$
16	*S. granitata*	" "	$26.0 - 28.5\mu \times 19.0 - 21.0\mu$	$27.0 \times 20.0\mu$
17	*E. acrea*	" "	$27.5 - 39.5\mu \times 20.0 - 32.0\mu$	$32.0 \times 24.0\mu$
18	*E. crepuscularia*	" "	$24.0 - 32.0\mu \times 15.5 - 21.0\mu$	$28.0 \times 18.5\mu$
19	*A. rubicunda*	*E. tenthredinis‡*	$25.5 - 39.5\mu \times 18.5 - 27.5\mu$	$31.5 \times 22.0\mu$
20	*N. canosaria*	" "	$27.5 - 39.5\mu \times 20.0 - 27.5\mu$	$33.0 \times 23.0\mu$

* *E. thaxteriana.* Conidia nearly spherical or broadly ovoid, with a papillate base which is sometimes furnished with a sharp point, $30-40\mu \times 28-33\mu$ (22, p. 165).

† *E. grylli.* Conidia ovoid to pear-shaped, with a broad papillate base and evenly rounded apex, hyaline and containing one or more large fat globules, $30-40\mu \times 25-36\mu$; resting spores spherical, colorless, $30-45\mu$ in diameter (22, p. 159).

‡ *E. tenthredinis.* Conidia broadly ovoid, tapering slightly towards the apex and with a prominent, rather narrow papillate base, $35-55\mu \times 25-35\mu$ (22, p. 162).

32

contained spores that resembled *E. thaxteriano* (Thaxter) Petch (15 and 22). Some of its spores are nearly spherical (Fig. 4), others are not separable from those of *E. grylli*. Isolates from insect species 8 to 18 are mainly characteristic of *E. grylli* (Fig. 5) but those from 19 and 20 contained spores resembling *E. tenthredinis* Fres. (Fig. 6). This species, closely resembling *E. grylli*, is separated from it by a slight tendency of the spores to taper more equally from the middle towards the base and apex.

All of the spores from the above isolates contained a single centrally-located oil globule that ranged in diameter from 8 to 14μ. The variation in color was slight and in general ranged from pale cream to chestnut brown; in one species, that from *M. imitata*, a slight tinge of green was noted; this, however, was not regarded as a distinguishing characteristic.

Resting spores (zygospores or azygospores) were not developed by any of the *grylli* forms listed in Table II, with the exception of the isolate from *D. carolina*. These spores are azygospores, spherical, smooth-walled, and vary in diameter from 29.5 to 32.0μ, averaging 31.5μ (Fig. 8). Some chlamydospores were observed in *S. albescens* and ranged in diameter from 14.5 to 24.0μ, averaging 18.0μ (Fig. 9).

It was not surprising to find species of the *grylli* type on so many of the insects examined as it is one of the more widely distributed of the *Empusa* species and is generally abundant.

E. (= *Entomophthora*) *sphaerosperma* Fres., isolated from *P. mali* (4), *C. fumiferana*, *N. tsugae*, and *L. f. fiscellaria*, is another form known for its great diversity in host species. The four infected insect species contained both primary and resting spores. In each case the spores were fairly uniform in both size and shape. The conidia are long-elliptical to nearly cylindrical (Fig. 7), papillate at the base, and taper very slightly near the rounded apex, usually with a fine granular content. They range in size from 11.0 to 20.0μ by 4.5 to 9.0μ, averaging $18.0 \times 6.0\mu$. The resting spores, spherical and smooth-walled, resemble those of *E. grylli* and range from 18.5 to 31.0μ, averaging 25.5μ. Chlamydospores were also present in *C. fumiferana* and *N. tsugae*; they vary from 16.5 to 24.0μ in diameter, averaging 20.5μ. This species is also known to attack *H. punctata* (13), and *T. pomaria* (23).

Empusa erupta Dustan is parasitic on *L. communis* var. *novascotiensis*. Its conidia are more or less bell-shaped, and in this respect it resembles *E. muscae* Cohn (5).

Empusa muscae Cohn is parasitic on *M. domestica*. Its spores are characteristically bell-shaped (22).

Empusa aphidis Hoffman is one of the more common *Empusa* species parasitic on aphids. In this survey it was isolated from *M. albifrons*, *M. pisi*, and *M. solanifolii*. Its conidia are ovoid to elliptical (22).

While smooth-walled resting spores are associated with the *Empusa* species *erupta*, *muscae*, and *aphidis*, spores were not observed in any of the specimens infected with these species in the present survey.

TABLE III

Empusa SPECIES WITH ROUGH-WALLED RESTING SPORES

Species	Primary spores	Resting spores
E. reticulata	Conidia not observed. Host, Diptera	Zygospores, faint red in mass, spherical, 44–84μ epispore reticulated
E. coleopterorum*	Conidia not observed. Host, Coleoptera	Resting spores dark brown, thick-walled (up to 6μ), densely verrucose, globose, 35–50μ or broadly oval, 48–52 × 44–46μ, or sometimes pyriform, 56 × 44μ
E. megasperma†	Conidia not observed. Host, Lepidoptera (*Agrotis segetum*)	Azygospores, spherical, dark brown, 34–55μ, average 50μ, epispore with sinuous furrows
E. calliphorae	Conidia not observed. Host, Diptera (*Calliphora* sp.)	Resting spores, deep chestnut brown, spherical, 30μ
E. muscivora	Conidia ovoid, blunt papilla, 20–24 × 11–13μ. Host, Diptera (*Calliphora* sp.)	Resting spores, deep chestnut brown, spherical, 24–28μ, Syn. with E. calliphorae (22)
E. bullata	No formal description of conidia, but stated to be indistinguishable from those of E. americana‡ Thaxter, (18). Host, Diptera (*Calliphora* sp.)	Zygospores, subglobose, 30–50μ, epispore bullate
E. echinospora	Conidia ovoid, tapering to a papillate base, usually nearly symmetrical, containing one or more large oil globules, 20–25 × 10–14μ. Host, Diptera	Zygospores, spherical, 30–40μ, epispore spinose
E. atrosperma§	Conidia not observed. Host, Homoptera	Resting spores blackish-brown, globose, 38–45μ, epispore with spines (2μ in length)
E. coronata″	Conidia globose, prominent papilla at the base, 30μ. Host, Homoptera	Resting spores, globose with covering of blunt hair-like appendages on the entire surface

* In 1944 Petch (17) identified an isolate from Sitones flavescens as the conidial stage of E. coleopterorum. In this instance only conidia (narrow oval, 32–44 × 8–14μ) were present. The synonymy of these two forms is based upon their "hold-fast" the distinctive features of which have been used as criteria upon which to establish a number of species within this genus.

† The conidial stage of this species is believed by Thaxter (22, p. 178) to be E. (= Entomophthora) virescens Thaxter. "Conidia ovoid to oblong, of irregular shape, with bluntly rounded base and apex, the former often hardly papillate and not well distinguished from the apex, color greenish-yellow in dried material, containing numerous small, irregular often rod-like fat bodies, 16–36μ × 10–20μ, average 30 × 14μ. Host, Lepidoptera (Agrotis fennica)".

‡ Although E. americana has smooth-walled resting spores, its primary spores resemble those of E. muscivora except for a slight variation in size. In the former the spores are slightly larger.

§ Petch (14) also included Entomophthora (= Tarichium) lauxaniae Bubák in his list of entomogenous fungi of Great Britain, but without description. This fungus may also have rough-walled resting spores, since it was originally described as a Tarichium species.

″ According to Harris (9) conidia in older cultures are transformed into appendaged resting spores.

B. Forms with Rough-walled Resting Spores

At least 10 *Empusa* species (Table III) have been recorded in the literature as having rough-walled resting spores. A number of these are incompletely described, and therefore cannot at present be recognized with certainty. On the basis of current information, however, they appear to fall into three groups as follows:

1. Resting spore outer wall reticulate, verrucose, or with sinuous furrows. E. (= *Tarichium*) *reticulata* Petch (16), E. (= *Entomophthora*) *coleopterorum* Petch (14), and E. (= *Tarichium*) *megasperma* Cohn (3).

2. Resting spore outer wall with knob-like projections. *E.* (= *Entomophthora) calliphorae* Giard (8), *E.* (= *Entomophthora) muscivora* Schroeter (19), and *E.* (= *Entomophthora) bullata* Thaxter (18).

3. Resting spore outer wall with spines or hair-like appendages. *E.* (= *Entomophthora) echinospora* Thaxter (22), *E.* (= *Entomophthora) atrosperma* Petch (14), and *E.* (= *Entomophthora) coronata* (Cost.) Kevorkian (9 and 10).

In the present survey, rough-walled resting spores were found among three out of the 44 isolates examined, the first from adults of a *Calliphora* species, the second from adults of *S. aldrichi*, and the third from larvae of *M. disstria*, *M. americanum*, and *M. pluviale*.

The isolate from the *Calliphora* adults is characteristic of group 2, and appears to be identical with *E. bullata*. The resting spores are spherical, with knob-like projections, and vary in diameter from 42 to 60.5μ, averaging 52.5μ. The conidia are long-ovoid, with dimensions ranging from 17.5 to $27.5\mu \times 9.0$ to 18.5μ, averaging $22.5 \times 12.0\mu$, and have a broad, evenly-rounded apex.

The isolate from *S. aldrichi* also forms resting spores that resemble those of *E. bullata*. They vary in diameter from 39.5 to 60.5μ, averaging 46.5μ (Fig. 14); the epispore is thin and hyaline, and in mass displays a faint reddish-brown tinge. The conidia, however, are quite different. They are broadly ovoid to pear-shaped with a very rounded apex and a broad papillate base (Fig. 15), with dimensions ranging from 29.0 to $35.0\mu \times 22.0$ to 27.5μ, averaging $32.5 \times 25.0\mu$. The contents are evenly granular, without any large central globule, thus differing from *E. grylli*. This fungus may therefore be a new species, or a species already named but incompletely described.

One of the two isolates found on *M. disstria* (Table I) produced smooth-walled resting spores similar to those of *E. grylli*, while the other formed rough-walled spores. The latter was obtained also from larvae of *M. americanum* and *M. pluviale*. The resting spores resemble those of *E.* (= *Tarichium*) *megasperma*, described by Cohn (3) in 1875 from larvae of *Agrotis segetum*, and not reported since. There is no description of the conidia of *E. megasperma*, but in 1888 Thaxter (22) described the species *E. virescens* from heavily infected larvae of *Agrotis fennica* submitted by Mr. J. Fletcher of Ottawa, Canada. Only primary spores were found, but Thaxter suggested on the basis of the closely related hosts that *E. virescens* and *E. megasperma* might

---

Fig. 1. Coenocytic hyphae characteristic of *Empusa* infected insects. 550×.
Fig. 2. Unbranched, or simple conidiophores (*Empusa* species). 550×.
Fig. 3. Branched, or digitate conidiophores (*Entomophthora* species). Note that a cross-wall cuts off each branch from the main axis of the conidiophore. 550×.
Fig. 4. Conidia, nearly spherical (*E. thaxteriana*). 550×.
Fig. 5. Conidia, pear-shaped (*E. grylli*). 550×.
Fig. 6. Conidia, broadly ovoid, tapering slightly from middle toward base and apex (*E. tenthredinis*). 550×.
Fig. 7. Conidia cylindrical (*E. sphaerosperma*). 550×.
Fig. 8. Smooth-walled resting spores (*E. grylli*). 550×.
Fig. 9. Chlamydospore (*E.* species). 550×.

PLATE I

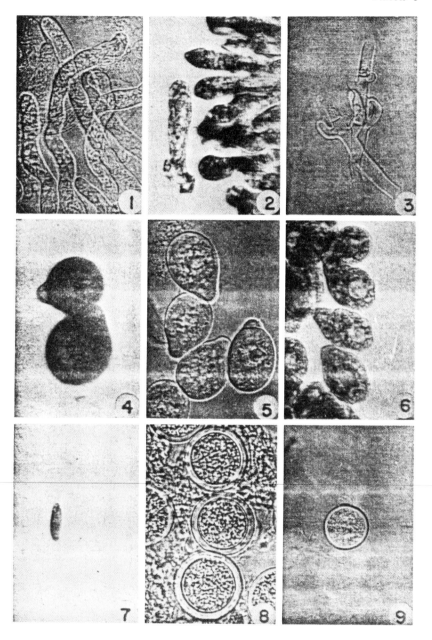

PLATE II

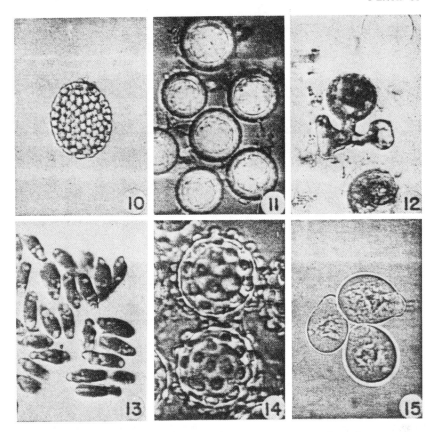

FIG. 10. Resting spores from external surface of *M. disstria* infected with *E. megasperma*, note rough surface. 550×.

FIG. 11. Resting spores found in *M. disstria* infected with *E. megasperma*, note sinuous outline. 550×.

FIG. 12. Zygospore from *E. megasperma* on *M. disstria*, note that resting spore is formed in an outgrowth at the point of conjugation between two hyphal cells. 550×.

FIG. 13. Conidia, ovoid to oblong from *M. disstria* infected with *E. megasperma*. 550×.

FIG. 14. Resting spores with knob-like projections from *S. aldrichi* infected with an *Empusa* species. 550×.

FIG. 15. Conidia resembling *E. grylli* from *S. aldrichi* infected with an *Empusa* species. 550×.

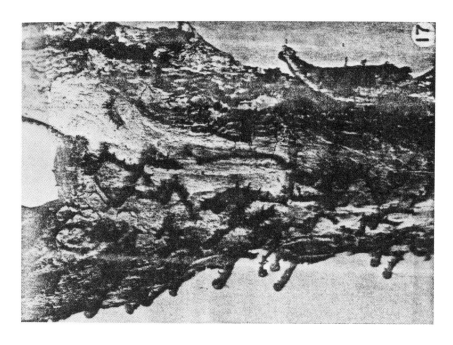

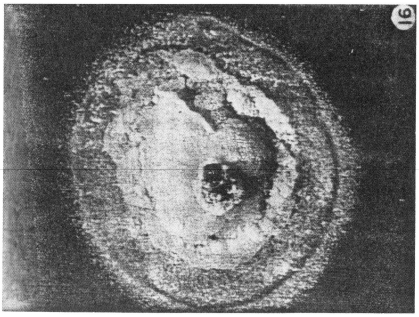

be synonymous, a point that can be determined with certainty, however, only when the resting spores of the former and the conidia of the latter become known.

With infected *Malacosoma* species, some resting spores develop among the mycelium on the external surface, but for the most part occur internally. The epispore of those occurring externally is verrucose, the projections, though they resemble those of *E. bullata*, are much less pronounced (Fig. 10). Among the internal spores the outer wall is wavy or sinuous in outline (Fig. 11), and not unlike the sinuous furrows described by Cohn for *E. megasperma*. This wavy outline is caused by the remnants of the disintegrated verrucose wall or epispore in which the spores were enclosed during development, and from which they can be liberated in most *Empusa* species through pressure. They also resemble *E. megasperma* in that they are spherical and brownish in color, but differ in that they are not azygo- but zygospores formed as a result of conjugation between hyphal bodies (Fig. 12) and being somewhat smaller in size, ranging in diameter from 24.0 to 31.0μ, averaging 27.5μ (Table III). In general the conidia resemble *E. virescens* (Table III), but differ in that they are hyaline, and smaller in size with dimensions ranging from 16.5 to 23.0μ $\times$ 6.5 to 10μ, averaging $18.5 \times 8.0\mu$ (Fig. 13).

The hosts of the above *Empusa* species belong to the order *Lepidoptera*, *Agrotis* species from the family *Phalaenidae*, and *Malacosoma* species from the family Lasiocampidae. Infected *Agrotis* species eventually become black and shrivelled, the fungus appearing as a greenish-yellow coating, while infected *Malacosoma* larvae turn brown to black, the fungus appearing as a fawn to dark brown coating. Infected larvae of the three *Malacosoma* species contained quantities of yellow crystals, variable in size and shape and of unknown composition.

It has been reported that in *E. echinospora* and *E. reticulata*, the outer wall surrounding the mature spore may be readily removed by pressure of a cover glass upon it, disclosing within a spore of the usual type, i.e. a smooth-walled resting spore identical with those of *E. grylli*. This was also found to be true for the *Empusa* species on the *Calliphora* species, but did not occur among the spores from *S. aldrichi*, or the *Malacosoma* species.

Effectiveness of *Empusa* Species as Insect Control Agents

The literature records that under favorable conditions, epizootics caused by *Empusa* species have reduced large and destructive outbreaks of insect pests in various countries throughout the world. In Canada *Empusa* species are indigenous and occur on a wide range of insect species from a number of orders,

---

FIG. 16. An *Empusa* species of the "*grylli* type" growing on Sabouraud maltose agar. The head (black spot) of a naturally infected *C. fumiferana* larva that had been used as a source of inoculum can be seen in the center of the colony. Note that fungus seems to grow in deep folds or convolutions which give the surface of the colony an unusual appearance. $2\times$.

FIG. 17. Naturally infected larvae of *M. disstria* destroyed by *E. megasperma*. $0.7\times$.

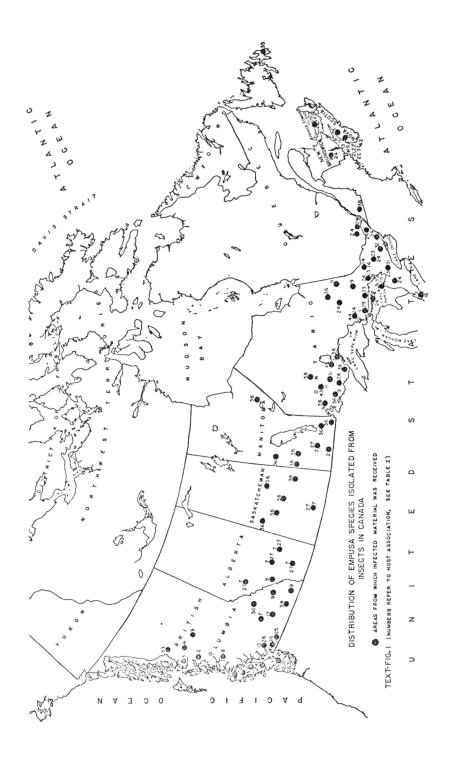

DISTRIBUTION OF EMPUSA SPECIES ISOLATED FROM
INSECTS IN CANADA

● AREAS FROM WHICH INFECTED MATERIAL WAS RECEIVED

TEXT-FIG. I (NUMBERS REFER TO HOST ASSOCIATION, SEE TABLE I)

of which members of the Lepidoptera seem to be most susceptible. Insects attacked by this fungus have been found in various localities (Text-fig. 1) in each of the provinces where insect collections have been made.

Of the two types (*E. grylli* and *E. sphaerosperma*) reported on *C. fumiferana*, the former is more prevalent and has been isolated from larvae collected in British Columbia, Ontario, and New Brunswick; the latter was restricted to larvae from British Columbia, and just inside the Alberta border on the Banff–Windermere Highway. These forms also occur on *L. f. fiscellaria* from British Columbia, but in this case *E. sphaerosperma* is the more important form.

Empusa thaxteriana, occasionally found on *M. disstria* larvae, is not as important in the control of this insect as is the *Empusa* species described in this paper. The latter caused high larval mortality at widely separated points in Ontario, from 1949 to 1952. In one specific area dead larvae (Fig. 17) were massed on the north side of the trunks of a series of trees examined in a mature hard maple woodlot that had been thinned by selective cutting.* Approximately 150 dead larvae were counted on one square foot of bark surface near the base of one of the trees in this area.

Dr. G. E. Bucher (personal communication) reported 94% mortality among laboratory reared samples of *C. pellucida*, collected from a population (20 per sq. yd.) infected with *E. grylli* at Darfield, British Columbia. Although the center of infection was found in a pasture of several acres, the disease was common in this area along the bottom flats for several miles.

Unfortunately *Empusa* species, while they are frequently an important agent in the control of harmful insects, occasionally attack beneficial ones as well. The effectiveness, for example, of *S. aldrichi*, one of the most important pupal parasites of *M. disstria* is lessened by an *Empusa* species that attacks it in the adult stage.

Acknowledgments

The writer wishes to express his thanks to Dr. J. MacBain Cameron for constructive criticism in the preparation of this paper, and to Mr. D. C. Anderson for the photographs.

References

1. BREFELD, O. A. Über die Entomophthoreen und ihre Verwandten. Botan. Ztg. 35 : 345-355, 368-372. 1877.
2. COHN, F. *Empusa muscae* und die Krankheit der Stubenfliegen. Nova Acta K. Acad. Caes. Leop.-Carol. Germ. Nat. 25 : 301-360. 1855.
3. COHN, F. Über eine neue Pilzkrankheit der Erdraupen. Beitr. Biol. Pflanz. 1 : 58. 1875.
4. DUSTAN, A. G. A fungus parasite of the imported apple sucker (*Psyllia mali* Schmid.). Artificial spread of *Entomophthora sphaerosperma.* Agr. Gaz. Can. 10 : 16-19. 1923.
5. DUSTAN, A. G. Studies on a new species of *Empusa* parasitic on the green apple bug (*Lygus communis* var. *novascotiensis* (Knight)) in the Annapolis Valley. Proc. Acadian Entomol. Soc. 9 : 14-36. 1924.
6. FITZPATRICK, H. M. The lower fungi Phycomycetes. 1st ed. McGraw-Hill Book Company, Inc., Toronto. 1930. pp. 331.

* *MacDonald, J. E. Annual Biology Ranger Report, Sault Ste. Marie District. p. 5. 1951 (unpublished).*

7. FRESENIUS, G.   Notiz, Insekten-Pilze betreffend.   Botan. Ztg. 14 : 882.   1856.

8. GIARD, A.   Deux espèces d'entomophthorées nouvelles pour la flore française et présence de la forme *Tarichium* sur un muscide.   Bull. sci. France et Belg. 11 : 353.   1879.

9. HARRIS, M. R.   A phycomycete parasitic on aphids.   Phytopathology, 38 : 118-122. 1948.

10. KEVORKIAN, A. G.   Studies in Entomophthoraceae.   I.   Observations on the genus *Conidiobolus.*   J. Agr. Univ. Puerto Rico, 21 : 191-200.   1937.

11. NOWAKOWSKI,   L.   Entomophthoraceae.   Przycrynek   doznajomości   pasorzytnych grzybków sprariajacyck pomór owadów.   Pamietnik Akad. Umiejejnósci zu Krakau, 8 : 153-183.   1884.   *Cited by* H. M. Fitzpatrick (6).

12. OLIVE, E. W.   Cytological studies on the Entomophthoraceae.   Botan. Gaz. 41 : 192-208, 229-261.   1906.

13. PARKS, T. H.   The clover leaf weevil (*Hypera punctata* F.).   J. Econ. Entomol. 7 : 297. 1914.

14. PETCH, T.   A list of the entomogenous fungi of Great Britain.   Brit. Mycol. Soc. Trans. 17 : 170-178.   1932.

15. PETCH, T.   Notes on entomogenous fungi.   Brit. Mycol. Soc. Trans. 21 : 34-67.   1937.

16. PETCH, T.   Notes on entomogenous fungi.   Brit. Mycol. Soc. Trans. 23 : 127-148.   1939.

17. PETCH, T.   Notes on entomogenous fungi.   Brit. Mycol. Soc. Trans. 27 : 81-93.   1944.

18. POVAH, A. H. W.   The fungi of Isle Royale, Lake Superior.   Papers Mich. Acad. Sci. 20 : 113-156.   1935.

19. SCHROETER, J.   Entomophthorei. kryptogamen-flora von schlesien.   Band 3.   Lieferung 2 (Pilze), 146.   Dresden, 1876.   *Cited by* R. Thaxter (22).

20. SCHWEIZER, G.   Über die Kultur von *Empusa muscae* Cohn und anderen Entomophthoracean auf kalt sterilisierten nährböden.   Planta, 35 : 132-176.   1947.

21. SMITH, M. C. W.   The nutrition and physiology of *Entomophthora coronata* (Cost.) Kevorkian.   Dissertation Abstr. 13 : 648-649.   1953.   *Cited from* Rev. Appl. Mycol. 33 : 441.   1954.

22. THAXTER, R.   The Entomophthoreae of the United States.   Mem. Boston Soc. Natural Hist. 4 : 133-201.   1888.

23. WINGARD, S. A.   Parasitism of the apple leaf hopper, *Typhlocyba pomaria* Mca., by *Entomophthora.*   Phytopathology, 26 : 113.   1936.

24. WOLF, F. T.   The cultivation of two species of *Entomophthora* on synthetic media.   Bull. Torrey Botan. Club, 78 : 211-220.   1951.

POLLINATION OF ALFALFA AND RED CLOVER[1]

George E. Bohart

The subject of insect pollination is a large one with
several rather distinct phases investigated by different
authors. A voluminous literature has developed on floral
biology with emphasis on the adaptions of flowers to particular insect visitors. Workers in this field have usually been botanists -- C.R. Darwin, P. Knuth, and F.E.
Clements -- to name a few. The golden age for this group
was in the last half of the nineteenth century. Entomologists, "behaviorists," and a few botanists have studied the
instincts and adaptions of insects for utilizing floral
products. Felix Plateau, August Forel, Karl von Frisch,
and C.G. Butler typify this group. The greatest volume of
literature in this field appeared in the first 30 years of
the present century. In the last 30 years applied research
directed toward improving seed and fruit production has
dominated the field. Agronomists, horticulturists, and
entomologists have joined forces in this effort. Insect
pollination of crops is itself a broad subject with more
than 50 crops involved, many of which have their own peculiar problems. This review will therefore be limited to
the two most important forage crops, alfalfa and red clover.

Pollination has frequently been the principal limiting
factor in the growing of alfalfa and red clover for seed.
Since these are the two most important legume seed crops in

[1] The survey of the literature pertaining to this review
was completed in June 1956.

ANNUAL REVIEW OF ENTOMOLOGY, 1957, Vol. 2, pp. 355-380.

the world, it is not surprising that their pollination has been studied intensively for many years. Among insects only bees serve as alfalfa pollinators to any extent. Many species of bees other than honey bees are highly efficient in this capacity, but the problem of supplying enough of them to pollinate large acreages is well nigh insurmountable in most areas. Honey bees can do a good job of alfalfa pollination under ideal conditions, but these conditions are difficult to meet and may be unattainable over certain broad regions where seed is grown. Red clover is pollinated efficiently by most kinds of bumble bees, but here again the most discouraging problem is that of supplying enough of them in the face of increasingly intensive cultivation. Fortunately, honey bees can pollinate red clover satisfactorily in most areas, providing that enough of them are used and competing bloom is not too abundant.

The research work discussed herein is concerned mainly with the manner in which the plants are pollinated, ways and means of increasing the number of honey bees and wild bees on the seed fields, and attempts to increase the efficiency of honey bees.

Valuable research on nutrition, communication, and foraging habits of honey bees; on the nesting habits, life histories, foraging habits of wild bees; and on nectar secretion is fundamental to all pollination research, but it would be impossible to discuss it properly in a review of this scope.

ALFALFA

Tripping

The peculiar mechanism of the alfalfa flower which trips, or "explodes," when a bee visits it for pollen was known at the time of Linneaus. In 1867 Henslow (1) described the flower, the forces that hold it together, and the tensions that release the sexual column at the moment of tripping. Further descriptions of the floral mechanism were made by Müller (2) in 1873, Burkill (3) in 1894, Piper *et al.* (4) in 1914, Lesins (5) in 1950, and finally Larkin & Graumann (6) in 1954. In spite of essential agreement among these authors, there is still some question as to the exact location and nature of some of the forces involved.

Our interest as entomologists is centered more on how the bee operates the floral mechanism. This has been described in detail many times, but a simple description by Vansell and Todd (7) will suffice:

> The pollen-collecting bee straddles the
> keel and extends its proboscis into the
> throat of the flower where the tripping
> mechanism is contacted. When the flower
> trips, the bee's head is momentarily
> caught between the standard petal and the

tip of the sexual column. A splotch
of pollen is entangled among the hairs
on the bee's head at precisely the spot
where the stigma of the next flower
tripped will strike.

Before the rank and file of agronomists were finally
convinced that alfalfa seed production is dependent on
bees, it was necessary to prove (a) that tripping is required for pod setting, (b) that commercially acceptable
varieties of alfalfa are largely cross-pollinated, and
(c) that only bees (and rarely certain other insects) can
accomplish both the tripping and cross-pollinating necessary for commercial seed production.

Müller (2) knew in 1874 that alfalfa pollen is shed in
the bud stage and covers the stigma before the flower is
open. His co-worker, Urban (8), found that in rare cases
an untripped flower will form a pod. This was confirmed
several times later, but Carlson (9) in 1930 reported as
much as 26 per cent under field conditions. Kirk & White
(10) in 1933, after experience with certain strains, considered that tripping was not necessary for fertilization.
Brink & Cooper (11) agreed with this view in their earlier
studies but later (12) retracted their statement. Most
other investigators have found that with rare exceptions
not more than 1 per cent of the flowers set pods without
tripping (Knowles (13)). According to Armstrong & White
(14), tripping is necessary to scarify or rupture the
stigmatic membrane and so release the moisture necessary
for pollen germination. Petersen (15) in Denmark verified
this and described the action of tripping on the membrane.

Various plant breeders (Knowles (13); Tysdal (16);
Jones & Olson (17); Burkart (18)) have generally obtained
figures for self-fertility ranging from 20 to 30 per cent,
but extremes are as low as 5 and as high as 60 per cent.
As Tysdal *et al.* (9) pointed out, even the self-fertile
strains are largely cross-pollinated under most field
conditions because of the prepotency of foreign pollen.

A number of plant breeders have tried to produce
satisfactory varieties of self-fertile alfalfa (Kirk (20);
Torssell (21)). However, the selfed progeny of the strains
studied have always decreased in both vigor and seed
productivity. Kirk (20) found that the forage yield of
Grimm fell from 100 per cent in the parent to 54 per cent
in the S_4 generation. Seed yields fell to 22 per cent in
the same number of selfed generations. Recently Lesins
et al. (22), working in both Sweden and Alberta, have been
trying to develop a moderately self-fertile variety for use
in areas where insect pollination is usually insufficient.
They are aiming for a plant that will trip automatically
and at the same time receive enough cross-pollination from
insects to retain its heterozygosity.

Automatic tripping and tripping induced by climatic
agencies have been discussed by a number of authors.
Interest in this subject was greatest when alfalfa was
considered to be largely self-fertile (Brand & Westgate (23);

Engelbert (24)). However, Tysdal (25) in 1946 in a careful study found that rain could increase tripping but would decrease pod set and that wind had no appreciable effect. Piper *et al.* (4) in 1914 observed that very high temperatures could cause automatic tripping and that automatic tripping could be induced by quickly moving a raceme from a shaded location into the full sunlight. Tysdal found that flowers trip more easily on warm, bright days than on cool, damp ones. Ufer (26) in Germany concluded that neither low humidity nor high light value alone could induce tripping but that these factors aided by heat could do so. Whether continuous exposures to temperatures well above 100°F (such as occur in Arizona and California) could cause much tripping does not seem to have been ascertained under field conditions.[2]

Interest in automatic tripping has been revived recently in far northern areas. Lesins *et al.* (22) stated that automatic tripping was less desirable than insect tripping because of the smaller seed set even in moderately self-fertile varieties. They suggested automatic tripping and self-fertility only for far northern areas where conditions seem to favor automatic tripping and discourage insect pollination. Petersen (15), Dwyer & Allman (27), and Lesins *et al.* (22) postulated that some cross-pollination might result from the stigma striking pollen grains already on the standard petal. They considered that grains left by nectar-collecting honey bees would be the most common, but also mentioned pollen propelled by the explosive action of tripping. However, their examinations of standard petals showed that the number of such cross-pollinations must be very low.

Calculations of Pollination Requirements

The populations of various pollinators necessary to set certain seed crops can be estimated from their tripping rate, their working hours, the proportion of the effective blossoming period in which they work, the number of flowers produced per unit area, the proportion of cross-pollinated flowers that set pods, the number of seeds per cross-pollinated pod, and the weight per seed. For example, Bohart *et al.* (28) calculated[3] that on a field with good agronomic potential for seed production six nectar-collecting honey bees per square yard tripping 1 per cent of the flowers visited could set about 350 pounds of seed per acre. Grandfield (29) calculated that one colony of bees tripping 2 per cent of the blossoms visited could set 120 pounds of seed. He also calculated that the nectar produced on a field is ample for at least three colonies per acre.

Although such figures are useful in showing orders of magnitude, they are subject to considerable error because

---

[2] F.E. Todd *in litera* states that alfalfa caged without bees sets no more seed in Arizona than in Utah.

[3] Adapted from original calculations by M.W. Pedersen.

of the variability of many factors involved. Flower populations vary greatly depending upon blooming conditions
and the length of the effective blooming season. For example, Pedersen & Stapel (30) estimated a total production
of 112,800 flowers per square meter on a field with good
bloom in Denmark, and Tysdal (25) estimated 218,034 on a
field in Nebraska. The proportion of cross-pollinated
flowers that sets pods is nearly as variable (Hadfield &
Calder (31); Tysdal (25); Petersen (15); Carlson (32)).
Pedersen *et al.* (33) showed that another cause for variability in this statistic is limitation in the ability of
plants to develop pods from cross-pollinated flowers when
pollination intensity is high. They found that when all the
flowers on one set of plants and one-third of the flowers
on another set were cross-pollinated, 46.7 per cent of the
former and 66.4 per cent of the latter set pods. Menke (34)
obtained similar data under field conditions. Such information shows that the effectiveness of each tripping must
be lowered gradually as the total amount of tripping increases, until it finally approaches zero when the plant
capacity is reached. According to Pedersen *et al.* (33),
seed weight varies somewhat according to pollination intensity. They found seed averaging 2.24 mg. for a low
intensity and 2.09 for a high intensity of pollination.
Petersen (15) in Denmark found an average of 3.9 seeds per
hand cross-pollinated pod and 1.6 per self-pollinated pod.
Lesins (5) agreed fairly well with Petersen, finding 3.5
seeds per cross-pollinated pod and 1.5 per self-pollinated
pod.

Another reason for caution in making theoretical calculations of the seed crop that a particular population of
pollinators could set is the variation between strains of
alfalfa in seed-setting potential (Petersen (15); Lesins (5)).
Finally, the calculations may be upset by indeterminate
amounts of automatic tripping.

Mechanical Pollination

Seed growers have always dreamed of producing alfalfa
seed without the aid of bees (Brand & Westgate (23)).
Silversides & Olson (35) in 1941 evaluated 10 devices
designed to trip the flowers and found that most of them
increased tripping but that all of them decreased seed set,
presumably because of injury to the plants. Several tripping machines have been built in recent years and placed on
the market or used for custom operations. Pharis & Unrau (36)
in 1952 tested a large machine with sponge-rubber-covered
rollers working in pairs. They found that it tripped a high
percentage of the flowers but failed to increase seed setting.
Hvistendahl (37) recently placed on the market a "mechanical
bee" designed to open the blossoms and dust the pollen ahead
of the tripping device so that the stigmata will contact
foreign pollen when they strike the standard petals. So
far, his claims have not been substantiated by scientific
investigators.

Importance of Bees

Urban (8) in 1873 concluded from the structure of alfalfa flowers that bees were the primary agents of pollination. At first, attention was centered on honey bees because of their abundance in alfalfa fields. However, when Henslow (1), Burkill (3), and Brand & Westgate (23) found that they tripped fewer than 1 per cent of the flowers they visited, honey bees fell into disrepute. In the United States Piper *et al.* (4) in 1914, Aicher (38) in 1917, and Sladen (39) in 1918 were among the first to emphasize that wild bees could be highly effective even when not particularly abundant. They observed species of *Megachile* tripping over 90 per cent of the flowers visited and at rates up to 25 per minute. Tysdal (16) in 1940 concluded from his studies that bumble bees were the most important pollinators in the Eastern States, leaf-cutting bees (*Megachile*) in the Great Plains area, and alkali bees (Nomia melanderi Cockerell) in the West. In regard to wild pollinators Tysdal's statement still holds true in a general way, but both he and his predecessors underrated the over-all importance of honey bees.

Pollination by Honey Bees

Müller (2) was the first to describe how nectar-collecting honey bees avoid the pollination mechanism of alfalfa by inserting their proboscis into the side of the flower between the standard and wing petals. Helmbold (40) observed in 1929 that some honey bees collect pollen from alfalfa and enter the flower in the normal manner.

The research in 1944-1945 by Vansell & Todd (7) and Hare & Vansell (42) in Utah laid the foundations on which the highly successful alfalfa pollination programs in California and certain other areas have been built (Townsend (43)). Vansell & Todd (7) found that honey bee populations on alfalfa fields could be classified primarily into three groups: pollen collectors, nectar collectors operating from the side, and nectar collectors operating from the front. On the basis of later research in California, Vansell (44) described bees of the second category as "experienced" nectar collectors and of the third as "inexperienced."

Nectar collectors.--Reinhardt (45), who worked with Vansell at Davis, California, made a study of the various responses of caged honey bees to alfalfa flowers. He classified the two types of nectar collectors as "side workers" and "nectar trippers" and showed how nectar trippers learn to be side workers and in the process lose their pollinating efficiency and nearly double their working speed. It took many of his bees several days to learn the side approach, but the scarcity of nectar trippers in the field suggests that they learn more rapidly in the open. Nectar trippers are usually observed when alfalfa first comes into bloom or when bees are first moved into the field (Pedersen & Todd (46)). At other times they generally make up less than 1 per cent of the population.

Vansell (44) recommended "overstocking" alfalfa fields with colonies of bees to increase the percentage of young bees working close to the hives. Vansell (in personal communication) considered that it would be feasible to use recently divided colonies with rapidly expanding populations. Another method would be to move in as replacements colonies with field forces that had never worked in alfalfa.

Experienced nectar collectors accidentally trip and pollinate a small percentage of the alfalfa flowers they visit. Tremendous amounts of data accumulated by Franklin (47) in Kansas; Tysdal (16) in Ohio, Nebraska, and Wyoming; Bohart and others in Utah and California (mostly unpublished); Hobbs & Lilly (48) in Alberta; Stephen (49) in Manitoba; and many others show that this accident rate varies from time to time and from place to place. It tends to be greatest in Oklahoma, Arizona, and southern California (about 2 per cent) intermediate in Kansas, Utah, and Nebraska (about 1 per cent), somewhat lower in southern Alberta (0.7 per cent), and still lower in Manitoba (0.3 per cent). Surprisingly, this trend does not coincide with published figures for automatic tripping which have sometimes been quite high in the North (Lesins *et al.* (22)).

Although the tripping rates of nectar collectors are low at best, large populations tripping at the higher rates can set a fairly good seed crop. Bohart *et al.* (32) calculated[3] that bees tripping 1.5 per cent of the flowers they visit can set about 35 pounds of seed per acre for each bee per square yard in a three-week period. From four to six bees per square yard can be concentrated on fields with abundant bloom, and in some areas the blossoming season can be extended considerably beyond three weeks. Where nectar collectors trip only 0.3 per cent of the blossoms visited, their value must be slight, as stated by Hobbs & Lilly (48) and Stephen (49). On the other end of the scale, Jones (50) claimed that on some California fields, with yields running up to 1500 pounds of seed per acre, nectar-collecting honey bees performed 99 per cent of the tripping. In this case there must have been an extraordinarily high percentage of nectar trippers or else there were brief but unobserved periods of pollen collection by honey bees or wild bees.

Nectar collectors trip some flowers by accidentally lodging their legs in blossoms while crawling over the racemes. In such cases the stigma usually misses the bee entirely, and the result is the same as automatic tripping. This form of tripping seems to be most prevalent percentage-wise in the North (Hobbs & Lilly (48); Stephen (49)). Pharis & Unrau (36) found that flowers tripped by honey bees produced fewer seeds per pod than flowers crossed by hand or tripped by leaf-cutting bees and bumble bees. However, Petersen (15) in Denmark found tripping with the legs to take place in only 0.1 per cent of all visits. Furthermore, he found no difference in seeds per pod between flowers tripped by honey bees and those crossed by hand.

There is some indication that the rate of accidental

tripping by nectar collectors differs between varieties of honey bees. Petersen (15) reports that in Denmark "*Apis mellifica*" (the native, dark German or Nordic bee) trips about 2.8 per cent of the flowers visited and "*Apis ligustica*" (the Italian variety) trips about 2.1 per cent. These are surprisingly high tripping rates, but they may include some activity by nectar trippers. Bieberdorf (51) in Oklahoma found indication that Caucasians were more effective trippers than Italians. Apparently, no one has done any work on this problem from the standpoint of bee breeding.

McMahon (52) in Saskatchewan made the unique observation that accidental tripping by nectar collectors increased from 0.3 per cent to 1.8 per cent when the removal of surrounding bloom greatly increased the bee population on the field. He found that when the field was "overstocked" the bees had to work the compactly clustered florets toward the apex of the raceme and in doing so were forced to enter many flowers from near the front, thus increasing the accident rate. McMahon suggested two methods of achieving such high populations: increasing the number of colonies per number of flowers and eliminating competing bloom. He failed to point out, however, that exceptionally high populations will not visit a field unless nectar production is also exceptionally high (Pedersen (53)).

Pedersen & McAllister (28) found that open stands had twice as much nectar per flower, twice as many bees per flower, and twice as much seed per acre as dense stands. It may well be that the principal value of open stands lies in the heavy concentrations of honey bees attracted by the copious secretion of nectar in well spaced plants.

Other methods of increasing the number of bees on the field have been suggested. Drake (54), on the basis of studies in Iowa and Nebraska, strongly recommended growing seed from part of the field as the first growth and staggering the cutting dates on the rest of the field to cause the appearance of second-crop bloom at different times over the field. Todd (55) suggested the same method of utilizing the bee supply more efficiently. In some areas staggering the cutting dates would increase weed and insect control problems. Soboleva (56) in Russia advocated feeding bees 50 to 100 gm. of alfalfa-scented sugar syrup per hive for 5 to 10 days at the time of mass flowering.

Vansell (44) and Jones (50) reported that when colonies of bees were first placed in central California alfalfa fields the population rose, but after about eight days it fell to near the original level. When these colonies were replaced by others, the same thing occurred. Levin (57,58) observed that bees from newly placed colonies visited alfalfa more freely than those from colonies already in the field, whether or not they had had previous experience with alfalfa. In general, the newcomers stayed with the alfalfa longer when moved from an area with abundant alfalfa to one with little alfalfa.

Åkerberg & Lesins (59) postulated another role for

nectar collectors, that of "setting up" the flowers for automatic tripping by their repeated visits. They found that when bee trippings were subtracted from total trippings in their unguarded plots the remainder was still greater than the amount of tripping in guarded plots. Pharis & Unrau (36) corroborated Lesins' findings in cages with and without honey bees. However, Piper *et al.* (4) concluded from experiments at Pullman, Washington, that nontripping insects had no effect on subsequent pod set. If such delayed-action tripping is prevalent, it might explain the difficulties that we in northern Utah have always had in trying to associate nectar-collecting honey bee populations with the number of tripped flowers from hour to hour. The Swedish investigators (59) believe that it may also explain the rather large quantity of selfed seed they harvest from fields where wild bees are scarce.

Pollen collectors.--Pollen-collecting honey bees are far more desirable on alfalfa seed fields than those in either of the nectar-collecting categories. Bohart *et al.* (28) pointed out that, since pollen collectors trip about 80 per cent of the blossoms they visit compared with 1 per cent for nectar collectors and visit slightly over half as many flowers per minute, they should be 45 times as valuable. However, since they "take time off" now and then to gather nectar for their own needs, their relative efficiency is probably somewhat less than this. Nevertheless a few pollen collectors added to a nectar-collecting bee population can make a big difference in the rate of pollination. The percentage of pollen-collecting honey bees found on different seed fields varies from 0 to 100. It may vary from 1 per cent to 50 per cent on adjacent fields depending upon the growing condition of the plants (unpublished observations). Table I shows the percentages of pollen collectors on alfalfa in various localities. These figures follow the same regional trend as those for tripping by nectar collectors. The reasons for this are not clear but they probably involve a combination of climatic effect on the plants and the nature and abundance of competing pollen sources (Bohart (61)).

Many investigators have stressed the importance of competing pollen sources (Linsley & MacSwain (62); Vansell and Todd (7); Hare & Vansell (42); Franklin (47); Hobbs & Lilly (48); and others. That honey bees can be forced to collect alfalfa pollen by caging them inside plots of alfalfa has been demonstrated by several workers (Akerberg & Lesins (59) in Sweden; Hobbs & Lilly (48) in Alberta; Reinhardt (45) in California; Levin & Pedersen (64) in Utah). Linsley & MacSwain (62) increased the number of pollen collectors on an alfalfa field by cutting an adjacent field of mustard but only after the entire field was cut. Similar trials in Utah failed (Bohart (61)). In this case the competition was in the form of continuous strips of roadside gumweed and sweet-clover, and the bees merely moved along the same strips to points beyond the mile zone of control.

There is some evidence that certain pollen sources for

honey bees such as sweetclover and mustard, are more potent as competitors than others such as greasewood (*Sarcobatus*) and various grasses (Hobbs & Lilly (48); Hare & Vansell (42)). The relative potency of the competing sources may be as important as their abundance in determining the degree to which they need to be controlled (Bohart (61)).

Climate and competition are not the only factors controlling abundance of pollen collectors on alfalfa. Hare & Vansell (42) were the first to note the importance of plant condition in attracting pollen collectors. Vansell (44) suggested that lush conditions on certain fields at Delta, Utah, were responsible for low amounts of tripping. Unpublished observations by the Legume Seed Research Laboratory at Logan, Utah, generally support the same conclusion. Pedersen & Bohart (65), in a study of the attractiveness of certain clones of alfalfa to pollen-collecting bumble bees, found nectar production to be the most highly associated. It might be expected, therefore, that high nectar production would be associated with the slightly dry condition that pollen-collecting honey bees seem to favor. However, other factors are probably involved because, according to Pedersen (unpublished data), only when the soil moisture is exceptionally high does nectar production decline.

Rudnev (41) claimed that he increased pollen collection by honey bees in Russia both by replacing pollen-filled combs with empty combs and by feeding syrup flavored with alfalfa pollen. The reported increases appear to have been for all pollen rather than alfalfa pollen alone. Butler & Simpson (66) failed to increase the collection of red clover pollen in the field by suspending red clover pollen in syrup fed to the bees. Consequently, they doubted that "training" would serve to increase pollen collection.

Recommendations.--Todd & Vansell (67) gave some practical advice for alfalfa seed growers interested in using honey bees for pollination. They recommended three colonies or less per acre for fields where pollen-collecting honey bees were abundant and six colonies or more for fields depending on nectar trippers.[4] They also recommended scattering the colonies in groups of 10 to 12 throughout the fields. To take full advantage of the higher tripping occurring around the incoming colonies, they suggested moving in the first colony per acre at the one-quarter bloom stage and the remainder at intervals of 7 to 10 days until five to six bees per square yard are present at the peak of bloom. Considering the tremendous variation in the working habits of honey bees on alfalfa, it is probably impossible to make satisfactory blanket recommendations for colony numbers. Bohart *et al.* (28) in 1955 recommended a formula similar to that of Todd & Vansell and further suggested methods by which the grower could check his progress and adjust the number of colonies.

---

[4] Experienced nectar collectors were not mentioned but may have been omitted by oversight.

TABLE 1

Percentage of Pollen-Collecting Honey Bees
in Various Localities*

Locality	Observers	Per cent of Pollen Collectors
Southern California	Linsley & MacSwain (62,	5-20
Southern Arizona	Bohart	4-100
North Central California	Linsley & MacSwain (62)	0-5
Central Utah	Vansell & Todd (7)	5-50
Northern Utah:		
Howell Valley	Bohart & Levin	1-50
Cache Valley	Bohart & Pedersen	
	Vansell & Todd (7)	0-5
Wyoming	Bohart	0-1
Washington	Menke (34)	0
Alberta	Hobbs & Lilly (48)	0
Manitoba	Stephen (49)	0
Minnesota	Haws (63)	0
Saskatchewan	Peck & Bolton (60)	0

*Figures given for Bohart and associates are taken from
unpublished data.

Where there is no pollen collection and tripping rates
range around 0.5 per cent, it seems to be doubtful whether
honey bees can be utilized on an economically sound basis
(Stephen (49)). Pengelly (68) suggested that in such areas
honey bees should not be used because they lower the attractiveness of the field and seriously compete with wild
bees in poor forage years and during a critical season. He
quoted an ecological paper by Pearson (69) to support his
belief. Peck & Bolton (60) expressed a similar view.
Bohart *et al.* (28) stated that heavy concentrations of
honey bees lower the attractiveness of alfalfa fields to
bumble bees and leaf-cutting bees but not to alkali bees.
They recommended that if the field normally attracts enough
wild bees (except alkali bees) to set a good seed crop,
honey bees should not be increased in the area. On the

other hand Jones (50) stated that honey bees do not depress populations of other bees.

The evidence in favor of Todd & Vansell's recommendation for scattering colonies throughout the fields is not yet conclusive. Vansell (44) reported that a field in California set 30 per cent more seed 100 feet from the colonies than 1,000 feet farther out. He attributed the phenomenon to greater numbers of young, inexperienced bees close to the colonies (personal communication). This belief is based on the assumption that young bees and bees recently moved into a field tend to work close to the hive. Members of the research group at Logan, Utah, are now attempting to verify this point.

Pollination by Bees Other Than Honey Bees

Judging from the 50 or more species of alfalfa-visiting bees found in Utah (Bohart (28)), the total number on alfalfa the world over must be several hundred. The problem of reviewing the scattered literature on the pollinating activities, populations, seasonal and geographic distributions, and methods of protecting, increasing, and utilizing even the most important members of this assemblage leaves me with a feeling of helplessness to say the least.

Linsley (70) in California wrote the first survey paper for the wild pollinators of any area. Subsequently Drake (54) in Iowa, Peck & Bolton (60) in Saskatchewan, Stephen (49) in Manitoba, Pengelly (68) in Ontario, Franklin (47) in Kansas, Fischer (71) in northern Minnesota, Bohart (72) in Utah, Menke (34) in Washington, and Hobbs & Lilly (73) in southern Alberta have made at least hasty surveys of local areas. As might be expected, the largest number of species are found in the bee-rich areas west of the Rockies. Lesins (5) in Sweden, Petersen (15) in Denmark, and Ufer (74) in Germany have published considerable information on the limited number of species of wild bees pollinating alfalfa in northern Europe. So far as I know, the wild bees visiting alfalfa in southeastern Europe and central Asia, where alfalfa supposedly originated, have not been surveyed.[5]

---

[5] Since writing the above, two important Russian articles by V.B. Popov have come to my attention. The first ("The Significance of Bees (Hymenoptera-Apoidae) in the Pollination of Alfalfa," *All-Union Entomol. Soc.*, 43, 65-82 (1952)) lists 22 important alfalfa pollinators in Central Asia as follows:

Halictus eurygnathus Bluthgen, *H. malachurus* (Kirby), *Andrena labialis* (Kirby), *A. flavipes* Panzer, *A. albofasciata* Thomson, *Nomia diversipes* Latreille, *Melitta leporina* (Panzer), *Melitturga clavicornis* (Latreille), *Megachile argentata* (Fabricius), *M. pilidens* Alfken, *M. maritima* (Kirby), *M. sausurei* Radoszkowski, *Eucera tuberculata* (Fabricius), *E. interrupta* Bär, *E. clypeata* Erichson, *E. nigrifascies* Lepeletier, *E. chrysopyga* Perez, *Tetralonia tricincta* Eversmann, *Amegilla magnilabris* (Fedtschenko),

Table 2 summarizes existing information concerning the species known to have at least local or sporadic importance. Obviously there are many unreported species of importance in seed-growing areas such as Argentina, southern Russia, and Australia. I have taken the liberty of "interpreting" some of the published data to make it conform to the headings used in the table. For example, my observations indicate that bumble bees and *Megachile* nearly always trip alfalfa flowers when they are seeking pollen. Consequently, when only 30 per cent of the visits of a species of these genera were reported as causing the flower to trip, the table shows that about 65 per cent were collecting nectar.

It can be seen at once that generalizations concerning pollination by wild bees are rather futile because of the great diversity among them. Even within a genus and in some cases a species, it is difficult to make valid generalizations. For example, *Megachile frigida* Smith is considered by Stephen (49) and Peck & Bolton (60) to be the most important alfalfa pollinator in Manitoba and Saskatchewan. Stephen claims that it prefers alfalfa to all other host plants. On the other hand, Hobbs & Lilly (73) say this species is rather common in southern Alberta but is almost never found on alfalfa. In Utah I have seen it commonly on hairy vetch and wild licorice (Glycorrihiza) but never on alfalfa. Stephen found *Megachile brevis* Say to be principally a nectar collector on alfalfa in Manitoba. Linsley (70) found it to be a consistent and efficient collector of alfalfa pollen in California.

In spite of these precautions, the following generalizations, compounded from the literature and personal experience, may be in order: (a) Wild bees more than three-eighths inch long are generally much more consistent trippers of alfalfa than are honey bees. Bees less than one-quarter inch long do not trip at all (Bohart *et al.* (28). (b) With the exception of *Nomia melanderi* Cockerell, wild bees rarely keep pace with expanding acreage of seed. Sooner or later the combined effects of reducing the nesting areas and spreading the existing population over more alfalfa reduces their effectiveness. (c) With the exceptions of *Nomia*

_____

5   *Bombus silvarum* (Linnaeus), *B. agrorum* (Fabricius), *B. terrestris* (Linnaeus).

The second ("Bees, Their Relations to Melittophilous Plants and the Problem of Alfalfa Pollination," *Entomol. Rev. U.S.S.R.,* 35, 528-598 (1956) summarizes knowledge on the distribution and biology of the most important species of central Europe and Asia. *Melitturga clavicornis* (Latreille) was considered the most valuable species. Honey bees were given little credit for alfalfa pollination in any part of Russia.

melanderi in suitable habitats and certain species of
Megachile in the cottonwood and aspen "bush country" of
Canada, we have no proven methods for large-scale increase
of wild alfalfa pollinators (Todd & Vansell (67)).
(d) Because wild bees often have short seasons and sporadic
or cyclical appearance from year to year, it is advantageous
in each area to have as many alfalfa-visiting species as
possible. Consequently, there should be great possibilities
for improving the pattern of wild bee pollination by making
suitable introductions (Piper *et al.* (4); Larkin (76)).

Among exceptions to point (a) are certain long-tongued
bumble bees and *Anthophora* that visit alfalfa largely for
nectar and avoid the pollinating mechanism in the same manner
as nectar-collecting honey bees (see Ufer (74) concerning
Bombus and Stephen (49) concerning *Anthophora*). Bees of
this sort can sometimes avoid tripping the flowers even
when they enter the throat of the flower. Small halictids
and andrenids often have great difficulty tripping the
flowers and spend much of their time looking for tripped
flowers (Franklin (47)). However, when they do succeed
in tripping, they do it more frequently than nectar-
collecting honey bees. In general, large size is correlated
with speed in tripping. Queen bumble bees work more rapidly
than workers (Franklin (47)), and large individuals of
Halictus rubicundus Christ trip more flowers than small ones
(unpublished data).

Linsley (70) suggested that the species of *Lasioglossum*,
Halictus, and *Hylaeus* that are too small to trip flowers may
be of benefit in cross-pollinating automatically tripped
flowers. Pengelly (68) discussed the same possibility.
However, Pedersen (verbal communication) concluded that
cross pollination after tripping probably occurs but rarely,
since the entire receptive surface of the stigma is tightly
appressed to the standard petal. If Linsley's hypothesis is
valid, tripping machines might be used to advantage in areas
where these bees are particularly abundant. In Utah it has
been observed that *Halictus provancheri arapahonum* Cockerell
often increases on a field as soon as large-scale tripping
takes place.

Stephen (49) described the usual history of seed
production in new areas. At first there are a few small
seed fields with exceptionally high yields; a period of
land expansion, clearing of burnt-over land, and thorough
cultivation follows; finally, within 4 to 10 years yields
drop from 1,000 pounds to 150 pounds or so, and seed production is no longer profitable. According to personal
communication from Wayne Wright, a large-scale seed grower
in northern Manitoba, the usual history has been interrupted
and perhaps even reversed in this territory by a process of
limiting fields to narrow strips surrounded by aspen and
cottonwood "bush." According to reports, the growers are
providing nesting sites for *Megachile* and bumble bees by
piling refuse timber around the edges of the fields. Obviously such a procedure is feasible only under special
conditions.

TABLE 2

Wild Pollinators of Alfalfa*

Species	Areas Important as Alfalfa Pollinators	Alfalfa a Preferred Host	Per Cent Collecting Nectar	Flowers Tripped by Pollen Collectors		Nesting Sites
				Per Cent	Number per minute	
Bombus terrestris (Linn.)	Northern Europe (L), (Pe), etc., New Zealand (Ha)	Yes (Le)	10-30 (Pe)	70-90 (Pe)	20 (Le)	Underground usually deep (Le)
occidentalis Greene	Great Basin, U.S. (B), Southern Alberta (H)	Yes (B)	0 (B)	90-95 (B)	15-18 (B)	Underground in rodent nests (P)
terricola Kirby	Manitoba (S), Minn. (Fi), Saskatchewan (P), Ontario (Pn)	Yes (S)	30-40 (Pn)	85-90 (S)	12-28 (P)	Underground long tunnel (Pl)
distinguendus Morawitz	Central Denmark (Sk)	No (Sk)		86 (Sk)		Underground (Lo)

57

TABLE 2 (cont.)

borealis Kirby	Saskatchewan (P)		60± (Pn)		12-27(P) 19+ (Pn)	Underground (Pl)
morrisoni Cresson	Great Basin of U.S. and Southern Utah	Yes (B)	5-10 (B)	80-95 (B)	16-22 (B)	Above ground in buildings etc.
crotchii Cresson	California (L)					
huntii Greene	Great Basin of U.S. (B)	No (B)	20-40 (B)	80-90 (B)	14-18 (B)	Underground in rodent nests (B)
griseocollis DeGeer	Utah and Idaho (B)	Yes (B)	10-20 (B) 40-50 (Pn)	90± (B)	15-20 (B)	Above ground or at surface (B)
ternarius Say	Manitoba (S), Ontario (Pn)		55± (S) 40-50 (Pn)		20-24 (Pn)	Underground in long tunnels (Pl)

TABLE 2 (cont.)

Species						
impatiens Cresson	Iowa (D), Ontario (Pn)	No (Pn)	20-25 (Pn)		16-22 (Pn)	Underground in long tunnels (Pl)
vagans F. Smith	Manitoba (S), Saskatchewan (P)	No (P)	80± (S)		15-16 (S)	Some surface some underground (P)
californicus F. Smith	California (L)					
sonorus Say	California (L)					
americanorum (Fabricius)	Kansas (F), Ontario (Pn)		50± (F)	80 (Pn)	16-20 (Pn)	Above ground or shallow underground
ervidus (Fabricius)	Manitoba (S), Ontario (Pn)	No (B)	90± (B) 50± (B)	80-90 (B)	21 (B) 14-28 (Pn)	Near surface of ground: above or below

TABLE 2 (con't)

Species	Location					
fraternus (F. Smith)	Kansas (F)		50±			
rufocinctus Cresson	Manitoba (S), Saskatchewan (P)	No (P)	60± (S)		12-27 (P)	Above ground or at surface (Pn)
auricomus (Robertson)	Iowa (D)					Shallow underground
Anthophora furcata terminalis Cresson	Saskatchewan (P), Ontario (Pn)	No (Pn)	60± (Pn)		12 (B) 14-17 (Pn)	Decayed wood (B)
urbana Cresson	California (L), Southern Utah (B)	No (B)	40±	86 (B)	10-14 (B)	Sandy soil usually Gregarious
californica Cresson	Southern Calif. (L)	No (L)				
walshii Cresson	Iowa (D)					Soil (B)
Tetralonia edwardsii Cresson	Utah, Idaho (B)	Yes (B)	0 (B)	97 (B)	14-16 (B)	Soil-hidden in grass

TABLE 2 (Con't)

Eucera longicornis (Linnaeus)	Northern Europe (Le), (Pe), etc.		0 (Le)		7-15 (Le)	Soil (Le)
Melissodes agilis Cresson	California, Kansas (L), (F)	No (L)	40 (B)	60-85 (B)		Soil (B)
timberlakei Cockerell	California (L)		30 (B)		16-19 (B)	Soil-- under chips or other objects
obliqua Say	California (L), Kansas, (F)	No (B)				Soil -- in sparse grass (B)
Florilegus condignus Cresson	Nebraska (La), Iowa (D), Kansas (F)	No (La)	$60^{\pm}$ (D)	95 (La)	20 (La)	Soil (B)
Xylocopa virginica (Linnaeus)	Kansas (F), Iowa (D)					Dead wood (B)
varipuncta Patton	California (L)					Dead wood (L)

TABLE 2 (Con't)

Species	Locality					Nest site
californica arizonensis Cresson	Southern Utah (B)	Yes (B)	0 (B)	90± (B)	23-30 (B)	Dead wood and yuca
sp.	Israel (me)					
Megachile brevis (Say)	Calif. (L), Utah (B), Alberta (H), Manitoba (S), Ontario (Pn)	Yes (B), No (S)		99-100 (Pn)	16-20 (Pn)	Hollow and pithy stumps (B)
onobrychidis Cockerell	Utah (B), Calif. (L)	Yes	0 (B)	98 (B)	18-21 (B)	Soil cracked under clay stones (B)
gentilis Cresson	Utah (B), Calif. (L)					Soil (B)
coquilletti Cockerell	Utah (B), California (L)			98± (B)		Probably (B)
mendica Cresson						
texana Cresson	Utah (B), Ontario (Pn), Kansas (F)	Yes (B)	0	95 (B), 85-95 (F)	16-20 (B), 18-22 (Pn)	In soil

TABLE 2 (Con't)

perihirta Cockerell	Western U.S., Western Canada	Yes (B)	0 (B)	98 (B)	19-24 (B)	In soil, between hay, in gravel (B)
dentitarsus Sladen	Utah, Idaho, Alberta	Yes (B)	0 (B)	95$\pm$ (B)	18-26 (H)	In soil with light vegetation (H)
latimanus Say	Minn. (Fi), Man. (S), Saskatchewan (P), Ontario (Pn)	Yes (P)	0 (P)	95 (P)	16-22(P) 12.2(Fi) 19-28(Pn)	In soil
relativa Cresson	Minn. (F), Man. (S), Saskatchewan (P)	No (P)	40 (S)		"rapid" (P)	Tunnel in possibly wood also
nivalis Friese	Saskatchewan (P)	No (P)			"rapid" (P)	Beetle cottonwood
inermis Provancher	Manitoba (S), Saskatchewan (P)	No (Pn)	0 (Pn) 60 (S)	95 (Pn)	16-22 (Pn) 8-27 (P)	Old cottonwoods (P)
melanopnaea Smith	Manitoba (S), Saskatchewan (P), Ontario (Pn)	No (S)	40 (S) 0 (Pn)	100 (Pn)	13-16 (Pn) 15 (P)	

TABLE 2 (Con't)

Species						Nesting site
gemula Cresson	Minn. (Fi), Saskatchewan (P)	No (P)			11.4 (Fi)	
integra Cresson	Kansas (F)		5 (F)	85 (F)		
willughbiella (Kirby)	Northern Europe (Le), (Pe)		0 (Le)	100 (Le)	20 (Le)	Gravel holds soil (Le)
Diceratosmia subfasciata punctata Michener	Imperial Co., Calif. (L)	Yes (L)		High (L)		Beetle burrows, wood-willow, thickets, etc. (L)
Osmia seclusa Sandhouse	Utah, Idaho (B)	Yes (B)	0 (B)	95 (B)	12-14 (B)	Soil in nests of *Diadasia* (B)
Anthidium edwardsii Cresson	California (L)	No (B)	0 (B)	95 (B)	14-18 (B)	Shallow burrows in soil (L)

TABLE 2 (Con't)

Halictus farinosus Smith	California (L), Utah (B)	No (B)	0 (B)	60-90 (B)	6-9 (B)	Hard-packed Cells 4-15 in. deep (B)
Halictus rubicundus Christ	Utah (B)	No (B)	0 (B)	10-60 (B)	1-5 (B)	Hard or medium soil. Cells 12 in. (B)
ligatus Say	California (L)	No (B)	0 (B)			Hard-packed (L)
parallelus Say	Iowa (D)	No (D)	0 (B)			Hard-packed (B)
Lasioglossum athabascense Sandhouse	Ontario (Pn)		0 (Pn)	"low" (Pn)	"low" (Pn)	
sisymbrii Cockerell	Utah (B)	No (B)	0 (B)	30-60 (B)	3-8 (B)	Soil (B)
Rophites canus Eversmith	Central Europe (U), (Le)	Yes (U)	0 (U)	90-95 (U)		Soil (U)

TABLE 2   (Con't)

Nomia *melanderi* Cockerell	Western U.S. (B), etc.	Yes (B)	0 (B) Except Males	90-95 (B) (males 40-70)	10-14 (B)	Moist, alkaline soil. Cells in. (B)
Nomia *nevadensis* Cresson	Southern Calif. (L)	No (B)	0 (B)	90± (B)	10 (B)	Moist, usually alkaline soil. Cells 6-20 in. deep (L)
Agapostemon *cockerelli* Crawford	Utah (B), Calif. (L)	No (B)	0 (B)	40-80 (B)	6-10 (B) Males 1-5	Deep in (L)
melliventris Cresson	Southern Calif. (L)	No (B)	0 (B)			Soil (L)
virescens (Fabricius)	Iowa (D), Utah (B)	No (B)	0 (B)	50-80 (B)	8-10 (B) Males 1-5	Deep in soil sometimes in lawns (B)

66

TABLE 2 (Con't)

Species	Location	Social				Substrate
Adrena wilkella (Kirby)	Indiana, Ontario (Pn)		0 (B)	40-60 (Pn)	11-18 (Pn)	Soil (B)
prunorum Cockerell	Utah, Idaho (B)	No (B)	0 (B)	40-60 (B)	4-8 (B)	Loose soil
Nomadopsis scutellaris (Fowler)	Utah (B)	No (B)	0 (B)	5-40 (B)	1-5 (B)	Hard-packed often moist
Calliopsis andreniformis (Smith)	Nebraska (La, Cr)		0 (Cr)			Hard-packed (Cr)
Melitta leporina (Panzer)	Northern Europe	Yes	0 (Le)	90-100 (Le)	15 (Le)	Soil, entrance concealed
Macropis labiata (Fabricius)	Central Europe (J)					Soil (Lo)
Campsomeris plumipes (Drury)**	Southern Utah (B)	No (B)	Eat pollen nectar (B)	52 (B)	4-9 (B)	Parasite of scareb larvae in soil (B)

TABLE 2   (Con't)

			Predator on etc. (B)
tolteca (Saussure)**	Calif. (L), (Hu)		
Chauliognathus pennsylvanicus DeGeer***	Iowa (D)	No (D)	Predator on etc. (B)

* L=Linsley (70), Pe=Petersen (15), Ha=Hadfield & Calder (31), Sk=Skovgaard (75), Bohart (mostly original), F=Franklin (47), S=Stephen (49), Fi=Fischer (71), P=Peck & (60), D=Drake (54), Le=Lesins (5), La=Larkin (76), Me=Melamed (*in lit.*), U=Ufer (74), Pengelly (68), Pl=Plath (78), Lo=Loeken (*in lit.*), Hu=Hurd (140).

** Scoliidae

*** Cantharidae

The usual history has likewise been altered in certain seed-growing districts of the Northwest where conditions are favorable for *Nomia melanderi*. The early expansion of seed production in these areas, instead of reducing *Nomia* populations, has actually increased them by providing large amounts of sweetclover, alfalfa, and other plants to replace the former meager forage (Bohart (79)). Futhermore, irrigation has greatly increased areas of alkaline, water-logged land suitable for their highly gregarious nesting. In such areas many seed growers are protecting their nesting sites and certain farmers are developing new nesting sites (Menke (34,80); Bohart (79,81,82,); Bohart & Cross (83)).

General rules for making the best use of wild bees were summarized by Bohart *et al.* (28) as follows: (a) Time the bloom with the period of their greatest abundance. (b) Plant seed alfalfa in areas where alfalfa-pollinating species are known to be abundant (McMahon (84)). (c) If wild bees are setting most of the crop, don't expand the acreage beyond the capacity of the bees to pollinate it (Stephen (49); Bohart (85)). (d) Reduce competing bloom in the area during the period the seed crop is in bloom. (e) Provide spring and early-summer bloom for bumble bees, leaf-cutting bees, and other species with long seasons (Pengelly (68); Bohart & Knowlton (86)). (f) In areas with natural timber growth, provide nesting sites for leaf-cutting bees by cutting and piling trees (especially poplars, willows, and aspens) near the alfalfa field. The timber should be piled loosely for aeration and availability to beetles and bees. (g) Search for nesting sites of gregarious species and keep them in an unaltered condition.

Highlights

The highlights of alfalfa pollination may be summarized as follows: (a) Existing commercial varieties depend upon bees to trip and cross-pollinate enough flowers to produce a commercial seed crop. However, some efforts are still being made to develop satisfactory self-tripping and self-fertile varieties. (b) Honey bees are efficient alfalfa pollinators when they collect pollen but inefficient when they collect nectar (except during a brief learning period). (c) In areas where the weather is cool or humid or both, or where strongly competing pollen sources are abundant, honey bees rarely collect alfalfa pollen. (d) Pollen collecting can be encouraged in suitable areas by spacing the plants and not irrigating heavily after the bloom begins. (e) Nectar-collecting bees can set a good seed crop if sufficiently abundant on the field. If they trip many fewer than 1 per cent of the flowers, the population sufficient for setting a good seed crop may be unattainable. (f) Most species of wild bees are highly efficient pollinators when they visit alfalfa, but in most areas they are too scarce to set good seed crops. Practical methods for conserving and increasing them are still undeveloped except in the cases of *Nomia melanderi* in the northwest and timber-inhabiting *Megachile* in the cottonwood and aspen zones of Canada.

RED CLOVER
Tripping

The floral structures of red clover and alfalfa differ significantly with respect to their tripping mechanism. In alfalfa, if cross-pollination doesn't take place during the single act of tripping, it is not likely to take place at all. The pollinating mechanism of red clover is of the piston type. Pressure against the standard and wing petals operates a lever which forces the stigma and anthers upward and out of the enclosed keel petals. When the pressure is released the sexual parts revert to their former position. There is no naturally occurring side opening that bees can use for stealing nectar without tripping the flowers. Therefore, any insect that applies sufficient pressure to the petals when seeking either nectar or pollen serves as a pollinator. With few exceptions, only bees apply such pressure. Müller (87) described the floral mechanism in considerable detail.

Darwin (88) popularized red clover pollination with his assertion that cats increase red clover seed yields by catching mice that destroy nests of the bumble bees that pollinate red clover. Hardly an article on red clover seed production neglects to mention Darwin's concept, although it is based on two controversial assumptions, (a) that red clover depends upon bumble bees for pollination and (b) that mice reduce bumble bee populations.

Darwin's insistence that red clover requires insect pollination was disputed by Meehan (89) but was later dramatically proven, by the introduction of bumble bees into New Zealand and the subsequent abrupt increase in seed production. Since honey bees were already present this event also seemed to confirm Darwin's belief that honey bees are of little value to red clover.

Until the intensive studies of Westgate & Coe (90) in 1915, opinion was about equally divided as to whether red clover is self-sterile or self-fertile. The need for insect pollination was well recognized, and the predominance of bumble bees as pollinators was accepted by all except a few workers such as Hopkins (91) in 1896 and Pammel & King (92) in 1911. Westgate & Coe showed that all commercial varieties of red clover were self-sterile, but they failed to convert many workers to the view that honey bees are important as pollinators. As late as 1925 Plath (93) reported seeing no honey bees in a four-year study of a red clover field near Boston

Pollination by Honey Bees

More recent workers have been generally in agreement that honey bees are efficient red clover pollinators under the proper conditions. The first reason advanced for the reluctance of honey bees to visit red clover was the long,

narrow corolla tube of the plant in comparison to the
length of the honey bee's proboscis (Pammel & King (92)).
Martin (94) in 1938 calculated that with corolla tubes
8.5 mm. in length honey bees could just touch a nectar
column 1 mm. high. This, he said, placed most American
varieties out of the reach of honey bees for nectar collection. However, Pedersen (95) found that the height of the
nectar column varies from 0 to 1.5 mm. in bee-visited flowers and from 0 to 3.5 mm. in isolated flowers. Wexelsen (96)
pointed out that the value of honey bees was reduced by
their habit of seeking out old florets, incapable of fertilization but wilted enough for the bees to reach the
nectar. Another drawback of honey bees is their habit of
"stealing" nectar from the holes cut in corolla bases by
certain species of bumble bees (Pedersen (95); Schelhorn
(97)).

Investigators have perceived three obvious approaches
to the problem of fitting honey bees to red clover flowers:
(a) shorter corolla tubes, (b) more nectar, (c) longer-
tongued bees. Linhard (98) and Kratochvil & Snoflak (99)
obtained greater yields from short-tubed red clovers than
from long-tubed varieties. On the other hand, Wilsie &
Gilbert (100) found the latter more attractive to honey bees
and higher in seed production. This discrepancy may have
been associated with holes that short-tongued species of
bumble bees in Europe had cut in the corollas of long-tubed
strains. Starling *et al.* (101) on the basis of earlier
studies and a genetic study concluded that the short-tubed
strains had no advantage over the long-tubed ones in seed
setting and that they were lower in general growth and vigor.
In spite of these results Akerberg *et al.* (102) consider
the development of a good short-tubed variety a major objective.

Cultural rather than genetic attainment of a plant
with short corolla tubes has been more widely accepted. As
early as 1906 Fruwirth (103) quoted Schachinger as saying
that corolla tubes are shorter in the second crop than in
the first. Akerberg (104) found a direct correlation between
hot, dry weather and short corolla tubes. Pedersen (95) in
Denmark, Akerberg *et al.* (102) in Sweden and Dunham (105)
in Ohio reported a greater visitation of honey bees to the
short-tubed flowers of second crop. Pedersen's data indicate three other possible reasons: (a) There was slightly
more nectar per floret in late clover. (b) There were more
flower heads per unit area and more florets per head on late
clover. (c) There were only half as many bumble bees on
late clover. This reduced the competition, thus allowing
for an increase in honey bees. It also reduced the number
of holes cut in the corollas by bumble bees. In spite of
such evidence in favor of growing second crop for seed,
Wilsie & Gilbert (100) and Starling *et al.* (101) found no
increase in seed setting of the second crop over the first.
Hammer in 1949 (106) and Shuel in 1951 (107) found that red
clover secretes nectar more copiously in hot weather and
that the sugar concentration is highest in hot, dry weather

(through increased evaporation). Since the atmosphere is generally hottest and driest in late July, more favorable nectar supply rather than shorter corollas may be the reason for the attractiveness of second-crop bloom to honey bees.

According to Stapel (108), Italian bees are more consistent visitors to red clover than northern European races because their tongues are slightly longer. Schwan (109) in Sweden found the short-tongued Nordic bees more disposed than Italian bees to use the holes cut by bumble bees. However, he found that Nordic bees collected red clover pollen more frequently than did the Italian bees. Pedersen (95) found that the Italian bees increased on second crop and the Danish bees decreased and that the Italian bees were less often nectar thieves on both crops. Data published in a 277-page symposium on red clover pollination edited by Gubin (110) showed that Ukrainian bees with slightly longer tongues than northern bees were slightly better pollinators and Caucasian bees with even longer tongues were nearly twice as valuable as the northern bees. Their findings were based on relative rates of increase in yields as one approached the apiary. Hunkeler (111) in Germany stated that Carniclan bees were ousting northern bees in red clover districts because they gathered more red clover honey and did a better job of pollination. In North America there has been little effort to evaluate or use one strain of bees over another for red clover pollination. Perhaps in areas where bumble bees cut few holes in the corolla tubes, the question of honey bee races is of minor importance.

Training bees to red clover is another approach to increasing their nectar visits. Von Frisch (112) placed hives close to red clover fields and fed the bees in front of the hives with sugar water. The bees had to creep through a layer of fresh red clover flowers to reach the syrup. Afterward they danced in the hive and other bees, perceiving the odor of the flowers on the dancers' bodies, searched for the red clover. Von Frisch tried 12 paired experiments in different localities, and in every one visitation was higher to red clover fields adjacent to trained than to untrained colonies. Several Russian investigators tried similar experiments. As early as 1930 they simply steeped the florets in the feeding solution. In 1933 Gubin & Romashov (113), using extracted perfume, trained one group of colonies to red clover and another to willow herb and then reversed the training of both groups. Most Russian investigators now advocate this method of increasing honey bee nectar visits to red clover. Czech research workers, following up on the Russian experiments, sprayed hives and red clover fields with fennel (*Foeniculum officinale*) and aniseed (*Pimpinella asisum*) oils in sugar syrup (Cumakov (114)). On the other hand, Minderhoud (115) in Holland and Valle (116) in Finland tried similar methods (using extracts as well as florets) without clear-cut results. Minderhoud claimed some success with spraying the crop with saccharose instead of plain sugar syrup. However, MacVicar and associates (117) in Canada sprayed honey on red clover without benefiting pollination.

Zivov & Skvorcov (118) surrounded plots of red clover with sowings of *Trifolium ambiguum* and harvested the latter when the red clover was in good bloom. They claimed excellent results with this method in commercial seed fields of four provinces in Russia. Apparently this procedure has not been tried in other countries or, if tried, was found unsuccessful and remained unreported.

Honey bees collect pollen as well as nectar from red clover. According to Skovgaard (119) the pollen collectors have two advantages over nectar collectors: (a) they pollinate about twice as fast, and (b) there are no "inferior" pollen-gathering races. (This was said in defense of the northern races of bees, usually considered inferior in nectar collecting). Schwan (109) in Sweden went a step further by showing a higher percentage of pollen collectors and more rapid pollen visits for the Nordic bees in comparison with Italian strains. Another obvious advantage of pollen collectors (not seen in the literature) is that they nearly always enter the flower from the top instead of using the side entrances made by bumble bees. The percentage of pollen gathers on red clover is variable but usually quite substantial.

Skovgaard (119) stated that the percentage of pollen gathers on red clover is associated with the pollen needs of the colonies involved. He did not state how the association was determined. In his studies pollen collectors averaged 30 per cent on early clover and 20 per cent on late clover. This difference may merely be an expression of the greater number of nectar collectors on the late clover. Butler (120) found an average of 40 per cent pollen collectors on red clover and concluded that visitation of both pollen and nectar collectors was determined by the height of the nectar in the corolla tubes. Woodrow (121) stated that most of the honey bees on red clover in Ohio collect pollen. He did not make a sharp distinction between pollen and nectar collectors, stating that the pollen collectors seem to receive the pollen unintentionally while probing for nectar. Dunham (122) stated that honey bees devote practically all their time on red clover bloom to collecting pollen.

Such discrepancies in observation probably result from variable complexes of competing bloom as well as variations in the nectar content of red clover. Wilsie & Johnson (123) concluded that red clover does not compete well with most other nectar-bearing plants for nectar-collecting honey bees but holds its own with all but the most attractive pollen plants for pollen collectors. MacVicar *et al.* (117) studied pollen-trap collections from an area where many sources of pollen were available and found red clover to be the dominant pollen in nearly every sample. Others have made similar findings (Braun *et al.* (124); Bohart (unpublished data)). It is easy to see why the number of nectar collectors fluctuates widely from time to time and place to place, but the occasionally reported absence or near absence on red clover of honey bees of any kind (Plath (93); Valle (125)) is hard to understand. Perhaps the fields were very small and surrounded by strongly competing pollen sources.

Most observers have found a negative relationship between red clover seed yields and distance from colonies of honey bees. Wilsie (126) in a three-year study of two areas with fields extending as far as 16 miles from major bee yards, found significant decreases in seed yields at the greater distances. Walstrom *et al.* (127), working more intensively with smaller distances, found a distinct break in seed yields between 400 and 600 feet. MacVicar *et al.* (117) found a similar break between 500 and 800 yards away from the colonies. Braun *et al.* (124), found a break in both honey bee populations and seed yields between 800 and 1200 feet and progressive declines up to 2000 feet. However, Harrison *et al.* (128) in Michigan found no significant differences in seed yields as the distance from the apiary was increased up to 1 mile.

Pollination by Wild Bees

All students of red clover have unanimously accorded bumble bees the highest place in red clover pollinating efficiency. Apparently the long-tongued species of bumble bees and red clover are "made for each other" (Brian (129)). A number of observations on the working speed of bumble bees indicate that the queens pollinate about four times as many florets per minute as pollen-collecting honey bees and the workers from two to three times as many (Schwan (109)). Pedersen (95) gave bumble bees 2.5 "bee units" in comparison with 1.0 for honey bees. With this as a basis he calculated that 0.5 bee unit per square meter should be able to pollinate enough red clover flowers to set a seed crop of 1000 to 1200 kg. per hectare.

The principal trouble with bumble bees as red clover pollinators seems to be their scarcity in most localities. Valle in Finland (116), Schwan in Sweden (109), Benoit & Gillard in Holland (130), and Bird in Quebec (131) have noted great population fluctuations from year to year, making seed production without honey bees very unreliable.

A shortcoming of bumble bees that applies principally to certain short-tongued species is their habit of cutting holes in the bases of the corollas to secure the nectar more easily (Brian (129)). These holes are then used by other bees, and the flowers remain unpollinated. *Bombus terrestris* (Linnaeus) is the most common nectar thief in Scandinavia (Schwan (109); Pedersen (95)). *Bombus terricola* Kirby and *B. occidentalis* Greene are well-known nectar thieves in North America. Unfortunately, when three species of bumble bees were introduced into New Zealand, *B. terrestris* was included (Cumber (132)).

Williams (133) in Wales and Morrison (134) in Ontario are among those reporting the importance of timing the bloom for seasonal peaks of bumble bee populations. In such northern latitudes they reported a small peak in June when the queens foraged and a much larger peak in late July when the workers appeared in large numbers. On the other hand, Pedersen (95) found twice as many bumble bees on the first crop as on the second. Apparently, timing the crop for bumble bee pollination must be done on the basis of local conditions.

Other pollinators are usually unimportant on red clover. However, as reported by Folsom (135) first-crop red clover may be pollinated in the Midwest to an important degree by species of *Tetralonia*, and the early second crop by species of *Melissodes*. Yamada & Ebara (136) reported *Eucera sociabilis* Smith as an important red clover pollinator in Japan, and Benoit & Gillard (130) give some credit to *Andrena wilkella* (Kirby) in Holland.

Many agronomists, entomologists, and naturalists of various kinds have studied the biology of bumble bees and methods of domesticating them. It appears that no one has yet demonstrated any advantage to keeping bumble bees for pollination except for small-scale work in enclosures (Bohart & Pedersen (137)). However, Hasselrot (138) in Sweden and Valle (139) in Finland have made efforts to develop bumble bee keeping for pollination on a field scale.

To summarize, nearly all authors are now in agreement on the following points concerning red clover pollination: (a) Red clover is self-sterile and requires pollination by bees. (b) Bumble bees, except for a few nectar-thieving species, are ideal pollinators although their populations are unpredictable and usually insufficient. (c) Honey bees are satisfactory pollinators providing that they are sufficiently concentrated in the area and competing pollen and nectar sources are kept at a minimum. (d) As a pollen source, but not as a nectar source, red clover competes well with other plants for the attention of honey bees. (e) Honey bee pollination is generally better on second-crop than first-crop bloom. (f) Nectar production and sugar concentration in red clover are greatest in warm, dry weather.

There is still disagreement as to the value of long-tongued honey bees, short-tubed flowers, scent training of nectar gathers, and attracting bees with attractive flowers prior to red clover bloom.

The foregoing review should at least make it clear that a great deal of work is going on at the present time in the field of legume pollination. Experimental pollination studies are difficult and often costly because of the wide-ranging foraging habits of most pollinators and the large number of species involved. Some of the more complex problems such as the nature and significance of competition between pollinators will probably never be completely answered.

LITERATURE CITED

1. Henslow, G., *Proc. Linnean Soc. Botany*, 9, 327-29 (1866)
2. Müller, H., *Die Befruchtung der Blumen durch Insekten und die gegenseitigen Anpassungen beider* (Leipzig, Germany, 1873)
3. Burkill, J.H., *Proc. Cambridge Phil. Soc.*, 8, 142-53 (1873)
4. Piper, C.V., Evans, W.M., McKee, R., and Morse, W.J., *U.S. Dept. Agr. Bull.*, *No. 75*, 32 pp. (1914)
5. Lesins, K., *Ann. Roy. Agr. Coll. Sweden*, 17, 441-83 (1950)
6. Larkin, R.A., and Graumann, H.O., *Botan. Gaz.*, 116, 40-52 (1954)
7. Vansell, G.H., and Todd, F.E., *J. Am. Soc. Agron.*, 38, 470-88 (1946)
8. Urban, J., *Verhandl. Botan. Verein Provinz Brandenburg*, 15, 13-16 (1873)
9. Carlson, J.W., *J. Am. Soc. Agron.*, 22, 780-86 (1930)
10. Kirk, L.E., and White, W.J., *Sci. Agr.*, 13, 591-93 (1933)
11. Brink, R.A., and Cooper, D.C., *Am. J. Botany*, 23, 678-83 (1936)
12. Cooper, D.C., and Brink, R.A., *J. Agr. Research*, 60, 453-72 (1940)
13. Knowles, R.P., *Sci. Agr.*, 24, 29-50 (1943)
14. Armstrong, J.M., and White, W.J., *J. Agr. Sci.*, 25, 161-79 (1935)
15. Petersen, H.L., *Årsskrift. Kgl. Vet.--og Landbohøjskole*, 138-69 (1954)
16. Tysdal, H.M., *J. Am. Soc. Agron.*, 32, 570-85 (1940)
17. Jones, L.M., and Olson, P.J., *Sci. Agr.*, 23, 315-21 (1943)
18. Burkart, A., *Anales acad. nac. cienc. exact fis. y nat. Buenos Aires*, 12, 39-57 (1947)
19. Tysdal, H.M., Kiesselbach, T.A., and Westover, H.L., *Neb. Agr. Expt. Sta. Bull. No. 124*, 46 pp. (1942)
20. Kirk, L.E., *Proc. Worlds Grain Exhibition and Conference, Canada*, 2, 161-67 (1933)
21. Torssell, R., *Beretn. Nord. Jordbrugsforskn. Kongr. i Helsingfors, København*, IV, 666-69 (1929)
22. Lesins, K., Åkerberg, E., and Bojtos, Z., *Acta Agr. Scand.* 4, 239-56 (1954)
23. Brand, C.J., and Westgate, J.M., *U.S. Dept. Agr. Bureau of Plant Industry Circ.* 24, 23 pp. (1909)
24. Engelbert, V., *Sci. Agr.*, 12, 593-603 (1931)
25. Tysdal, H.M., *J. Am. Soc. Agron.*, 38, 515-35 (1946)
26. Ufer, M., *Der Züchter*, 5, 217-21 (1933)
27. Dwyer, R.E.P., and Allman, S.L., *Agr. Gaz. N.S. Wales*, 44, 363-71 (1933)
28. *Utah Agr. Expt. Sta. Circ.* 135, 60 pp. (1955)
29. Grandfield, C.O., *What's New in Crops and Soils*, 2, 18-19 (1950)

30. Pedersen, A., and Stapel, C., *Tidsskr. for Frøavl København*, 17, 176-82 (1945)
31. Hadfield, J.W., and Calder, R.A., *New Zealand J. Agr.*, 57, 28-33 (1936)
32. *Utah Agr. Expt. Sta. Circ.* 125, 72 pp. (1950)
33. Pedersen, M.W., Peterson, H.L., Bohart, G.E., and Levin, M.D., *Agron. J.*, 48, 177-80 (1956)
34. Menke, H., *Washington Agr. Expt. Sta. Bull.*, No. 555, 24 pp. (1954)
35. Silversides, W.H., and Olson, P.J., *Sci. Agr.*, 22, 129-34 (1941)
36. Pharis, R.L., and Unrau, J., *Can. J. Agr. Sci.*, 33, 74-83, (1953)
37. Hvistendahl, D., *Ten Principles of Alfalfa Seed Growing* (Mechanical Bee Corporation, Worthington, Minn., 11 pp., mimeo., 1955)
38. Aicher, L.C., *Idaho Agr. Expt. Sta. Bull.* No. 101 (1917)
39. Sladen, F.W.L., *Can. Entomol.*, 50, 301-4 (1918)
40. Helmbold, F., *Z. Pflanzenzücht.*, 14, 113-74 (1929)
41. Rudnev, W., *Sozializtichezkoye Zernovoye Khozhaiztvo*, 2, 141-44 (1941)
42. Hare, Q.Z., and Vansell, G.H., *J. Am. Soc. Agron.*, 38, 462-69 (1946)
43. Townsend, G.F., *Can. Bee J.*, 60, 14-17 (1955)
44. Vansell, G.H., *U.S. Dept. Agr. Circ.* 876, 11 pp. (1951)
45. Reinhardt, J.F., *Am. Naturalist*, 86, 257-75 (1952)
46. Pedersen, M.W., and Todd, F.E., *Agron. J.*, 41, 247-49 (1949)
47. Franklin, W.W., *Kansas Agr. Expt. Sta. Bull.*, No. 70, 64 pp. (1951)
48. Hobbs, G.A., and Lilly, C.E., *Can. J. Agr. Sci.*, 35, 422-32 (1955)
49. Stephen, W.P., *J. Econ. Entomol.*, 48, 543-48 (1955)
50. Jones, L.M., *Rept. 12th Alfalfa Improvement Conf.*, 38-40 (1950)
51. Bieberdorf, G.A., *Proc. Oklahoma Acad. Sci.*, 49-51 (1949)
52. McMahon, H., *2nd Ann. Rept., Plant Industry Branch, Saskatchewan Dept. Agr.*, 314-15 (1953)
53. Pedersen, M.W., *Botan. Gaz.*, 115, 129-38 (1953)
54. Drake, C.J., *J. Econ. Entomol.*, 41, 742-50 (1949)
55. Todd, F.E., *Iowa: Report State Apiarist for year ending December 31, 1950*, 104-8 (1951)
56. Soboleva, E., *Hlopkovodstvo*, 4, 32-34 (1954)
57. Levin, M.D., *J. Econ. Entomol.* (In press)
58. Levin, M.D., *J. Econ. Entomol.*, 48, 484-85 (1955)
59. Åkerberg, E., and Lesins, K., *Kgl. Lantbruks-Högskol. Ann.*, 16, 630-43 (1949)
60. Peck, O., and Bolton, J.L., *Sci. Agr.*, 26, 388-417 (1946)
61. Bohart, G.E., *Rept. 14th Alfalfa Improvement Conf.*, 24-26 (1954)
62. Linsley, E.G., and MacSwain, J.W., *J. Econ. Entomol.*, 40, 349-57 (1947)

63. Haws, B.A., *Iowa: Report State Apiarist for year ending December 31, 1950*, 57-58 (1950)
64. Levin, M.D., and Pedersen, M.W., *Agron. J.*, 47, 387-88 (1955)
65. Pedersen, M.W., and Bohart, G.E., *Agron. J.*, 45, 548-51 (1953)
66. Butler, C.G., and Simpson, J., *Rept. Rothamsted Expt. Sta.*, 167-75 (1953)
67. Todd, F.E., and Vansell, G.H., *Proc. 6th Intern. Grasslands Congr.*, 1, 835-40 (1952)
68. Pengelly, D.H., *84th Ann. Rept. Entomol. Soc. Ontario*, 101-18 (1954)
69. Pearson, J.F.W., *Ecol. Monographs*, 3, 373-441 (1933)
70. Linsley, E.F., *J. Econ. Entomol.*, 39, 18-29 (1946)
71. Fischer, R.L., *Minnesota Branch Station Conf.*, 3 pp. mimeo. (1952)
72. Bohart, G.E., *Rept. 11th Alfalfa Improvement Conf.*, 57-65 (1948)
73. Hobbs, G.A., and Lilly, C.E., *Ecology*, 35, 453-62 (1954)
74. Ufer, M., *Der Züchter*, 4, 281-86 (1932)
75. Skovgaard, O.S., *Tidsskr. for Frøavl*, 17, 9-13, 211-14 (1947)
76. Larkin, R.A., *Agron. J.*, 44, 216-18 (1952)
77. Crandall, B.H., and Tate, H., *J. Am. Soc. Agron.*, 39, 161-63 (1947)
78. Plath, O.E., *Bumblebees and Their Ways* (Macmillan & Co. Ltd., London, England, 201 pp., 1934)
79. Bohart, G.E., *Utah Agr. Expt. Sta. Farm & Home Sci.*, 16, 23-24, 39 (1955)
80. Menke, H.F., *What's New in Crops and Soils*, 4, 36-37 (1952)
81. Bohart, G.E., *Rept. 12th Alfalfa Improvement Conf.*, 32-35 (1950)
82. Bohart, G.E., *Utah Agr. Expt. Sta. Farm & Home Sci.*, 8 13-14 (1948)
83. Bohart, G.E., and Cross, E.A., *Ann. Entomol. Soc. Amer.*, 48, 403-6 (1955)
84. McMahon, H., *Rept. 12th Alfalfa Improvement Conf.*, 36-37 (1950)
85. Bohart, G.E., *What's New in Crops and Soils*, 8, 12-13, 26 (1955)
86. Bohart, G.E., and Knowlton, G.F., *J. Econ. Entomol.*, 45, 890 (1953)
87. Müller, H., *The Fertilization of Flowers* (Thomson, D.W., Trans., Macmillan & Co., Ltd., London, England, 669 pp., 1883)
88. Darwin, C.R., *The Origin of Species by Means of Natural Selection* (Modern Libraries, Inc., New York, N.Y., 1000 pp., 1936)
89. Meehan, T., *Proc. Natural Sci. Philadelphia*, 108-12 (1876)
90. Westgate, J.M., and Coe, H.S., *U.S. Dept. Agr. Bull., No. 289*, 31 pp. (1915)

91. Hopkins, A.D., *Proc. 17th Ann. Meeting Promotion Agr. Sci.*, 35-40 (1896)
92. Pammel, L.H., and King, C.M., *Proc. Iowa Acad. Sci.*, 18, 35-45 (1911)
93. Plath, O.E., *Am. Naturalist*, 59, 441-51 (1925)
94. Martin, J.N., *Am. Bee J.*, 78, 102-4 (1938)
95. Pedersen, A., *Årskrift. Kgl. Vet.-og Landbokøjskole*, 59-138 (1945)
96. Wexelsen, H., *Nord. Jordbrugsforskn.*, 17, 478-88 (1935)
97. Schelhorn, M. von, *Pflanzenbau*, 18, 311-20 (1942)
98. Lindhard, E., *Tidsskr. Planteavl*, 27, 653-80 (1921)
99. Kratochvil, J., and Snoflak, J., *Acta Univ. Agr. Brno. Bull. C. 39*, 30 pp. (English Summary) (1948)
100. Wilsie, C.P., and Gilbert, N.W., *J. Am. Soc. Agron.*, 32, 231-34 (1940)
101. Starling, T.M., Wilsie, C.P., and Gilbert, N.W., *Agron. J.*, 42, 1-8 (1950)
102. Åkerberg, E., Bingefors, S., and Lesins, K., *Sveriges Utsådesförenings Tidskr.*, 3, 1-29 (1947)
103. Fruwirth, C., *Die Züchtung der landwirtschaftlichen Kulturpflanzen*, 3 (Paul Parey, Berlin, Germany, 1906)
104. Åkerberg, E., *Meddelande N:02 Från Sveriges Fröodlareforbund*, 16-33 (1952)
105. Dunham, W.E., *Ohio Farm & Home Research*, 44-45 (May-June, 1955)
106. Hammer, O., *Oikos*, 1, 34-47 (1949)
107. Shuel, R.W., *Nord. Jordbrugsforskn.*, 508-16 (1935)
108. Stapel, C., *Nord. Jordbrugsforskn.*, 17, 508-17 (1955)
109. Schwan, B., *Meddelande N:02 Från Sveriges Fröodlareforbund*, 34-61 (1953)
110. Gubin, A.F., *Medomosnye pchely i opylemie kransogo klevera* (Moskva Scl'Rozgiz, Moscow, U.S.S.R., 227 pp., (1947) (In Russian with English Summary)
111. Hunkeler, M., *Bienen Zeitung*, 46, 179-88 (1943)
112. Frisch, K. von, *Bees, Their Vision, Chemical Senses and Language* (Cornell University Press, Ithaca, N.Y., 119 pp., 1950)
113. Gubin, A.F., and Romashov, G., *Opileniye kransnovo klevera i pooti klevernove semenovogstva* (Shizu I Znanie, Moscow, U.S.S.R., 1933)
114. Cumakov, V., *Za sotisialisticheskoe zemledelie*, 5, 747-54 (1955)
115. Minderhoud, A., *Mededeel. dir. Tuinbouw*, 11, 381-92 (1948)
116. Valle, O., *Ann. Entomol. Fennici 14, Liite-Suppl.*, 225-31 (1947)
117. MacVicar, R.M., Braun, E., Gibson, D.R., and Jamieson, C.A., *Sci. Agr.*, 32, 67-80 (1952)
118. Zivov, V., and Skvorcov, S., *Selektsiia i Semenovodstvo*, 18, 63-64 (1951)
119. Skovgaard, O.S., *Tidsskr. Planteavl*, 55, 449-75 (1952)
120. Butler, C.G., *Ann. Appl. Biol.*, 28, 125-35 (1941)
121. Woodrow, A.W., *J. Econ. Entomol.*, 45, 1028-29 (1953)

122. Dunham, W.E., *J. Econ. Entomol.*, 32, 668-70 (1939)
123. Wilsie, C.P., and Johnson, I., *Federation News Letter, National Federation Beekeepers' Assoc.* (May 2-3, 1946)
124. Braun, E., MacVicar, R.M., Gibson, D.R., Pankiw, P., and Guppy, J., *Can. J. Agr. Sci.*, 33, 437-47 (1952)
125. Valle, O., *Beretn. Nord. Jordbrugoforskn. Kongr. i København*, 9 pp. (1935)
126. Wilsie, C.P., *Agron. J.*, 41, 545-50 (1949)
127. Walstrom, R.J., Paddock, F.B., Park, O.W., and Wilsie, C.P., *Am. Bee J.*, 91, 244-45 (1950)
128. Harrison, C.M., Kelty, R.H., and Blumer, C., *Mich. Agr. Expt. Sta. Quart. Bull.*, 28, 35-89 (1945)
129. Brian, A., *Bee World*, 35, 61-67, 81-91 (1954)
130. Benoit, P., and Gillard, A., *Mededel. Landbonwhogeschool en Opzoehings-stas. Staat Gent.*, 13, 297-346 (1948)
131. Bird, J.N., *J. Am. Soc. Agron.*, 36, 346-57
132. Cumber, R., *New Zealand J. Sci. Technol.*, 34, 227-40 (1953)
133. Williams, R.D., *Welsh Plant Breeding Station Bull., Ser. H.*, No. 4 (1925)
134. Morrison, F.O., *73rd Ann. Rept. Entomol. Soc., Ontario*, 16-20 (1943)
135. Folsom, J.W., *Ann. Entomol. Soc. Am.*, 15, 181-84 (1922)
136. Yamada, I., and Ebara, E., *Hokkaido Nat. Agr. Expt. Sta. Rept.*, 45, 1-33 (1952) (In Japanese with English Summary)
137. Bohart, G.E., and Pedersen, M.W., *Agron. J.*, 42, 608 (1950)
138. Hasselrot, T.B., *Medd. N:02 Fran Sveriges Fröodlareforbund*, 62-68 (1953)
139. Valle, O., *Acta Agral. Fennica*, 83, 205-20 (1955)
140. Hurd, P.D., *Bull. Calif. Insect Survey*, 1, 141-52 (1952)

Fungus-Growing Ants

Neal A. Weber

The fungus-growers are a New World tribe of myrmicine ants, the Attini, that has developed a unique relation with saprophytic plants. The ants eat only the fungus that they culture, and it is not found outside the ant nest. Many animals feed on fungi, and certain beetles and termites grow them in their nests, but the culturing of fungi as described here is believed to be unique. In this process a flourishing growth of one fungus is produced, and of this fungus only, although the medium on which it grows (the substrate) is suitable for the growth of many other kinds of organisms. When the ants are removed, these other organisms multiply and replace the fungus.

The vital part of the attine nest is the fungus garden. It is the abode of the queen and brood as well as of the fungus. Despite the diversity in morphology of the species, the development and care of the garden are fundamentally similar for all varieties.

Fungus-growing is distinguished from leaf-cutting. All members of this tribe subsist solely, in nature, on the fungus that they culture, but some are leaf-cutters and others are not. The latter pick up vegetal particles of suitable size, or insect excrement, and grow the fungus on these. The leaf-cutters go in files, often on well-formed trails, and cut leaves, flowers, or stems. They are most commonly members of the largest species and belong to the genera *Acromyrmex* and *Atta.* Inconspicuous *Trachymyrmex* and *Sericomyrmex* species may also cut leaves and flowers.

It is the purpose of this article to

SCIENCE, 1966, Vol. 153, pp. 587–604.

review the chief features of the life of these ants and of the fungus on which they depend. Because of the economic importance of the large species of *Atta*, and particularly of *Atta sexdens* L. in Brazil, a considerable body of literature has grown up, here summarized, and *A. sexdens* may be taken to represent a high expression of this symbiosis. Studies of other species and genera have made significant contributions to the knowledge of the biological role of the attines and are here reviewed.

Species of this tribe were listed by Linnaeus in 1758, and the type genus *Atta* was named by Fabricius in 1804. Latreille called such ants *Oecodoma* in 1818, and this name was used by the early naturalists, such as Bates, Belt, and Smith in Latin America, for the conspicuous leaf-cutters with soldiers now known as *Atta*. Mayr, from 1862 to 1865, originated the generic names *Cyphomyrmex*, *Apterostigma*, *Sericomyrmex*, and *Acromyrmex*, and he has been the chief contributor to the generic classification. Outlines of the wings, heads, and side views of the ants show differences characteristic of the genera (Figs. 1–4).

The tribe has a wide distribution, from approximately 40° north latitude to 44° south latitude (Fig. 5). The economically important *Atta* species have smaller ranges (Figs. 6 and 7). Their general distribution in South American countries is known, although incompletely in Andean areas.

Thomas Belt, who arrived in Nicaragua in 1868, discovered the fungus-growing role of the ants (*1*). He did not realize the full extent of the ant-fungus relationship, thinking that the fungus grew naturally in the damp underground chambers of the ant nest. Belt greatly stimulated Alfred Moeller (*2*), who quoted Belt's conclusions on the frontispiece of his publication. Moeller and then von Ihering, Sampaio, Goeldi, and Huber (*3*, *4*) showed the dependence of the ants on the fungus and how this dependence was transmitted from one ant generation to another. Moeller first produced evidence that there could be a fungus sexual or fruiting stage; to this stage he gave the name *Rozites gongylophora*. His careful mycological studies were basic to later work.

Specimens of *Atta cephalotes* L. and *A. sexdens* had been brought from Guiana to Europe in the 18th century. Their long trails, thronged with workers, had been confused with the files of army ants, *Eciton*, in the popular accounts brought back to Europe from Tropical America. The ants also figured in Central American mythology (*5*).

Almost as soon as the Spanish arrived in the New World they made note of the depredations of ants, which probably were *Acromyrmex* or *Atta*. Bartolome de las Casas in 1559 described the failure of the Spaniards in Hispaniola to grow cassava and citrus trees because of ants whose nests, at the bases of the trees, were "white as snow" (probably the fungus gardens and brood). Article 19 of the cedula proclaimed by the King of Spain on 20 November 1783 for opening Trinidad to immigration states that "the Government was to take the utmost care to prevent the introduction of ants into Trinidad" (see *6*). The ants, of course, had been there all along.

The importance and conspicuousness of *Atta* are attested by the common names which are in general use by the people of various Latin-American countries and used in official publications by their ministries or departments of agriculture (*7*).

Latin-American countries have passed national laws classifying certain ant species as plague animals because of their concentration on economically important plants. For example, Argentina, in Law 4863 of 27 July 1909, considered "*hormigas coloradas*" and

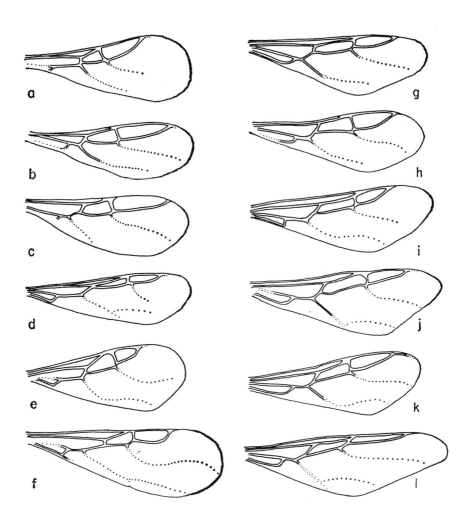

Fig. 1   Wings of representative genera. (*a*) *Cyphomyrmex rimosus* Spinola. (*b*) *C. bigibbosus* Emery. (*c*) *Mycetophylax conformis*. (*d*) *Mycocepurus manni* Weber. (*e*) *Myrmicocrypta buenzlii* Borgmeier. (*f*) *Apterostigma robustum* Emery. (*g*) *Sericomyrmex urichi*. (*h*) *Trachymyrmex cornetzi* Forel. (*i*) *T. urichi* Forel. (*j*) *Acromyrmex (Moellerius) landolti pampanus* Weber. (*k*) *A. (A) octospinosus* Reich. (*l*) *Atta sexdens*.

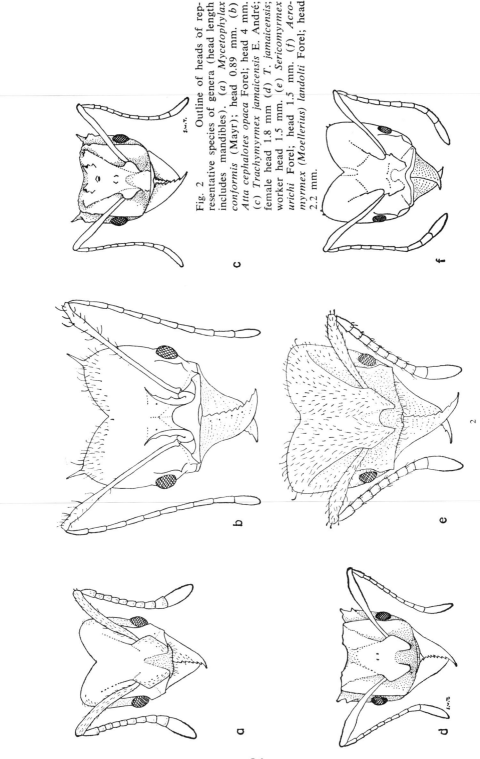

Fig. 2 Outline of heads of representative species of genera (head length includes mandibles). (a) *Mycetophylax conformis* (Mayr); head 0.89 mm. (b) *Atta cephalotes opaca* Forel; head 4 mm. (c) *Trachymyrmex jamaicensis* E. André; female head 1.8 mm (d) *T. jamaicensis*; worker head 1.5 mm. (e) *Sericomyrmex urichi* Forel; head 1.5 mm. (f) *Acromyrmex (Moellerius) landolti* Forel; head 2.2 mm.

84

"*hormigas negras*" to be plagues. These were later identified as *Atta sexdens* and *Acromyrmex lundi* (Guer.). When the ants are legally classified among the plague animals, the government usually undertakes to carry out extermination methods at the expense of the person occupying or owning the land, if he does not do it himself. The government also surveys yearly the incidence of the animals and the damage done by them and freely disseminates the information. In many countries experts experiment with all control products as they are developed (*8, 9*). A method of controlling *Atta* that is effective in one country will have a calculable probability of success against *Atta* in another country, based on differences in soil, climate, and other variables. No one product has had such complete success in any country that it has replaced all other control methods for very long. People still have difficulty in practicing agriculture in some primitive areas (see *10*).

The Indians of Central and South America have long used the large females of *Atta* as food, and there is no doubt that the gasters filled with eggs have nutritional value. I tried them raw and found them to have a pasty consistency and a bland flavor.

Of even greater importance is the impact of these ants on soil nutrition (*11*). In tropical rain forest areas few animals and few roots of trees go much below the soil surface. In such sites a large *Atta* nest contains far more organic matter, in the form of hundreds of fungus gardens, than any other agency in the soil. This organic matter makes possible the multiplication of great quantities of bacteria, nematodes, insects, and other organisms that can only exist deep underground in such numbers because the ants have carried substrate there.

More pervasive, if less dramatic, is the influence of the nests of smaller and less conspicuous attines. Recent studies of these species in Trinidad showed that there was an average of a nest every 2 square meters in one area (*12*). The size and numbers of the fungus gardens showed that the total impact of these ants on soil nutrition was considerable. They were the only burrowers in the area to construct large underground chambers. These were filled with gardens, as in *Atta*. On the fertile pampas of Argentina the presence of nests of *Acromyrmex* is marked above ground by a richer growth of plants (*11*).

Atta sexdens

The best known and economically most important South American attine is *Atta sexdens* L., together with its subspecies *A. rubropilosa* Forel. This has been the species most commonly studied in Brazil.

Huber (*3*) observed in detail the early stages of colony foundation and watched the female, larvae, and first brood consuming the eggs that she had laid. He estimated that 90 percent of the eggs laid in the approximately 40 to 60 days before the first workers appear were consumed; about 50 eggs were laid daily in this period. Among these Autuori (*13*) clearly distinguished eggs of two kinds, alimentary and reproductive, and he produced an excellent photographic record. The alimentary eggs, laid in the early stages of colony formation, are markedly larger and more globular than the reproductive eggs. The female eats the alimentary eggs herself or feeds them to the first larvae. The internal anatomy of the female gaster (*14*) and the histological basis for the two egg types (*15*) have been described. The spermatheca of the newly fertilized female has been shown to contain some 200 to 300 million sperm as a result of

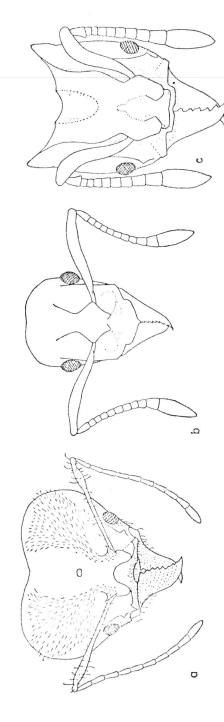

Fig. 3. Outline of heads of representative species of genera (head length includes mandibles). (a) *Atta cephalotes opaca*; soldier head 5.8 mm. (b) *Apterostigma calverti* Wheeler; head 1.6 mm. (c) *Cyphomyrmex bigibbosus* Emery; head 1.3 mm.

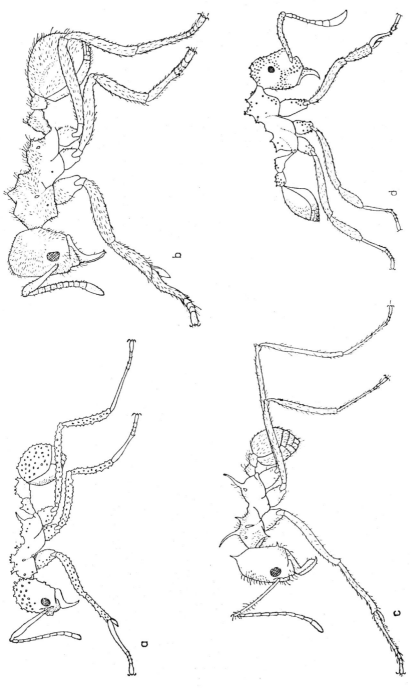

Fig. 4. Outline of representative workers in side view (thorax length is measured from anterior pronotal to posterior epinotal angle). (a) *Trachymyrmex arizonensis* Wheeler; length 4.5 mm (thorax 1.5 mm). (b) *Sericomyrmex urichi*; length 3.5 mm (thorax 1.6 mm). (c) *Atta cephalotes opaca*; length 7 mm (thorax 2.8 mm). (d) *Myrmicocrypta ednaella* Mann; length 2.3 mm (thorax 0.85 mm).

probable fertilization by from three to eight males (16).

Autuori has also graphically portrayed the reproductive potential and size of mature nests.

In five successive years the nuptial flights and preparation of the initial nest of the females were noted, then the emergence of the first workers. The average interval between the nuptial flight and the emergence of these workers was 87.2 days, varying from 72.0 days in 1938 to 93.9 days in 1937. Temperatures must have been a significant factor in the time required for development, and Eidmann (14) gives these as 18.5° to 25.3°C in the mature garden, according to the depth. The workers used the original nest opening first made by the female.

From examination of a number of young colonies, the average developmental times were found to be as follows: pre-oviposition period, 5 days; incubation, 22 days; larval period, 22 days; pupal period, 10 days.

The appearance of a second nest opening marked the next significant stage. This took place, on the average, 443 days after the appearance of the first opening (minimum 421, maximum 561 days).

The full size range of worker castes appeared between the 4th and 10th month, the soldier caste not appearing until the 22nd month.

The number of entrances to the nests rapidly increased in the second year to 63, 113, and 53, respectively, in three colonies. In the 38th month the numbers had increased to 853, 984, and 1071, respectively. Betancourt (17) used the data in estimating the size of the colony. He maintained that the numbers of openings can be plotted as a logistic curve

$$N = \frac{1000}{271737e - 0.42\ t + 1}$$

where N = monthly average total openings, e = natural logarithmic base, t = number of months from the start of nest building, and 1000 = the theoretical upper asymptote. The maximum size of 1000 openings approximately coincides with the beginning of the production of sexual forms.

A nest of 47 months was opened by Autuori on the day before its second nuptial flight. This nest had 1027 chambers, of which 390 had fungus gardens and ants. There were 38,481 males and 5339 females, a proportion of males to females of 7.2 to 1 [Eidmann (14) had given the ratio as 10:1]. An enormous chamber at a depth of 125 centimeters was used as a refuse site and cemetery. It was 90 centimeters high and 120 centimeters in diameter. This contained 1491 adult Coleoptera, 15 adult Diptera, 56 Hemiptera, 40 Mollusca, 4 Reptilia, and 1 Pseudoscorpionida.

Autuori followed one nest for 77 months. It produced a nuptial flight in its third year and annually thereafter. The loose soil on the surface of the nest was measured before the nest was excavated; it amounted to 22.72 cubic meters and weighed approximately 40,000 kilograms. There were 1920 chambers in this nest, 296 containing refuse, 157 with loose soil, 248 with gardens, and 1219 empty. The empty chambers were believed to have been used for sheltering the sexual forms after they matured and before they left on their nuptial flight. The weights of 184 fungus gardens varied from 15 to 2250 grams, a common weight being 300 grams. It was calculated that, during the life of the colony, 5892 kilograms of vegetation had been used in the nest, with an estimated ratio of 12.4 parts fresh substrate to 1 part discarded substrate.

The mortality of females following their nuptial flight was determined by excavating the nest sites after the resulting colonies had opened the entrance. Autuori concluded that as many as 97.5 percent of the queens died within 100 days. Of the young nests, 99.95 percent were destroyed by natural causes within 15 months. The critical period in colony life was divided into four phases: (i) descent from nuptial flight to ground, 30 to 60 minutes; (ii) excavation of the tunnel and first chamber, 6 to 8 hours; (iii) queen remains in chamber, rearing first brood, 80 to 100 days; (iv) from opening of first entrance to opening of second, 15 months.

Mammals, birds, and other insects, including other genera of ants, were significant predators.

In a later study it was concluded that it was impossible to rid extensive areas of *Atta* colonies. The best that could be expected was the eradication of nests in limited areas that could be thoroughly examined every 3 to 6 months.

Second in importance in Brazil and of primary importance northward to tropical Mexico is *Atta cephalotes*. Where the ranges of the two come together, in Surinam (*18*), British Guiana (*19*), Venezuela (*10*), Peru (*20*), and Panama (*21*), the species show ecological differences, *A. cephalotes* often inhabiting more densely forested areas.

The nests of *Atta cephalotes* are similar to those of *A. sexdens*. There is an extensive system of canals to permit air exchange, with one or more very large chambers (*Abraumgruben*), a meter or more in height, that may be used for refuse. Of 75 fungus gardens found in a mature nest, 44 weighed between 100 and 300 grams (*18*). In appearance, the gardens and the fungus are identical to those of *A. sexdens*. The trails may be well developed (Fig. 8).

Recent studies of young colonies of *A. cephalotes* of known age in Trinidad permit a cataloging of the stages (*12*). These stages show an acceleration in development over those for *A.*

sexdens in South Brazil (*22*), due probably to somewhat higher temperatures and higher rainfall. In Trinidad the temperature was 25° to 26°C at the 10- to 50-centimeter depths, under shade, where the young colonies were located (*23*).

Atta cephalotes Nest Stages

Stage 1. The reopening of the initial tunnel made by the female is marked at first by a scattering of soil grains about the entrance, then by the formation of a low tumulus or crater that is often 5 to 8 centimeters in diameter. Trail-making activity starts. Stage duration, 1st and 2nd months (see *10*, plate 2; *22*).

Stage 2. Externally the nest has a small turret of soil grains (10 to 15 centimeters high) and can be distinguished from turrets of other insects and other animals by the large size of the opening. There is a single underground chamber at first, then a second may be started. Only the smallest-to-medium-sized workers are produced. Small trails may extend in all directions. Duration, 2nd to 4th month (see *24*, Figs. 1 and 2; *22*).

Stage 3. The original chimney has now grown to a crater or cone because of the increase in amount of soil excavated. There is still only one entrance. The soil is dumped in the immediate vicinity of the original opening. The two underground chambers are increased to three or four. By this time the colony consists of several thousand workers, some of which are small soldiers. Fewer and more definite trails are formed. Duration, 4th to 7th month.

Stage 4. The number of craters is increased from one to two or three or more. None of these is a turret; they are, rather, low craters of the type many ant species construct, ex-

89

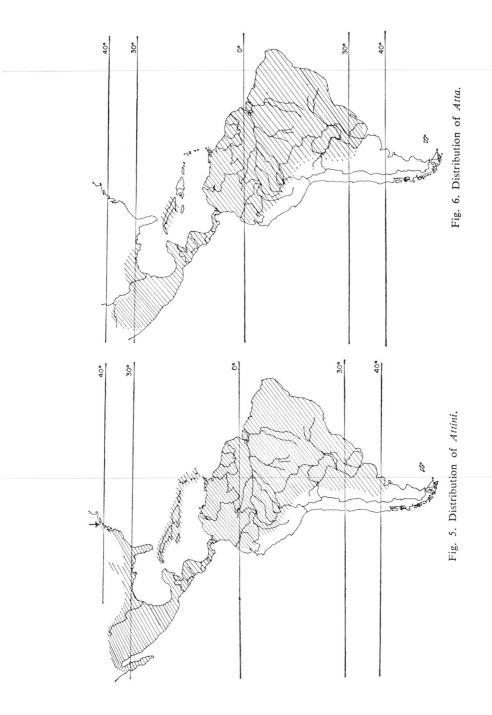

Fig. 5. Distribution of *Attini*.

Fig. 6. Distribution of *Atta*.

cept for their size, 20 to 40 centimeters in diameter. Each crater surrounds an entrance to the nest. Full-size soldiers are being produced. Duration, 7th to 11th month.

Stage 5. A score or two of craters, and a corresponding number of entrances and fungus gardens (similar to those of *A. sexdens*), characterize a fifth stage. Duration, 11th to 16th month.

Stage 6. From now on the colony increases to hundreds of thousands of workers. Sexual broods are produced annually at the appropriate season. Many scores of craters and fungus gardens are developed. It is this mature stage that has been well described in South America and Louisiana (*13, 14, 18, 25, 26*) (Figs. 9 and 10) for several *Atta* species.

The nests of the other species of *Atta* are known chiefly in their mature phases. Those of *A. vollenweideri* and *A. laevigata* in Argentina have been described (*26, 27*). The nest of the Panamanian *A. colombica tonsipes* Santschi is much like that of *A. cephalotes isthmicola* Weber in the same forest (*21*).

General Characters of Attines

Anatomical features that are significant in the life of all fungus-growers include the adult mouthparts, essential to grooming and feeding on the fungus, the infrabuccal pocket that receives dirt from the grooming as well as strands of the fungus, and the pecten or comb used in grooming (*28*; see also *10, 29*) (Fig. 11). Males, females, and workers all use those structures throughout their adult life.

If the ants found in files are strongly polymorphic, they belong to *Acromyrmex* or *Atta*. Characteristically the size range of the worker is continuous, from the smallest, or minima caste,

through a series of castes of intermediate size, or media, to the largest, or maxima caste. The extreme in the nonreproductive of *Atta* is usually called the soldier caste and has a disproportionately large head. Such an *Atta* size series (Fig. 12) then would be: (i) minima (total body length, 2 millimeters); (ii) media; (iii) maxima, including soldier caste (total body length, 14 millimeters).

The first two are the only worker castes found in *Atta* nests in the first several months of colony life. A few workers of the maxima sizes are produced during the first 6 months in *Atta cephalotes*, then an occasional soldier will appear (*30*). A large number of soldiers characterizes a mature colony.

The castes of *Atta* and *Acromyrmex* show a division of labor. The minima are largely confined to the fungus gardens and are effective in culturing the fungus and caring for the eggs and small larvae. The minima are so closely attached to the garden that, if a piece of the latter is removed, the minima flatten closely to the irregularities and do not leave the fragment. Workers of the media sizes also tend the gardens and brood, but in addition they cut leaves. The maxima cut leaves and protect the colony. The *Atta* soldiers tend to remain in the garden, often in the vicinity of the queen and brood, and come out mostly when the nest is disturbed. Their mandibles will, with one cut, produce a 5-millimeter cut in human skin; they can cut half-moon sections out of one's leather shoes.

The species of the other attine genera are largely monomorphic. There may be feeble polymorphism in such *Trachymyrmex* as *T. urichi* and *T. septentrionalis*. Laboratory colonies of these, especially of *T. septentrionalis*, may rear progressively smaller workers as the colony deteriorates or, in the latter species, after the height of summer

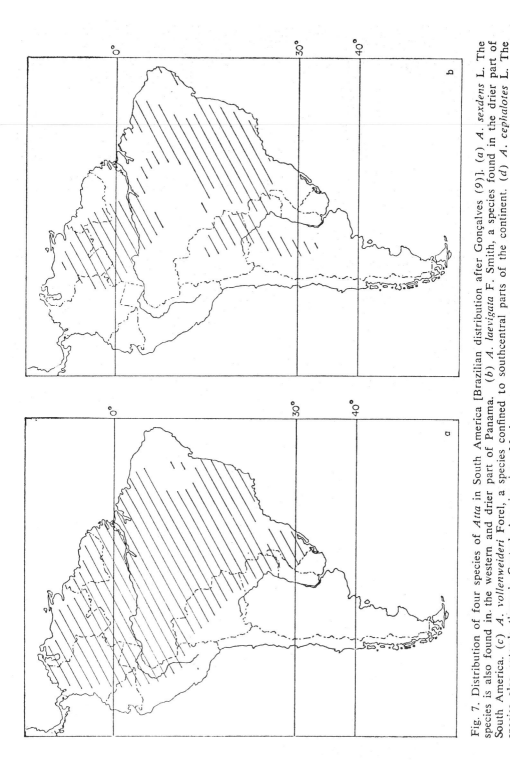

Fig. 7. Distribution of four species of *Atta* in South America [Brazilian distribution after Gonçalves (9)]. (a) *A. sexdens* L. The species is also found in the western and drier part of Panama. (b) *A. laevigata* F. Smith, a species found in the drier part of South America. (c) *A. vollenweideri* Forel, a species confined to southcentral parts of the continent. (d) *A. cephalotes* L. The species also extends through Central America into Mexico.

92

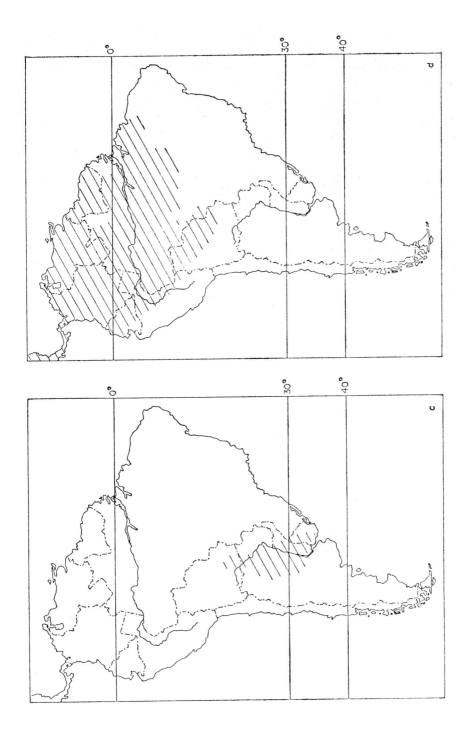

brood raising.

Communication among the members of a colony is accomplished by various means. Studies at the turn of this century indicated that stridulation is an important factor in maintaining co-operation between widely separated ants in underground chambers and that the vibrations are perceived by the ants through the soil (5). Recently these vibrations in *Atta cephalotes* have been clearly recorded (31).

Tactile communication is indicated whenever two ants of a colony meet. In all species the ants advance with antennae widespread and directed toward the other ant. Then the apices of the antennae meet, and the ants may maintain this position for a second or two, then continue with their previous activities. If the ants are of different species they merely approach without touching antennal apices, then generally act hostile. In these cases the responses may be chemical.

Wilson has shown that the general method of communication is chemical (32). The number and complexity of the chemicals are now being effectively studied. The general term for these substances is pheromone, defined as a chemical signal used in communication among members of the same species. He recognizes, among ants generally nine categories of responses: alarm, simple attraction, recruitment, grooming, exchange of oral and anal liquid, exchange of solid food particles, facilitation, recognition, and caste determination. My observations of numerous attine species indicate that, of these nine, the first four and the last three are the usual responses. A further modification of the chemicals would enable the ants to distinguish their own colony mates from other members of the same species.

A special use of pheromones is their use in making a scent trail (33). Ants of several attine species have been shown to follow one another by this means. The ants deposit droplets at intervals. These droplets form the trail, and other ants follow. The trail, in nature, may be invisible to the human eye, as reported for *Trachymyrmex isthmicus* (21). An alarm pheromone in mandibular glands of *Atta sexdens rubropilosa* has been isolated (34).

Visual means of communication have been little studied. Workers and soldiers of *Atta* will respond to a waving of the finger on the outside of the glass or plastic tube in which they are confined. Both males and females, especially males, have large eyes, and it seems possible that it may be a combination of chemical, auditory, and visual stimuli which brings the sexes together in the nuptial flight.

The Brood

The attine brood is normally covered by the mycelium of the garden, contrary to the impression given by photographs of the brood in the early stages of *Atta* colony formation (13). In these early stages the garden has not yet attained its luxuriant hyphal development. The eggs are especially difficult to distinguish in their mycelial mesh. The *Atta* queen lays eggs unassisted at first; after the workers mature, they remove the eggs as they appear at the cloaca. The female of the more primitive species like *Myrmicocrypta buenzlii* lays eggs unassisted during the entire life of the colony.

Soon after the larvae emerge they rotate so that the mouthparts are uppermost. For the duration of its life the larva lies on its side or dorsal surface, so that the head capsule is exposed. When the mouthparts are protruded ("pouting"), the nursemaid workers respond by placing a cluster (staphyla or "kohlrabi" of older authors) (Fig. 13, *b, d, g*) of inflated hyphae or a

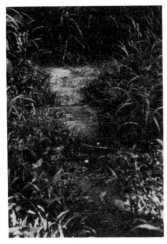

Fig. 8 (left). Forking trail made by a large colony of *Atta cephalotes* coming from the foreground and extending into areas where leaves were being cut. Parts of the trail were 30 centimeters wide. Trinidad.

Fig. 9 (center). Nest of *Atta vollenweideri* at the southern margin of the distribution of *Atta*, Santa Fe Province, Argentina. [Photograph by Bonetto]

Fig. 10 (bottom). A nest of *Atta vollenweideri* in cross section. [Photograph by Bonetto]

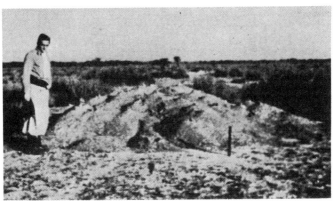

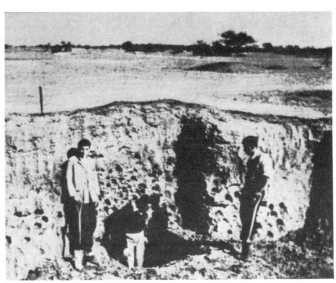

95

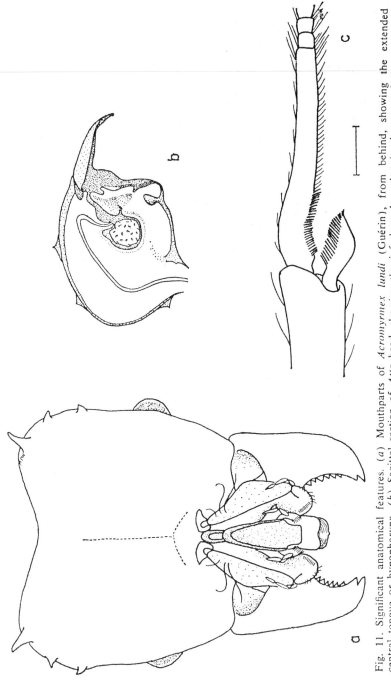

Fig. 11. Significant anatomical features. (*a*) Mouthparts of *Acromyrmex lundi* (Guérin), from behind, showing the extended central tongue or hypopharynx. (*b*) Sagittal section of *Atta* head, showing the infrabuccal pocket in the rear of the mouth. It contains a fungal mass that will be the nucleus for the new garden when the female leaves the parental nest [after Huber]. (*c*) Part of the foreleg of an *Atta* worker, showing the pecten used for cleaning the appendages. The bar represents 0.25 millimeter.

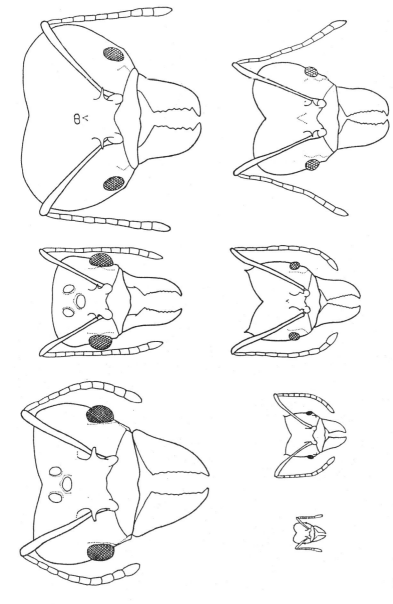

Fig. 12. *Atta cephalotes*. Outline of heads of castes, to scale. Lengths include the mandibles; width between eyes, in millimeters, given in parenthesis. (Top row, left to right) Female, 5.8 mm (3.92); male, 4.1 mm (2.28); soldier, 5.8 mm (3.54). (Bottom row left to right) Minima worker, 0.9 mm (0.58); media worker, 1.8 mm (1.16); media worker, 3.5 mm (2.03); maxima worker, 4.3 mm (2.53).

tuft of ordinary hyphae on them. Slender hairs posterior to the head capsule on the ventral surface of the body help to hold the fungus in place. The larval mandibles are minutely spinulose and puncture the fungal cells.

The distension of the body and increasing opacity of the skin signifies the semipupal stage. The *Atta* semipupa is bean-shaped, and the appendages may be faintly seen through the larval skin (Fig. 14). The pupa (Fig. 15) is naked, with segments and appendages clearly outlined. The compound eyes darken early, then general pigmentation proceeds in a sequence that is useful for determining ages.

The pupa later starts moving its appendages. Anterior legs and antennae are the first to move slightly, and there are slight body tremors. The mouthparts, which are extended throughout pupal life, start moving. Meanwhile the workers have been in attendance, licking the skin intently. The ant cannot emerge from the pupa without this assistance, although it can start to emerge anteriorly from the exuviae.

The callow stage of the adult is reached when the ant is out of the exuviae and can stand unsteadily on its legs. It is markedly paler than the mature ant, and the legs are pale brownish yellow in all castes in various species. The workers continue to groom it and assiduously lick the wings of the young male or female. The callow can feed by itself, taking a staphyla or a few strands of the fungus between the mandibles.

The highly developed social nature of the attine colony is well shown by this brood care and complete dependence of the larvae and adults on the fungus.

Indispensable to studies of the brood and to many other attine studies is some type of observation nest in which the ants can live normally and still be examined under the microscope. A type used for many species is shown in Fig. 16.

Other Colony Characters

Most of the year the fungus-growing ants have adequate food, thus insufficiency of food is not one of the hazards they face. But these ants are subject to predation, parasitism (as from mites and phorid flies), and such other ordinary dangers as accidental injury. Workers of the larger species that go long distances in files may become lost. They may drop from trees into unfavorable sites or be diverted away from their trail. Individual workers are known to have lived 19 months in the laboratory (*29*). The males usually live only a few weeks after maturity, dying the day of their nuptial flight, while fertilized females (which are easily distinguished) are perhaps the longest-living adult insects. Brazilian authorities believe 20 years may be a possible life span for the *Atta* queen (*35*), and a female *Trachymyrmex zeteki* is known to have lived more than 5 years (*36*). Individual workers marked with colored lacquer have lived in the Swarthmore laboratory for between 1 and 2 years. These are *Myrmicocrypta buenzlii* and *Trachymyrmex septentrionalis*; two living females of the latter species are now 4 years old.

The size of the colony has a bearing on the size of the garden or gardens that can be cultivated. A score of workers, or a few score, cannot maintain a garden larger than a few cubic centimeters because of inability to give all parts the requisite care. Colonies with the smallest populations appear to be those of certain *Cyphomyrex* and *Apterosigma* species, with 100 or 200 workers (*21, 37*). Representative colonies of three Trinidad species of other genera were far larger. One of *Myrmi-*

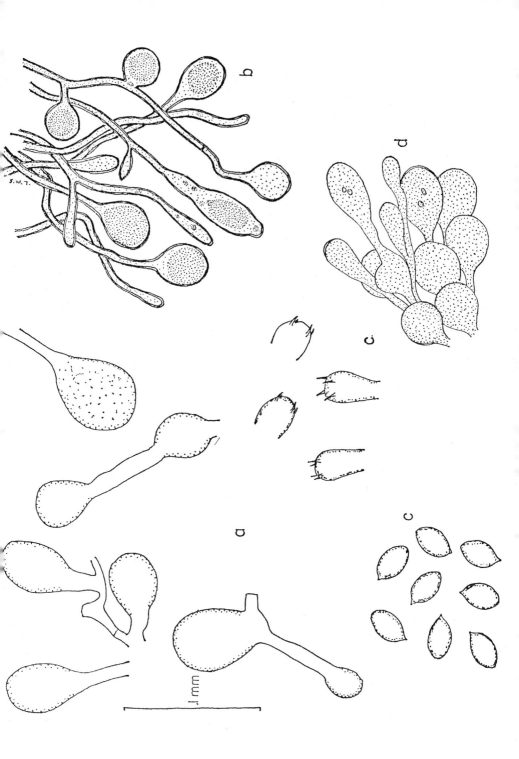

99

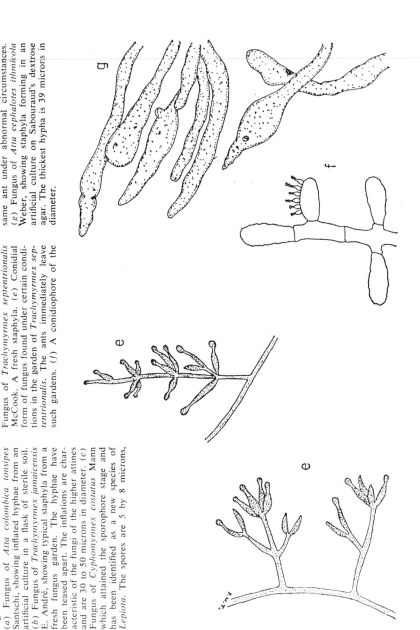

Fig. 13   Forms of ant fungi. (a) Fungus of *Atta colombica tonsipes* Santschi, showing inflated hyphae from an artificial culture in a flask of sterile soil. (b) Fungus of *Trachymyrmex jamaicensis* E. André, showing typical staphyla from a fresh fungus garden. The hyphae have been teased apart. The inflations are characteristic of the fungi of the higher attines and are 30 to 50 microns in diameter. (c) Fungus of *Cyphomyrmex costatus* Mann which attained the sporophore stage and has been identified as a new species of *Lepiota*. The spores are 5 by 8 microns, and the basidia are 10 microns thick. (d) Fungus of *Trachymyrmex septentrionalis* McCook. A fresh staphyla. (e) Conidial form of fungus found under certain conditions in the garden of *Trachymyrmex septentrionalis*. The ants immediately leave such gardens. (f) A conidiophore of the fungus found in another colony of the same ant under abnormal circumstances. (g) Fungus of *Atta cephalotes ithmicola* Weber, showing staphyla forming in an artificial culture on Sabouraud's dextrose agar. The thickest hypha is 39 microns in diameter.

100

cocrypta buenzlii, with a single garden 8.5 by 7.5 by 5.0 centimeters, had 1558 workers. One of *Sericomyrmex urichi*, with seven gardens varying from 3.4 by 7.0 by 1.0 to 11.5 by 8.0 by 5.0 centimeters had 1691 workers. One of *Trachymyrmex urichi*, with six gardens varying from 4.5 by 3.0 by 3.0 to 8.5 by 11.4 by 12.0 centimeters, had 763 counted workers, and those missed in the count brought the estimated total to 1000 (*11*). An *Acromyrmex octospinosus* colony had 7160 workers (*38*).

The Nest and Garden

The nest is large and conspicuous only in *Atta*. In some species of *Acromyrmex* a large colony may be hidden under what appears to be a pile of trash at the base of trees (*19, 38*). Other species of *Acromyrmex* may form a turret constructed of soil and grass sections (Fig. 17) or a dome of thatch (Fig. 18), beneath which are the garden or gardens.

The external indication of nests of species of other genera may be a low, semicircular crater (Fig. 19) or a circular crater (Fig. 20), which is frequently blown away in windy sites, where the ants habitually nest. Other types of nests and entrances have been sketched or photographed (see *10, 19, 21, 37*). In many cases the type of nest structure is a valid species character based on behavior.

The largest gardens are those of the genera of largest ants, *Acromyrmex* (Fig. 21) and *Atta*. The former may have a single very large garden (40 to 50 centimeters in diameter), or it may have a number of smaller gardens (25 to 30 centimeters). Those of *Atta* appear to be more consistently globular and some 20 to 30 centimeters in diameter.

The gardens of *Trachymyrmex* tend

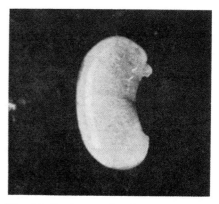

Fig. 14. Semipupa of a large worker of *Atta cephalotes* faintly showing ventral appendages under the taut larval skin. The head capsule is at upper right, the anal hillock at lower right. About 7 millimeters long. Trinidad.

to have a laminated structure, the septa being hung from rootlets entering the ceiling of the chamber. Some gardens rest completely on stones on the floor of the excavation.

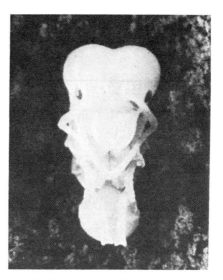

Fig. 15. Pupa of the soldier caste of *Atta cephalotes*. Legs and antennae are folded ventrally. The white skin and beginning pigmentation of the eyes show that this pupal form is a few days old; 12 millimeters long. Trinidad.

101

Gardens of *Sericomyrmex* tend to be disproportionately large. In *S. amabalis* and *S. urichi* the substrate is often pale brown and fruity.

The gardens of *Cyphomyrmex*, other than *C. rimosus*, are small (20 to 50 millimeters in diameter), corresponding to the size of the ant. Those of *Mycocepurus smithi* Forel are approximately 20 to 25 millimeters in diameter. The gardens of the small ants of *Myrmicocrypta buenzlii* Borgmeier (Fig. 22) are often 50 to 80 millimeters in diameter. All three genera have gardens with cells a few millimeters in diameter. The gardens consist of fragments of vegetal matter and of the antfungal mycelium. Sometimes carcasses of insects are incorporated as substrate. Certain *Apterostigma* gardens may be enclosed in a mycelial veil (Figs. 23 and 24).

The most fragile gardens are those of species like *Mycetophylax conformis* (Fig. 25) and *Acromyrmex (Moellerius) landolti* when the ants use grass for substrate. The pieces are relatively long and narrow, creating an irregular mesh of cells, and the mycelium is scanty. The weight of fresh leafy substrate necessary to build up one fungus garden (about 1200 cubic centimeters, weighing approximately 130 grams) in *Atta cephalotes* has been determined (*39*). In a young, vigorous colony 670 grams of substrate was used, in the course of 9 months, before any was cast out. The second garden was built in the next 3 months, when a total of 2060 grams for the two gardens had been taken in. It may be expected that a mature colony will use, in nature, fully 1 kilogram of fresh leaves for a garden of this size. Many gardens in nature have twice this bulk and must take fully 2 kilograms.

Among the interrelated factors involved in maintaining the fungus garden are behavioral, fungistatic, bacteriostatic, and, perhaps, growth promoting factors. These are promising lines of study currently being investigated and not hitherto fully appreciated. The evidence so far is mostly suggestive, and the need for experimentation is obvious.

The early investigators of *Atta* described the behavior of the new queen and first broods in caring for the fungus (*3, 4*). The female feels the fungus almost continually with her antennae and deposits anal droplets on the garden. This behavior has been shown to be universal among the attine workers (*40*).

If the ants are leaf-cutters the procedure is as follows: The cut leaf sections are brought into the nest. These sections may be placed at the base of the garden, or they may be brought to the sides and top. Next comes the cutting into much smaller pieces, a millimeter or two in diameter. Before or during this process the pieces are licked all over. The ants then press along the edges of the pieces with the sharp

Fig. 16 (top). A small colony of *Trachymyrmex septentrionalis* in standard Plexiglas observation nest. Each of the three chambers is connected to the others by a tunnel. This colony has cast out sand in the form of a semicircular crater, as it would have in nature. Soil is always removed from the vicinity of the fungus garden. Inside dimensions, 205 by 152 by 18 millimeters.

Fig. 17 (center). External indication of the nest of *Acromyrmex (Moellerius) landolti* Forel in the form of a turret, characteristic of the species, of soil and grass stems (*Trachypogon plumosus*). Such a turret, on the llanos of Venezuela, tends to reduce evaporation from the underground gardens constructed on the same grass. Card, 76 by 127 millimeters.

Fig. 18 (bottom). Mound nest of *Acromyrmex (Moellerius) heyeri* Forel. Thatch covers the single chamber, which contains one large fungus garden. The 15-centimeter ruler is covered with ants. Uruguay.

102

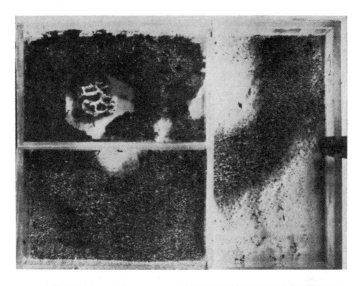

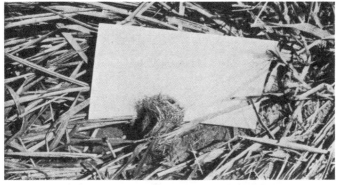

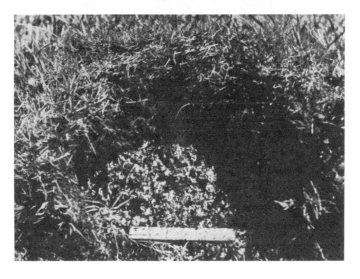

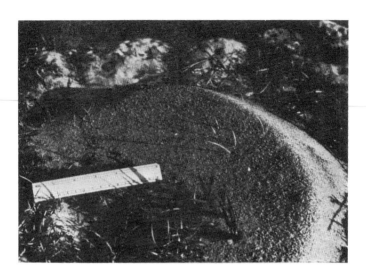

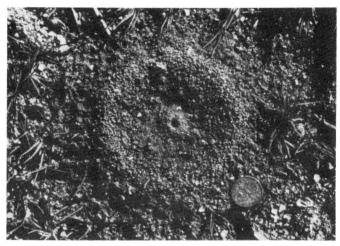

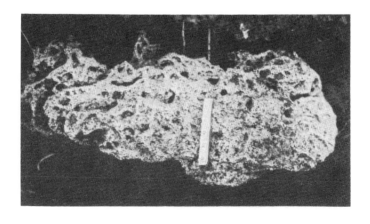

mandibles so that they become wet and pulpy. An ant may take the piece and place it under its body, curve the tip of the abdomen (gaster) forward, and deposit a clear anal droplet. The leaf piece is then inserted into the garden. The ant uses its forelegs with a side-to-side motion and forces the piece into place with the aid of the mandibles. An ant then picks up tufts of the fungal mycelium and places them at intervals on the prepared substrate (41). The hyphae grow out in all directions from the tuft.

If the ants are not leaf-cutters, the procedure may differ only in preliminary details (29). Caterpillar excrement may be broken into the original leaf sections, which are then planted in the garden. Woody particles or other vegetal debris and white cassava starch granules may be dragged to the garden, defecated on, then planted with the mycelium. I have dyed individual cassava particles with neutral red or nigrosine black in order to follow their history in the garden. Small attines may drag parts of insect carcasses to the nest and scatter them over the garden

Fig. 19 (top). External indication of the nest of *Trachymyrmex septentrionalis* in the form of a lunate crater characteristic of the species. The single entrance is below the middle of the 15-centimeter ruler. Florida.

Fig. 20 (center). Crater entrance, characteristic of the genus, to the nest of *Mycetophylax conformis* on the coast of Trinidad. Crater, 7 centimeters in diameter. Constant trade winds tended to blow away the excavated soil, and showers in the rainy season washed it away, but the ants repeated this pattern of crater formation.

Fig. 21 (bottom). Fungus garden of *Acromyrmex octospinosus* shown with a centimeter ruler. The garden was about 31 centimeters long and 11.5 centimeters high and was under a 3-meter log in a cavity in sand. Trinidad.

(19, 21, 29). These, too, acquire islands of mycelial growth.

All attines tend the garden similarly. The ants walk over all exposed parts and down into the cells, using the apices of the antennae as probes to determine the condition of the fungus. They lick the hyphae and occasionally eat them. It appears that droplets are normally deposited only on the garden. A garden fragment placed, with ants, on a nutrient agar plate will be maintained despite surrounding contaminants (Fig. 26).

A fungistatic factor is indicated by the fact that only one recognizable fungus is present in the normal garden. The older assumption that other fungi are weeded out may be valid only to a limited extent (40, 42). What is true is that spores of other fungi are brought into the garden on substrate but do not proliferate.

A selective bacteriostatic factor, like a fungistatic factor, is indicated by the control of bacterial growth. Some types of growth may normally be present, others may be harmful. When the ants are removed (18, 29, 40), the garden quickly degenerates, either becoming a slimy mass from bacterial action or becoming overgrown with sporulating alien fungi.

A growth-promoting factor is indicated by the growth of the ant fungus on the brood and on inert material like insect carcasses (19, 21, 29, 37). The brood, like the garden, is continually licked by the ants.

It appears probable that the products of the salivary glands and the anal droplets are of primary importance in creating the conditions described (29, 43, 44) (Fig. 27). These are consistently applied to the garden, in all species. The ants, in grooming, apply saliva copiously enough to keep the queen glistening (Fig. 28), and much of the time the workers are grooming one another. The combination of the two, or perhaps the products of the abdomen alone, are sufficiently pungent to give off an odor easily perceptible to blunted human senses. The odor of an *Acromyrmex lobicornis* colony in a confined observation nest was strongly ammoniacal. Species of *Atta* and *Acromyrmex octospinosus* have an entirely different odor. Ants preserved in ethanol for years will still give off the odor.

Some books containing chapters on the attines have errors that do not destroy their usefulness (see, for example, *45*). One of the chief myths is that the ant fungus does not develop the clusters of inflated hyphae (Fig. 13, *a, g*) in the absence of the ants. These clusters are produced in artificial culture containing no ants as well as in the absence of ants in nature (*18, 29, 43*). Wheeler suffered much abuse for casting doubt about Moeller's certainty that he had the true ant fungus in culture. Moeller was probably correct. He was cautious and his work was admirably thorough. One hopes that, after more than 70 years, his work in southern Brazil can be duplicated, or—better yet—his sporophores can be produced in artificial culture from the stage present in the normal nest. Forel referred to ants sowing spores; if spores are produced the ants never sow them but abandon that part of the nest. Forel's statement that indigenous vegetation (as contrasted with exotics), "gradually reinforced by natural selection, resists the attacks" of the ants does not correspond with the situation. His dismissal, as a myth, of the story of carpets of green leaf sections in garden chambers was premature. Such carpets may be found after times of abundant leaf-cutting.

The Fungus

Fungi associated with attine ants have been given a number of names

since Moeller described the first one as *Rozites gonglylophora* in 1893. A review appeared in 1938 (*46*). These fungi included *Xylaria, Bargellinia, Rhizomorpha, Locellinia, Poroniopsis, Lentinus*, and *Tyridiomyces* (Fig. 29) species belonging to the Ascomycetes, Basidiomycetes, and Fungi Imperfecti.

The assumption by investigators (*13, 18*) that the fungus grown by other *Acromyrmex* and *Atta* was the same as Moeller's *Rozites gonglylophora* of *Acromyrmex disciger* was challenged by Jacoby (*22*). The fungi are superficially much alike, as cultured by the ants, but Jacoby's experiments in which he exchanged gardens of the two fungus species resulted in rejection of each. I had performed this type of experiment earlier, in 1934–35 (*19, 37*), with many Trinidad species, and later with species of other countries. Where exchange of fungus gardens is attempted, a complication is the difference in pheromone substances of the two ant species, which the ants had added to the garden before the exchange; this difference may play a part in rejection. This complication is eliminated by using artificial cultures of the fungi (*19, 21, 29, 36, 41, 42*). Studies involving isolation of other fungi from

Fig. 22 (top). Fungus garden of *Myrmicocrypta buenzlii* in an observation nest of the type used in 1934–35 in Trinidad. This consists of a wood frame 2.5 centimeters high, with glass top and bottom. Needed moisture is brought in from the bottle by a paper wick.

Fig. 23 (center). Fungus garden of *Apterostigma dentigerum* Wheeler under a rotted log in rain forest, Panama. The garden, covered with a thin mycelial veil, has a single opening for the ants, at left. Forceps, 113 millimeters long.

Fig. 24 (bottom). The garden of Fig. 23 with veil torn aside to show the loose cells of insect excrement covered with the ant fungus.

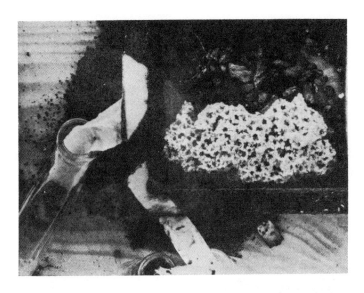

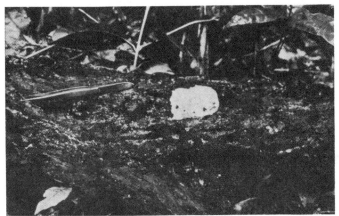

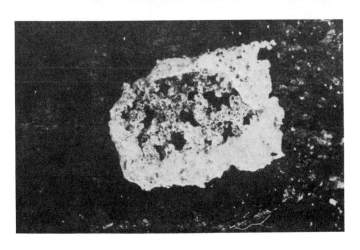

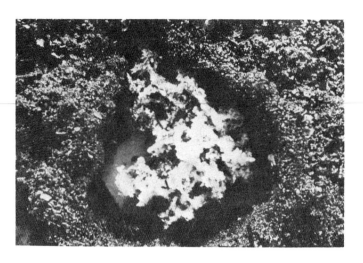

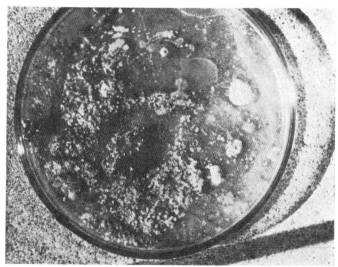

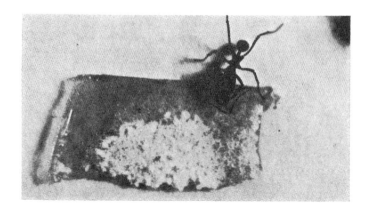

laboratory colonies should be carried out (27). Rarely, conidial forms may develop (Fig. 13, e and f).

Moeller's *Rozites* has been reexamined taxonomically in recent years and is now referred to as *Leucocoprinus gongylophora* (47) or *Leucoagaricus* or *Agaricus gongylophora* (48). Meanwhile I developed the first sporophore or fruiting body of an ant fungus to be produced in the laboratory, by starting with the stage cultured by the ants (29) (Fig. 13c). This was considered to be a new species of *Lepiota* by Locquin. In 1965 W. J. Robbins and his associates produced what is apparently the same species of *Lepiota* but from a culture from another ant species, which I submitted to him. Heim (47) considered the first *Lepiota* to be the same as Moeller's. I believe this to be unlikely. If they were the same, we would have one species of fungus cultured by *Acromyrmex discigera* in south Brazil, by *Cyphomyrmex costatus* in Panama, and by *Myrmicocrypta buenzlii* in Trinidad. It is more likely that Moeller's species of fungus belongs to a group of similar species that are cultured by *Acromyrmex* and *Atta*. My tests of fungus cultures of a number of *Lepiota* species submitted by Robbins showed acceptances for eating (not culturing) by several attine species (49).

The other fungus genera of the 1938 review may be dismissed as follows.

The *Poroniopsis bruchi* Spegazzini from discarded substrate of *Acromyrmex (Moellerius) heyeri* and *Atta vollenweideri* is the same as *Hypocreodendron sanguineum* P. Henning (50). It has not been proved to be a true ant fungus. Another synonym is *Rhizomorpha formicarum* Spegazzini (loc. cit.). The new name *Discoxylaria mirmecophila* Lindquist and Wright applies (51).

The *Locellinia Mazzuchii* Spegazzini from a nest of *Atta vollenweideri* is considered to be a species of *Agaricus* (47). It is in the same category as *Lentinus atticolus* Weber 1938, not proved to be a true ant fungus. In both cases large mushrooms or sporophores were growing over ant nests. The fact that hyphae grew down to abandoned fungus gardens is not conclusive evidence that the fungus cultured by the ants was the same.

The *Xylaria micrura* of Spegazzini and, later, of Bruch is still not proved to be an ant fungus.

The *Tyridiomyces formicarum* Wheeler 1907 is still classified as a member of the Fungi Imperfecti since no sexual stage has been produced. It is the yeast cultured by *Cyphomyrmex rimosus* Spinola (Fig. 29). The hyphal stage shown in Fig. 29 is new and hitherto undescribed.

Additional ant fungi that I have developed from new sources are as follows.

1) The fungus cultured from a 1957 Panamanian colony of *Apterostigma mayri* Forel. A fructification developed in an oak flask culture; the culture was

Fig. 25 (top). Fungus garden of *Mycetophylax conformis* after development on cassava granules. On the seashore, grass stems were generally used; these were retrieved from high tide level.

Fig. 26 (center). Fungus-garden fragment of a *Trachymyrmex septentrionalis* colony on nutrient agar in a Petri dish. Numerous bacterial and alien fungal colonies dot the agar, except in the vicinity of the garden. Here the ants (not shown) have cut the agar and piled the pieces at the side. These fragments, which have received some saliva in the cutting, do not grow alien organisms as fast as the untreated agar does and appear clean and shiny in contrast to adjacent contaminated agar surfaces.

Fig. 27 (bottom). Response of a worker of *Atta sexdens* to a culture of the fungus of *Trachymyrmex septentrionalis*. Fecal droplets (left) were soon deposited.

Fig. 28 (left). Queen of a young *Atta sexdens* colony on her fungus garden. The workers have kept her integument well licked. Panama.

Fig. 29 (below). The fungus of *Cyphomyrmex rimosus* Spinola growing as a yeast in the garden and as a mycelial growth on the brood or in artificial culture. The smallest cells are 8 microns in diameter, and hyphal projections are 2 to 3 microns wide. (*a*) Typical yeast form in a bromatium of the ant garden. (*b*) Yeast cells, one extending a hypha. (*c*) A cluster of seven cells from an ant larva skin, three of them extending hyphae. (*d*) Hyphae growing and forking from yeast cells. (*e*) Compact mass of cells and hyphae growing on the skin of an ant larva. (*f*) Yeast cells growing on cassava granules in an active ant observation nest.

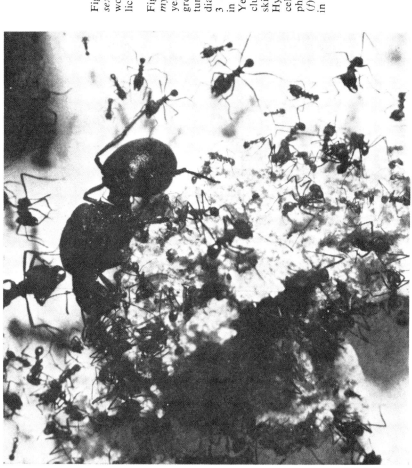

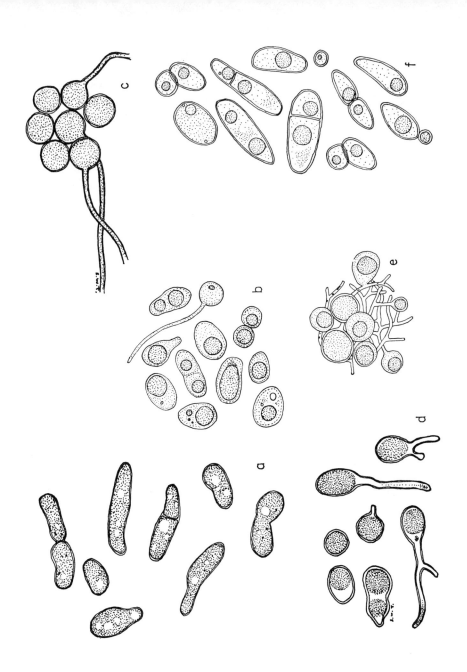

111

examined by Lekh Batra and submitted to G. W. Martin. The latter reported the fructification to be an *Auricularia*, perhaps *A. polytricha* (Mont.) Sacc., but, since it did not mature sufficiently, no further identification was possible.

2) The fungus cultured from a 1957 Panamanian colony of *Myrmicocrypta ednaella* Mann. A fructification developed in an oat flask culture but did not mature sufficiently for identification.

3) The fungus cultured from a 1957 Panamanian colony of *Cyphomyrmex rimosus* Spinola. Massive black sclerotia developed in a wheat flask culture; they were examined by W. C. Denison and Lekh Batra. The sclerotia were then sent to G. W. Martin, who characterized the subsequent culture and growth as that of a *Xylaria* with early similarities to *Daldinia*. The three mycologists agreed on its Ascomycetous nature.

In summary, the names presently applicable to ant fungi are as follows.

1) *Leucocoprinus, Leucoagaricus* or *Agaricus gongylophora* (Moeller 1893). Host ants: *Acromyrmex disciger*, possibly *Atta*.

2) *Tyridomyces formicarum* Wheeler 1907 (possibly a *Daldinia* or *Xylaria*). Host ant: *Cyphomyrmex rimosus*.

3) *Lepiota* n. sp. (Weber 1957, Robins 1965. Host ants: *Cyphomyrmex costatus, Myrmicocrypta buenzlii*.

4) *Auricularia* sp. Host ant: *Apterostigma mayri*.

Summary

Fungus-growing ants (Attini) are in reality unique fungus-culturing insects. There are several hundred species in some dozen genera, of which *Acromyrmex* and *Atta* are the conspicuous leaf-cutters. The center of their activities is the fungus garden, which is also the site of the queen and brood. The garden, in most species, is made from fresh green leaves or other vegetal material. The ants forage for this, forming distinct trails to the vegetation that is being harvested. The cut leaves or other substrate are brought into the nest and prepared for the fungus. Fresh leaves and flowers are cut into pieces a millimeter or two in diameter; the ants form them into a pulpy mass by pinching them with the mandibles and adding saliva. Anal droplets are deposited on the pieces, which are then forced into place in the garden. Planting of the fungus is accomplished by an ant's picking up tufts of the adjacent mycelium and dotting the surface of the new substrate with it. The combination of salivary and anal secretions, together with the constant care given by the ants, facilitates the growth of the ant fungus only, despite constant possibilities for contamination. When the ants are removed, alien fungi and other organisms flourish.

A mature nest of *Atta sexdens* may consist of 2000 chambers, some temporarily empty, some with refuse, and the remainder with fungus gardens. Thousands of kilograms of fresh leaves will have been used. A young laboratory colony of *Atta cephalotes* will use 1 kilogram of fresh leaves for one garden. The attines are the chief agents for introducing organic matter into the soil in tropical rain forests; this matter becomes the nucleus for a host of other organisms, including nematodes and arthropods, after it is discarded by the ants.

One ant species cultures a yeast; all others grow a mycelium. In the higher species the mycelium forms clusters of inflated hyphae. Mycologists accept as valid two names for confirmed fruiting stages: *Leucocoprinus* (or *Leucoagaricus*) *gongylophora* (Moeller 1893) and *Lepiota* n. sp.

112

References and Notes

1. T. Belt, *The Naturalist in Nicaragua* (Murray, London, 1874).
2. A. Moeller, *Schimper's Botan. Mitt. Tropen* **6**, 127 (1893).
3. I. Huber, *Biol. Centralbl.* **25**, 606 (1905); *Smithsonian Inst. Ann. Rep.* **1907**, 355 (1907).
4. E. Goeldi, *Compt. Rend. Congr. Intern. Zool., 6th, Berne* (1905), p. 457; ———, *ibid.*, p. 508; ———, *Bol. Museu Nacl. Rio de Janeiro Geol. No. 5* (1908), p. 223; H. von Ihering, *Briefl. Mitt. Mundoro* **1**, 156 (1881); ———, *Berlin. Entomol. Z.* **39**, 321 (1894); ———, *Zool. Anz.* **21**, 238 (1898); A. G. Sampaio de Asevedo, *Saúva ou Manhúaára* (monograph) (São Paulo, 1894).
5. W. M. Wheeler, *Bull. Amer. Museum Nat. Hist.* **23**, 69 (1907).
6. E. Williams, *Documents of West Indian History* (PNM Publishing Co., Trinidad, 1963), vol. 1, 1492-1655; *History of the People of Trinidad and Tobago* (Praeger, New York, 1964).
7. Vernacular names for *Atta* are as follows. Cuba, *bibijagua*; Mexico, various, including *sonteta* and *hormiga arriera*; Central America, *zompopas*; Panama and Colombia, *hormiga arriera* or *podadora*; Venezuela, *bachaco*; Trinidad, *bachac*; British Guiana, *cuschi* or *acuschi*; Surinam, *parasolmieren*; Brazil, *saúva* or *saúba*, also *hormiga mineira, carregadeira*; Peru, *coqui*; Paraguay, *hormiga minera*; Uruguay and Argentina, *hormiga isaú.*
8. L. F. Byars, *J. Econ. Entomol.* **42**, 545 (1949); R. W. Neelands, *Forests and People* **1959**, No. 4, 1 (1959); C. P. Kennard, *Exp. Agr.* **1**, 237 (1965).
9. C. R. Gonçalves, *Divulgaçe Agron.* **1**, 2 (1960); ———, *Studia Entomol.* **4**, 113 (1961).
10. N. A. Weber, *Bol. Entomol. Venezuela* **6**, 143 (1947).
11. This role is emphasized in N. A. Weber, "Actas del Primer Coloquio Latinoamericano de Biología del Suelo" (Proceedings 1st Latin American Colloquium on Soil Biology) (UNESCO, Montevideo, in press).
12. Field work with students in Trinidad, W.I., in 1964 and 1965 was under the auspices of the National Science Foundation Undergraduate Research Participation Program. The students were Peter Delmonte, Stephen Hitchner, Mary Lewis, John Melbourne, Nancy and Peter Weber, and Gary Williamson. Various aspects of the study were aided by the Swarthmore Faculty Research Fund.
13. M. Autuori, *Rev. Entomol.* **11**, 215 (1940); *Arquiv. Inst. Biol. São Paulo* **12**, 197 (1941); ———, *ibid.* **3**, 67 (1942); ———, *ibid.* **18**, 39 (1947); ———, *ibid.* **19**, 325 (1950); ———, in *L'instinct dans le comportment des animaux et de l'homme* (Masson, Paris, 1956).
14. H. ' Eidmann, *Z. Angew. Entomol.* **22**, 185 (1935).
15. M. Bazire-Benazet, *Compt. Rend.* **244**, 1277 (1957).
16. W. E. Kerr, *Rev. Brasil. Biol.* **21**, 45 (1961).
17. A. A. Betancourt, *Arquiv. Inst. Biol. São Paulo* **14**, 229 (1941).
18. G. Stahel and D. C. Geijskes, *Rev. Entomol.* **10**, 27 (1939); ———, *ibid.* **11**, 766 (1940); ———, *ibid.* **12**, 243 (1941); ———, *Secr. Agr. Direc. Publ. Agron. São Paulo* (1943), p. 33; G. Stahel, *Ann. Primer Reun. Sul-Amer. Botan. Rio de Janeiro* (1938), vol. 1, p. 199; ———, *J. N.Y. Botan. Garden* **44**, 245 (1943). Sporophores growing wild from *Atta cephalotes* nests were considered by Stahel and Geijskes (1941) to be the same as *Rozites gongylophora.* Parts were cultured on nutrient agar, and staphylae appeared in 10 days. Stahel and Geijskes were unsuccessful in attempts to grow sporophores from these cultures. Dense fungal growths that did appear were removed from the sterile bottles and planted near ant nests. These degenerated or were cut and discarded by the ants. On other occasions conidial forms appeared in garden fragments of both *Atta cephalotes* and *A. sexdens.* In Surinam, as in south Brazil, sporophores that represent true ant fungi are exceedingly rare. Sporophores of unrelated fungi are not unusual. Whether any of the ant-nest-associated sporophores that were reported in the Argentine literature were indeed true ant fungi cannot now be ascertained, except in cases where it was found possible to rear viable spores from the original specimens.
19. N. A. Weber, *Rev. Entomol.* **17**, 114 (1946).
20. W. Weyrauch, *Bol. Direc. Gen. Agr. Peru* **15**, 204 (1942).
21. N. A. Weber, *Rev. Entomol.* **12**, 93 (1941); *Yearbook Amer. Phil. Soc.* (1956), p. 153.
22. M. Jacoby, *Rev. Entomol.* **6**, 100 (1936); *ibid.* **7**, 416 (1937); *Rev. Soc. Rural Brasil* **17**, 36 (1937); *Bol. Min. Agr.* **27**, 21 (1938); *ibid.* **32**, 55 (1943).
23. Trinidad subsurface temperatures under shade were taken by the method of N. A. Weber, *Ecology* **40**, 153 (1959), and were found comparable to temperatures for Panamanian *Atta.*
24. N. A. Weber, *Trop. Agr. Trinidad* **14**, 223 (1937).
25. J. C. Moser, *Ann. Entomol. Soc. Amer.* **56**, 286 (1963).
26. A. A. Bonetto, *Min. Agr. Ganad., Santa Fe, Argentina* (1959), p. 1; C. Bruch, *Ann. Soc. Cient. Argentina* **84**, 154 (1917); J. B. Daguerre, *Rev. Soc. Entomol. Argentina* **12**, 438 (1945); E. Lynch Arribalzaga, *Bol. Direc. Gral. Def. Agr. Argentina* (1910), p. 53; J. C. Otamendi, *Circ. Dept. Zool. Agr. Argentina* **17**, 11 (1945).
27. W. Goetsch, *Naturwissenschaften* **28**, 764 (1938); ———, *Tropenplanz.* **41**, 385 (1938); ———, *Zoologica* **35**, 1 (1939); ——— and R. Stoppel, *Biol. Zentr.* **60**, 393 (1940); W. Goetsch and R. Gruger, *Naturwissenschaften* **28**, 764 (1940); ———, *Rev. Appl. Mycol.* **20**, 257 (1941); ———, *Biol. Gen. Vienna* **16**, 41 (1942). South American colonies of *Atta sexdens* and *Acromyrmex striatus* were taken by Goetsch to Germany in 1938. He and Stoppel then repeatedly isolated *Hypomyces ipomoeae* and *Fusarium* spp. from the fungus gardens. The ants accepted these fungus species when they were in the company of other fungi, especially *Mucor.* Sugar juices were added, and the ants appeared to raise brood normally. The *Hypomyces* and *Fusarium* were said to thrive best in the saliva secreted by the ants. The saliva was toxic to other fungi. This interesting case does not alter the general conclusion that, in nature, an entirely different fungus has an obligatory relationship with the ants.
28. N. A. Weber, *J. Wash. Acad. Sci.* **45**, 275 (1955).
29. ———, *Ecology* **37**, 150 (1956); *ibid.*, p. 197; *ibid.* **38**, 480 (1957).
30. These castes were produced in the Swarthmore laboratory in colonies of known ages. The temperature was 24° to 26°C, and fungus gardens were maintained on fresh, leafy substrate. Autuori (*13*) found that *Atta sexdens*

colonies were much older than *A. cephalotes* when soldiers first appeared.

31. H. Markl, *Science* **149**, 1392 (1965).
32. E. O. Wilson, *Ann. Rev. Entomol.* **8**, 345 (1963); *Science* **149**, 1064 (1965).
33. J. C. Moser and M. S. Blum, *Science* **140**, 1228 (1963); M. S. Blum, J. C. Moser, A. D. Cordero, *Psyche* **71**, 1 (1964); G. W. K. Cavill and P. L. Robertson, *Science* **149**, 1337 (1965).
34. V. A. Butenandt and B. Linzen, *Arch. Anat. Microscop. Morphol. Exp.* **48**, 13 (1959).
35. E. Amanta, personal communication to J. C. Moser (1965).
36. N. A. Weber, *Ann. Entomol. Soc. Amer.* **57**, 87 (1964).
37. ———, *Rev. Entomol.* **16**, 1 (1945).
38. W. M. Wheeler, *Mosaics and Other Anomalies in Ants* (Harvard Univ. Press, Cambridge, 1937).
39. Unpublished data from the Swarthmore laboratory.
40. N. A. Weber, in *Proc. Intern. Congr. Entomol., 10th, Montreal* (1958), vol. 2, p. 459.
41. ———, *Anat. Record* **125**, 604 (1956).
42. ———, *ibid.* **128**, 638 (1957).
43. ———, *Science* **121**, 109 (1955).
44. ———, *Anat. Record* **120**, 735 (1954).
45. W. M. Wheeler, *Ants* (Columbia Univ. Press, New York, 1926); A. Forel, *The Social World of the Ants Compared with Man* (Boni, New York, 1929).
46. N. A. Weber, *Rev. Entomol.* **8**, 264 (1938).
47. R. Heim, *Rev. Mycol.* **22**, 293 (1957).
48. R. Singer, personal communication (1965).
49. N. A. Weber, unpublished work.
50. J. C. Lindquist and J. E. Wright, *Darwiniana* **11**, 598 (1959).
51. ———, *ibid.* **13**, 138 (1964).

INTRODUCTION TO SECTION II: TOXICOGENIC INSECTS

A number of insects with piercing-sucking mouthparts cause serious plant damage by injecting toxic salivary secretions into plants during feeding. These insects are said to be toxicogenic and the diseases they cause are termed phytotoxemias. The exact chemical nature of the toxic secretions is not known, but they are definitely capable of causing serious changes in plant growth and metabolism. Such changes are well illustrated in the paper by Byers and Wells (1966) on the injury produced by the two-lined spittlebug. The plant itself is also an important variable in disease production as demonstrated by Taliaferro et al. (1969) in their study of phytotoxemia tolerance in Bermudagrass clones. The difficulty of separating certain phytotoxemias from virus diseases has been long recognized. The paper by Gardener and Cannon (1972) illustrates some reasons for this problem. We have also included the classic paper on psyllid yellows of potato by Richards and Blood (1933) because it provides details and insight into another of these very important diseases.

Phytotoxemia of Coastal Bermudagrass Caused by the Two-Lined Spittlebug, *Prosapia bicincta* (Homoptera: Cercopidae)

R. A. BYERS AND HOMER D. WELLS

The two-lined spittlebug, *Prosapia bicincta* (Say), caused extensive damage to Coastal bermudagrass, a cultivar of *Cynodon dactylon* (L.) Pers. (Beck 1963, Byers 1965). Since leaf spot and stolen rotting organisms are frequently associated with spittlebug damage on Coastal bermudagrass, we wanted to ascertain if this spittlebug under controlled conditions and in the absence of known disease-producing organisms can produce the typical symptoms that are observed in the field. We wanted to know whether it causes phytotoxemia as described by Carter (1939, 1962) and Leach (1940) or serves as the vector for a virus or other type of pathogenic disease. If this spittlebug causes phytotoxemia, we need to determine the stage or stages in which the toxin is produced and investigate the feeding habits of the insect during its life cycle.

Experiments were conducted in which spittlebugs were reared to the various instars and to maturity on pearl millet [*Pennisetum typhoides* (Burm.) Stapf. & C. E. Hubb.], oats (*Avena sativa* L.), centipedegrass [*Eremochloa ophiuroides* (Munro) Hack.], and St. Augustinegrass [*Stenotaphrum secundatum* (Walt) Kuntze] and then used as test insects on Coastal bermudagrass. Histological studies were conducted on leaves, stems, and roots of the grass on which nymphs in the different instars and adults had fed.

MATERIALS AND METHODS

Female spittlebugs were collected from the field in October and November and the system described by Byers (1965) was used for procuring eggs for use in these experiments.

ANNALS OF THE ENTOMOLOGICAL SOCIETY OF AMERICA
Volume 59, Number 6, pp. 1067–1071, November 1966

Eggs in the eye-spot stage were placed in plastic culture dishes containing young pearl millet sprouts. The eggs hatched within 3 days; on the fourth to seventh days the young nymphs and accompanying spittle masses were transferred to disease-free Coastal bermudagrass, pearl millet, or oats growing in 4-in. clay pots. The pots were covered with tight-fitting aluminum wire cages; then covered with plastic bags, to maintain high humidity; the plastic bags were removed during the nymph's third instar. The clay pots were maintained in individual steel saucers which were kept full of water. Nitrate of soda was added at intervals throughout the period to keep the grasses in a vigorous state of growth. The grasses were cut to a height of 4 in. at frequent intervals. Eggs in the eye-spot stage were placed directly on the base of the plant of centipedegrass or St. Augustinegrass in 8-in. pots in the greenhouse. The grasses were watered at regular intervals and caged with tight-fitting plastic screen soon after the nymphs entered the 4th instar. Newly emerged adults were confined with an aluminum screen wire cage (1 adult/pot) on disease-free Coastal bermudagrass in 4-in. clay pots in the greenhouse and allowed to feed for various periods (Table 1). Each feeding period was replicated 8 times except the 96- and 168-hr periods, which were replicated 7 and 6 times, respectively.

Nymphs in the first and second instars were transferred to disease-free Coastal bermudagrass grown in 4-in. clay pots in the greenhouse. The nymphs were allowed to mature on Coastal bermudagrass and the adults were removed as they emerged. The plants on which nymphs and adults were confined were observed daily for the development of symptoms which were described and categorized as to types. Maerz and Paul (1930) color charts were used to determine the colors in the description of symptom complexes.

Another test (replicated twice) consisted of 4 adults confined to a single stem of Coastal bermudagrass for 48 hr.

Four adults were confined in small aluminum-wire cages, 1 in. high, for 24 hr to each of the 3 following Coastal bermudagrass stem loci on which leaf sheaths had been removed: (1) from ground level to 1 in. above; (2) 1-in. area in the middle of a simple stem; and (3) 1-in. area above the fork of a divided stem. Each treatment was replicated twice. Patterns of symptom development were observed over a period of 7 days.

Two-lined spittlebug adults were restricted to the base of Coastal bermudagrass stems on which leaf sheaths had been removed. Several days later, the living leaves showing varying symptoms were sectioned by hand (with a razor blade) and studied microscopically to determine the tissues affected. Live portions of stems on which nymphs in each of the 4 instars and the adult had fed were sectioned by hand and examined microscopically to determine the tissue or tissues in which this spittlebug feeds.

Table 1.—Leaf symptoms of Coastal bermudagrass resulting from confinement of adult *P. bicincta* for varying lengths of time.

No. hr confined	Mean no. of damaged leaves/plant			Duncan's multiple range[a]
	Stippled	Streaked	Brown	
1	0.12	0.37	0.37	a
2	.00	.37	.75	a
4	.25	1.00	.37	a
8	.50	.75	.50	a
16	.00	1.00	.87	a
24	.12	1.37	2.00	b
48	.12	1.00	3.12	b
96	.29	1.28	4.14	c
168	.33	1.16	5.00	c

[a] Duncan's multiple range established only for leaves that were brown. Means with same letter not significantly different at P 0.01.

RESULTS

No symptoms developed on any of the Coastal bermudagrass on which only nymphs were allowed to feed.

Symptoms developed within 1–3 days after adults began feeding (Fig. 1). The first symptoms appeared on the leaves as White stippled areas, arranged in broken rows parallel to the leaf veins. In many instances, the stippled areas later coalesced to form Ivory (10B2) to Sea Foam Y (17C2) streaks. Some leaves remained stippled or streaked, but the most severe or advanced symptoms so progressed that entire leaves turned Vanilla Brown (10C3) and died. The individual stems on which 4 adults were confined for 48 hr did not become stippled or streaked, but they withered and died within 4 days. The severity of damage was directly proportional to the length of time the adult was confined to the plant (Table 1). Some plants developed symptoms after the adult was confined on them for 1 hr. All plants on which adults were confined for 2 hr and longer developed symptoms. The symptom expression was fully developed by 14 days. In instances where the above-ground portion of the plants was not killed, new leaves ap-

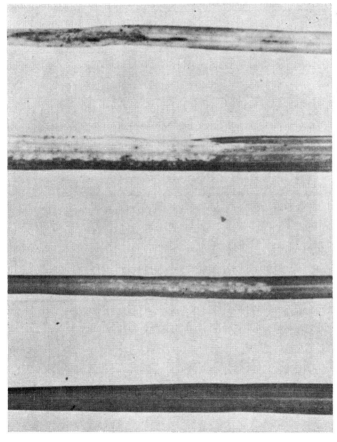

Fig. 1.—Symptoms of damage by *P. bicincta* on Coastal bermudagrass leaves. Leaves from left to right show: (1) normal, disease-free; (2) stippled; (3) streaked; and (4) brown or dead. Approximately ×3.

peared above the damaged leaves and were normal in every respect. All plants in which all the above-ground growth was killed developed new normal-appearing growth from the rhizomes.

Plants on which adults had been confined for 24 hr on stems (leaf sheaths removed) within 1 in. of the soil surface developed symptoms on the leaves. Plants on which adults had been confined for 24 hr within a 1-in. length on the middle of the stems (leaf sheaths removed), developed leaf symptoms above and below the point of confinement. Forked plants on which adults had been confined for 24 hr on a 1-in. length of stem (leaf sheaths removed) above the fork developed leaf symptoms above and below the point of feeding but not on the other arm of the fork.

Cross sections of leaves above areas with macroscopic stippling showed slight damage. In many instances, 1 or 2 cells of the border parenchyma adjacent to xylem elements were discolored, and a slight chlorophyll reduction was evident in the adjacent mesophyll (Fig. 2). A cross section through the stippled areas showed that the cell walls of the border parenchyma around many of the vascular bundles were brown and the border parenchyma cells were void of chlorophyll. Most mesophyll in the vicinity of the damaged border parenchyma was also void of chlorophyll. The chlorophyll content of mesophyllic cells increased with distance away from the affected vascular bundles. Cross sections of leaves showing severe stippling and streaking revealed collapsed border parenchymal and mesophyllic cells around most vascular bundles with only very little chlorophyll remaining in isolated cells (Fig. 3).

Cross sections of stems above and below feeding points of both adults and nymphs had randomly distributed discolored vascular bundles. In many instances, both phloem and xylem were collapsed. Since these observations were not made from serial sections, the relationship of discolored bundles to points of feeding was not established. Cross sections of stems through numerous feeding tunnels made by nymphs and adults, revealed no differences in the type of tunnel; both nymphs and adults probe into the xylem. In some instances the probe extended through 1 vascular bundle on into the xylem element of a deeper or adjacent vascular bundle. In several cases the feeding tunnel was forked, with each arm of the fork ending in the xylem element of separate vascular bundles (Fig. 4). Feeding tunnels varied from 30–45μ in width. New feeding tunnels were not discolored, whereas older feeding tunnels were bordered by brown dead cells, and the vascular bundles into

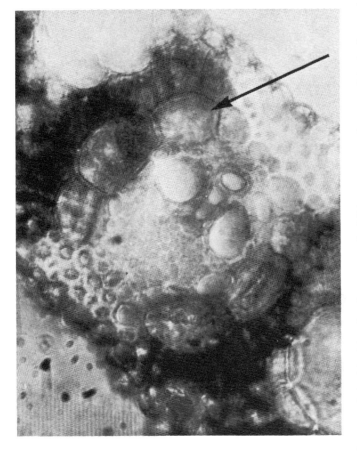

Fig. 2.—Cross section of leaf bundle above area of visible symptoms. Arrow points to damaged parenchymal cell adjacent to xylem. ×100.

which the insect probed were also brown.

DISCUSSION AND CONCLUSIONS

The most striking result of these experiments was that the nymphs failed to cause any macroscopic symptoms on Coastal bermudagrass, even though they were allowed to feed on the same plants continuously from the age of 4–7 days until they emerged as adults some 35–60 days later, whereas the newly emerged adults often caused symptoms after being confined to a pot of Coastal bermudagrass for only 1 hr. Beck (1963) reported some damage from nymphs. However, since the newly emerged adults can cause symptoms by feeding for no longer than 1 hr, it is plausible that in his tests some nymphs may have matured and fed before they were removed. The habit of feeding could not be used as an explanation for the failure of nymphs to produce symptoms because both nymphs and adults feed in the xylem, and cross sections of their respective feeding tunnels were identical under microscopic examination.

The stippling and streaking observed during these tests had not been observed by us previously or, insofar as we can ascertain, reported in the literature. However, after observing the stippling and streaking in the greenhouse, we have found them in abundance in the field. Perhaps these symptoms were overlooked in the past because no one suspected such manifestations to be a part of the symptom complex caused by the two-lined spittlebug.

Our experiments, which were designed to determine if the damage to Coastal bermudagrass is caused by feeding of a toxicogenic insect or whether the insects serve only as vectors for pathogenic organisms (such as a virus), wholly support our theory that the damage results from the feeding of a toxicogenic insect. After removal of the insects, the damaged plants always recovered and new growth appeared normal in every respect. The severity of damage was related to length of feeding time and degree of infestation. The insects were capable of producing damage even though they had been reared on disease-free Coastal bermudagrass, pearl millet, oats, St. Augustinegrass, and centipedegrasses.

The only possibility that could not be excluded in these tests is that the damage might be caused by a virus transmitted through the egg, but which the insect was not able to transmit until it became an adult. However, if this were a virus, it would have to be one which causes severe initial symptoms and then,

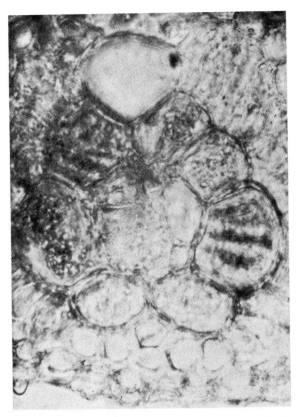

Fig. 3.—Cross section of leaf bundle in the area of visible symptoms. ×100.

in the absence of the insects, permits the plant to return to normal and thereafter serve only as a symptomless carrier. Such is not the case, because other experiments we have conducted here at Tifton have indicated that when new insects are placed on recovered plants, typical symptoms reappear. Also our arguments are in substantial agreement with those proposed by Carter (1939, 1962) and Leach (1940) in differentiating phytotoxemia from a virus, and

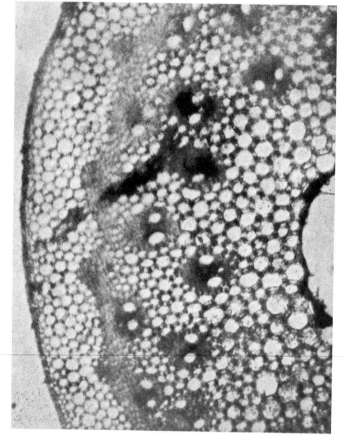

Fig. 4.—Cross section of Coastal bermudagrass stem, showing the adult feeding tunnel of *P. bicincta* ending in the xylem. ×100.

parallel those of Williams (1921) and Withycombe (1926), who concluded that sugarcane blight is a disease caused by a toxicogenic spittlebug, *Aeneolamia varia saccharina* Distant. Therefore, we conclude that *P. bicincta* causes phytotoxemia of Coastal bermudagrass.

Confining the spittlebug to various portions of the stem demonstrated that the toxic principle is translocated in the plant. Since symptoms appear in the leaves both above and below the points of feeding, it is evident that the toxin moves both up and down the stem.

Histological studies indicated that the toxic substance moves in the xylem. Feeding tunnels always ended in xylem elements. Cross sections of leaf tissue above macroscopically visible stippled areas, showed that cells of border parenchyma adjacent to xylem elements must be damaged before the adjacent mesophyllic tissue showed any effects from the toxin. In the stippled areas, the damage to border parenchyma was more severe than to the adjacent mesophyll, and the damage became less as the distance from the vascular bundles increased. Cross sections of stems indicated that the sclerenchymous sheaths surrounding the vascular bundles were impervious to the toxin, thus forcing it to move into the leaves before "breaking out" through the more pervious parenchymous sheaths. Some discoloration occurred along the sides of the feeding tunnels, possibly a reaction to wounding rather than an effect of a toxin.

Since symptoms resulted only from adult feeding, the nymph apparently does not produce the toxin, or if it does, it is produced in such small quantities that no visible symptoms develop on the plant.

In these studies, the first indication of damage to both parenchymal and mesophyllic cells was the loss of chlorophyll, an indication that the toxin may break down chlorophyll or interefere with chlorophyll synthesis. Since both border parenchymal and mesophyllic cells were also killed, it is evident that the toxin interferes with additional vital functions in cell metabolism. It is interesting to note that the tops of Coastal bermudagrass plants could be completely killed by the toxin and new growth would be initiated from below ground. Future studies should be designed to determine if the toxin fails to be translocated below the ground in the same quantities as above ground, or if schlerenchymous tissue prevents it from entering into the various tissues in the roots and rhizomes.

125

Beck, E. W. 1963. Observations on the biology and cultural-insecticidal control of *Prosapia bicincta,* a spittlebug, on Coastal bermudagrass. J. Econ. Entomol. 56: 747–52.

Byers, R. A. 1965. Biology and control of a spittlebug, *Prosapia bicincta* (Say), on Coastal bermudagrass. Univ. Georgia Agr. Exp. Sta. Tech. Bull. N.S. 42. 26 p.

Carter, W. 1939. Injuries to plants caused by insect toxins. Bot. Rev. 5: 273–326.

1962. Insects in Relation to Plant Disease. Interscience Publishers, New York and London. 705 p.

Leach, J. G. 1940. Insect Transmission of Plant Diseases. McGraw-Hill Book Co., Inc., New York. 615 p.

Maerz, A., and M. R. Paul. 1930. Dictionary of Color. McGraw-Hill Book Co., Inc., New York. 207 p.

Williams, C. B. 1921. Froghopper blight of sugar cane in Trinidad. Mem. Dep. Agr. Trinidad and Tobago 1: 1–170.

Withycombe, C. L. 1926. Studies on the aetiology of sugarcane froghopper blight in Trinidad. I. Introduction and general survey. Ann. Appl. Biol. 13: 64–108.

Tolerance of Cynodon Clones to Phytotoxemia Caused by the Two-lined Spittlebug

C. M. Taliaferro, D. B. Leuck and M. W. Stimmann

THE two-lined spittlebug, *Prosapia bicincta* (Say), sporadically inflicts severe damage to 'Coastal' bermudagrass, *Cynodon dactylon* (L.) Pers., and other bermudagrass cultivars in the southeastern U. S. (1, 2). Symptoms of spittlebug injury to bermudagrass are characterized by initial chlorotic stippling and streaking of leaves, with these areas subsequently coalescing to produce brown leaves. Spittlebug populations can increase rapidly in bermudagrass fields under some environmental conditions and entire fields of grass can be quickly and completely browned-off.

Recent investigations indicate that spittlebug damage to bermudagrass results from a toxicogenic substance injected into plant stems as the sucking-type insects feed (3). The vascular tissues transport the toxin up ond down the stems and into the leaves, where it escapes through the border parenchyma into the mesophyll, causing loss of chlorophyll and later, death of mesophyll parenchyma cells. Nymphs and adults feed in the same manner, but only the adults cause visible injury to the grass.

The largest spittlebug populations and resultant severe damage to bermudagrass generally occur in years with high spring and summer rainfall; however, varying numbers of these insects are present each year and cause an insidious amount of damage. Regrowth from browned-off bermudagrass fields is generally

The authors gratefully acknowledge the assistance of Dr. Glenn W. Burton, Geneticist, Crops Research Division, ARS, USDA, and the Georgia Coastal Plain Experiment Station, Tifton for making much of the plant material available.

Reprinted from CROP SCIENCE
Vol. 9, Nov.-Dec. 1969, p. 765-766

initiated from underground reproductive organs as insect-population size diminishes. Research indicates that spittlebug toxin has little, if any direct adverse effect on underground plant parts, but that root production and sod reserves are greatly reduced in damaged fields, due to the cessation of photosynthesis and other essential life processes in injured top growth (6). Thus, spittlebug damage to bermudagrass results in an immediate loss of available forage, plus a probable reduction in its future productivity and persistence.

The desirability of forage and pasture crop insect control through host-plant resistance has been elaborated on by Painter (4, 5). The importance of bermudagrass as a pasture and forage crop in the southern U.S.A. (grown on 6-10 million acres), and the need for an effective and inexpensive spittlebug-control method, led us to screen diverse *Cynodon* plant material for spittlebug resistance. The purpose of this paper is to report the results of initial screening tests.

MATERIALS AND METHODS

Source plant material for our spittlebug screening tests came from a nursery of highly variable *Cynodon* plant accessions maintained at Tifton, Georgia. Since the majority of these were obtained as vegetative sprigs and all are maintained vegetatively, individual entries will be referred to herein as "clones." The material tested totalled 398 clones.

In initial screening tests, a single 10 cm diam cup-cutter plug of grass was taken from each clone and planted in flats of steam-sterilized soil. Each flat contained 12 entries, including Coastal bermudagrass, which was used as a standard for comparison. Top growth was clipped from the plugs of grass and fertilizer applied to hasten new growth. When all grass plugs were growing well, the flats were placed on greenhouse benches, over which insect-proof, screen-wire cages had been constructed. Daytime greenhouse temperatures were maintained at 29 to 32 C with evaporative water coolers; and the screen-wire cages and grass provided sufficient shade for a near-normal spittlebug environment. Insect infestation was accomplished by placing 3 or 4 adult, field-collected spittlebugs per grass clone in the cage. The spittlebugs were collected with sweepnets from a field of Coastal bermudagrass. Differences in clonal reaction to spittlebug attack were measured by allowing insects to feed on all grass clones until some clones exhibited an advanced stage of damage. At this time, we rated each clone visually and independently four times. A rating scale of 1 to 9 was used with 9 representing the maximum amount of injury.

In order to test the validity of the initial screening trials and to investigate the nature of the apparent resistance, we conducted a second nonpreference type experiment with 12 selected clones. Twenty-centimeter diameter plugs of each of the 12 clones were established in the greenhouse (by sodding directly into the soil-floor of the house) in randomized, complete blocks replicated four times. Adult field-collected spittlebugs were caged on each grass plug on September 12, 17, and 19, 1968, at the respective rates of 15, 20, and 25 insects per plug. Visual ratings of percent phytotoxemia were made for each grass plug 5, 7, 11, and 14 days after initial infestation. Previously described rating methods were used except that three rather than four independent ratings were made at each date. Independent ratings by individuals and ratings over replications were averaged and the results analyzed statistically.

RESULTS

Differences in clonal reaction to spittlebug feeding became evident 2 to 3 days after infestation, when chlorotic stippling and streaking appeared on the leaves of the more susceptible clones. Ratings were made 7 to 8 days after infestation, when obviously susceptible clones were almost completely brown and contrast in clonal reaction appeared to be maximal. Variability of symptomatic expressions at this time ranged from severely injured clones to those showing only few leaves with stippled or streaked areas.

Of the 398 clones screened for spittlebug resistance, approximately 5% (19 clones) had mean ratings of 3.0 or less (Table 1); 47% (189 clones) rated from 3.1-6.0; and the remaining 48% (190) had ratings between 6.1-9.0. The three classes were arbitrarily designated as highly tolerant, intermediate, and susceptible, respectively. All highly tolerant clones had some injury when rated; and subsequent routine observation indicated that all could eventually be browned-off by continued insect feeding. Coastal bermudagrass had a mean rating of 5.34 ± 0.18 for n = 35 observations (C.V. = 19.6%).

The 12 *Cynodon* clones, individually caged and infested with spittlebugs, differed significantly at each of four rating periods in the amount of phytotoxic injury sustained (Table 2). As in the initial tests, injury symptoms appeared on the more susceptible clones about 24 hours after infestation, whereas symptom expression on more tolerant clones was delayed until the 3rd or 4th day.

At the 1st and 2nd ratings, 5 and 7 days, respectively, after initial infestation, the relative resistance ratings of the clones agree rather well with those obtained in the nonreplicated screening tests. At the last two rating intervals all clones showed severe injury, although differences were still detectable. The amount of phytotoxic injury sustained by the clones increased with each successive rating interval except in two instances. Clones 620 and 33 had slightly lower ratings at the 2nd and 3rd rating respectively than they had at the 1st and 2nd intervals. These small differences undoubtedly reflect the inherent degree of error associated with judged visual ratings by individuals in tests of this nature.

DISCUSSION

The results of our screening experiments leave little doubt but that *Cynodon* genotypes differ signifi-

129

cantly in reaction to feeding by the two-lined spittlebug.

The rapid expression of injury symptoms on some
clones, and an equally rapid, subsequent increase in
severity of injury on these clones, suggest either pref-
erential feeding by the insects or a low level of plant
tolerance for the insect toxin. Results from the nonpreference experiment with 12 selected *Cynodon* clones
strongly indicates that plant tolerance of the insect
toxin is responsible for resistance in the clones studied.
Although all the *Cynodon* clones tested can be severely
injured by spitlebugs, some clones are apparently able
to withstand significantly greater amounts of the toxin

Table 1. **Cynodon Accessions with High Tolerance to Phyto-
toxin of the Two-Lined Spittlebug, *Prosapia bicincta* (Say).**

Clone	P.I. number	Species*	Origin	Rating†
363	206553	C. dactylon var dactylon*	Greece	2.2
14	224128	C. dactylon	S. Africa	2.8
343	224151	C. transvaalensis	S. Africa	3.0
33	225594	C. dactylon	Tanganyika	2.8
379	255447	C. dactylon	Kenya	3.0
137	289915	C. dactylon var dactylon*	S. Africa	2.5
279	289930	C. dactylon var dactylon*	S. Africa	2.3
239	289931	C. transvaalensis	S. Africa	1.7
139	290660	C. dactylon var dactylon*	S. Africa	2.3
142	290663	C. dactylon var elegans*	S. Africa	1.5
143	290868	C. dactylon var dactylon*	S. Africa	1.1
242	290875	C. dactylon*	S. Africa	1.5
287	290879	C. dactylon var dactylon*	S. Africa	2.2
253	290887	C. dactylon var dactylon*	S. Africa	1.5
265	290905	C. transvaalensis	S. Africa	3.0
150	291583	C. dactylon var dactylon*	Rhodesia	3.0
396	292233	C. dactylon var dactylon*	Ghana	2.7
355	292253	C. dactylon var dactylon*	Philippines	3.0
190	294465	C. dactylon	Taiwan	2.2

* Jack R. Harlan, Professor of Plant Genetics, University of Illinois, Urbana, and
associates are presently working on taxonomic revision of the genus Cynodon. Through
personal correspondence they very graciously supplied the species and variety names
of the accessions indicated by an asterisk. Those accessions not followed by an asterisk carry the name listed by the New Crops Research Branch, ARS, USDA. † Ratings
were from 1 to 9 (9 = maximum damage).

Table 2. **Reaction of 12 Cynodon Clones to Spittlebug Phyto-
toxin at 4 Periods Following Initial Insect Infestation.**

Clone	P.I. no.	Rating, days after initial infestation*				Mean rating
		5	7	11	14	
142	290663	1.50	2.35	5.42	6.92	4.05
143	290868	1.75	2.78	5.92	7.25	4.43
14	224128	2.00	3.50	4.83	6.50	4.21
137	289915	2.50	4.35	8.25	8.67	5.94
150	291583	2.75	3.28	6.84	7.75	5.16
586	224152	3.25	3.88	4.67	5.25	4.26
Coastal	---	4.00	4.03	5.67	6.92	5.16
Coastcross 1	---	4.75	4.98	6.75	7.00	5.87
33	225594	4.75	5.23	4.67	6.00	5.16
620	316417	4.75	4.33	6.17	7.08	5.58
590	315902	5.25	5.78	7.25	7.92	6.55
366	223249	6.50	7.28	8.33	9.00	7.90
Mean rating		3.65	4.31	6.27	7.19	
5% LSD		1.48	1.70	1.88	1.36	

* Ratings were from 1 to 9 (9 = maximum damage). Infestations of 15, 20 and 25 adult
spittlebugs per grass clone were made on 9/12/68, 9/17/68 and 9/19/68, respectively.

than can others. The cultivar, Coastal, which can be browned-off by spittlebugs is, however, appreciably more tolerant than many of the *Cynodon* accessions. Our observations indicate that very large spittlebug populations are required to cause extensive damage to fields of Coastal, however these populations do occur naturally.

Additional investigation is needed to clearly characterize the nature and extent of spittlebug resistance in the genus *Cynodon*, but the significant genotypic variations found in these investigations provides the essential factor necessary for genetically increasing resistance by breeding.

LITERATURE CITED

1. Beck, E. W. 1963. Observations on the biology and cultural-insecticidal control of *Prosapia bicincta*, a spittlebug on Coastal bermuda. J. Econ. Entomol. 56:747-752.
2. Byers, R. A. 1965. Biology and control of a spittlebug, *Prosapia bicincta* (Say), on Coastal bermudagrass. Univ. of Ga. Agr. Exp. Sta. Tech. Bull. N.S. 42, 26 p.
3. ————, and Homer D. Wells. 1966. Phytotoxemia of Coastal bermudagrass caused by the two-lined spittlebug, *Prosapia bicincta* (Homoptera:Cercopidae). Ann. Entomol. Soc. of Amer. 59:1067-1071.
4. Painter, R. H. 1951. Insect resistance in crop plants. The MacMillian Co., New York. 520 p.
5. ————. 1960. Possibilities and methods of breeding for resistance to insects in forage crops. Proc., 8th Intl. Grassl. Cong., p. 81-83.
6. Taliaferro, C. M., R. A. Byers, and G. W. Burton. 1967. Effects of spittlebug injury on root production and sod reserves of Coastal bermudagrass. Agron. J. 50:530-532.

Curly Top Viruliferous and Nonviruliferous Leafhopper Feeding Effects upon Tomato Seedlings

Donald E. Gardner and Orson S. Cannon

A high degree of resistance to curly top disease exists in the wild tomato variety *Lycopersicon peruvianum* var. *dentatum* Dun. (1). Resistance, however, may vary depending upon such variables as virulence of the virus strain used for inoculation, numbers of viruliferous leafhoppers to which plants are exposed, and age of plants at the time of feeding (2, 4, 5, H. L. Blood, *unpublished data*).

In our studies of curly top, an additional factor associated with breakdown of resistance in *L. peruvianum* var. *dentatum* has been observed. This is the apparent toxic effect of leafhopper feeding upon the plants. Carter (3) listed general chloroses, veinbanding, chlorotic streaking, and wilting among known symptoms of insect-caused systemic phytotoxemias. Several genera of leafhoppers were noted as incitants of such effects. Carter stated that such feeding effects of virus vectors are sometimes easily separated from symptoms of the disease itself on the basis of different effects that each would have produced separately, but in many cases this separation is difficult. In addition, much difficulty is encountered in extraction of such toxins and in the reproduction of toxin-induced symptoms experimentally. Randall (5) reported that a number of tomato varieties exhibited leafhopper feeding injury that could not be separated from curly top symptoms.

This study was undertaken to further evaluate the early feeding effects of viruliferous and nonviruliferous leafhoppers on seedlings of *L. peruvianum* var. *dentatum* and *L. esculentum* Mill.

MATERIALS AND METHODS.—*Inoculation.—* Seeds of *L. peruvianum* var. *dentatum* and curly top-susceptible *L. esculentum* (unnamed breeding line VF7) were germinated in sand. Two to 3 days after emergence, seedlings were transplanted to soil or sand in flats, or were placed between sheets of moist absorbent paper and clamped between two small boards. With the latter arrangement, the pairs of

PHYTOPATHOLOGY, 1972, Vol. 62, pp. 183-186.

boards, with seedlings between, were placed in shallow pans containing a weak aqueous fertilizer solution. This provided a continuous source of moisture and nutrients to the roots. A similar solution was also used to water seedlings transplanted to sand.

The transplanted seedlings were placed in an inoculation cage comprised of cheesecloth and polyethylene plastic. A 500-w incandescent light in the cage top provided supplementary illumination. Five to seven leafhoppers/plant (depending upon the particular test) carrying a virulent isolate of the virus were introduced into the cage, and were allowed to feed for specific lengths of time. Depending upon the treatment, inoculation was begun 4 to 9 days after transplanting to determine the relationship of plant age to leafhopper-feeding effects.

Identical inoculation procedures were followed using nonviruliferous insects which were placed into a separate cage containing seedlings. Control treatments were established under the same environmental conditions without leafhoppers.

External and anatomical studies.—Seedlings to be examined were carefully removed from the growth medium at specific intervals, usually 12 hr, beginning with feeding initiation. They were observed with a dissecting microscope. The seedlings grown between boards were examined in a similar manner. In the latter case, the entire set of seedlings was removed from the inoculation cage at 12-hr intervals, the roots and stems were observed, and the seedlings were returned to the cage for further leafhopper exposure.

Stem and root sections for microscopic examination were prepared by killing and fixing these parts in Formalin-alcohol-acetic acid solution. These were dehydrated in a tertiary butyl alcohol series; passed through paraffin oil; and infiltrated with, and embedded in, paraffin. Longitudinal sections 10 μ thick were cut with a rotary microtome. Sections were mounted on microscope slides, deparaffinized, and stained with safranin-fast green (6).

RESULTS.—Viruliferous and nonviruliferous leafhopper feeding caused rapid wilting and subsequent death of seedlings of *L. peruvianum* var. *dentatum* and *L. esculentum* exposed 4 days after transplanting. Commonly recognized curly top symptoms, including vein clearing and leaf yellowing, did not occur in the plants that died rapidly. The viruliferous and nonviruliferous treatments produced qualitatively indistinguishable wilting symptoms. However, wilting became evident consistently sooner among seedlings of the viruliferous leafhopper

133

TABLE 1. Effects of plant age and viruliferous and nonviruliferous leafhopper feeding (six leafhoppers/plant) on seedlings of *Lycopersicon peruvianum* var. *dentatum*

Leafhopper type	6 Days after feeding initiation				12 Days after feeding initiation			
	Total plants	No. wilted	% Wilted		Total plants	No. dead	% Dead	
Feeding initiated 4 days after transplanting								
Viruliferous	70	43	61		70	51	73	
Nonviruliferous	70	18	26		70	22	31	
Feeding initiated 9 days after transplanting								
Viruliferous	68	15	22		68	32	47	
Nonviruliferous	70	1	1.4		70	2	2.8	

treatment, and considerably greater numbers of plants were affected than with the nonviruliferous leafhopper treatment (Table 1).

Feeding effects upon seedlings of *L. peruvianum* var. *dentatum* were equal to or more severe than those exhibited by *L. esculentum* seedlings. Both tomato types, however, were definitely affected by each leafhopper treatment. With the viruliferous leafhopper treatment, wilting became evident in each plant type within 24 hr of feeding initiation, and occasionally within 12 hr. In no case did wilting begin as soon or affect as many seedlings in the nonviruliferous as in the viruliferous leafhopper treatment. The majority of seedlings that had not wilted and died 7 days after exposure to viruliferous leafhoppers exhibited definite stunting and dulling of color in contrast to surviving nonviruliferous-exposed seedlings. The stunted *L. peruvianum* var. *dentatum* seedlings not dead within 7 days after leafhopper feeding often recovered and assumed normal growth, whereas seedlings of *L. esculentum* so affected always eventually died. Any stunting resulting from nonviruliferous feeding was usually overcome by seedlings of both plant types. No wilting or other abnormalities were noted in control seedlings.

A substantial reduction in rapid wilting was exhibited by *L. peruvianum* var. *dentatum* seedlings exposed to leafhoppers 9 days after transplanting as compared with those exposed 4 days after transplanting (Table 1). Although the older seedlings surviving viruliferous leafhopper attack sometimes exhibited stunting, this effect was overcome soon after feeding ceased. A comparable increase in resistance to rapid wilting was also exhibited by older *L. esculentum* seedlings, although those seedlings exposed to viruliferous leafhoppers eventually developed typical curly top symptoms and succumbed to the disease.

Macroscopic and anatomical examination.—Inhibition of branch root initiation and growth, and stunting of primary root growth, occurred in seedlings of both leafhopper treatments. This effect became readily evident in seedlings collected 60 hr after start of feeding, and it was more severe in seedlings of each plant type exposed to viruliferous leafhoppers (Fig. 1). Examination under the dissecting microscope revealed that developing secondary root tips and primary root tips turned brown. In contrast, the root tips of control seedlings were white. No abnormalities were observed in stems of plants of either leafhopper-exposed treatment.

Microscopic examination of longitudinal root tip sections from leafhopper-damaged seedlings revealed

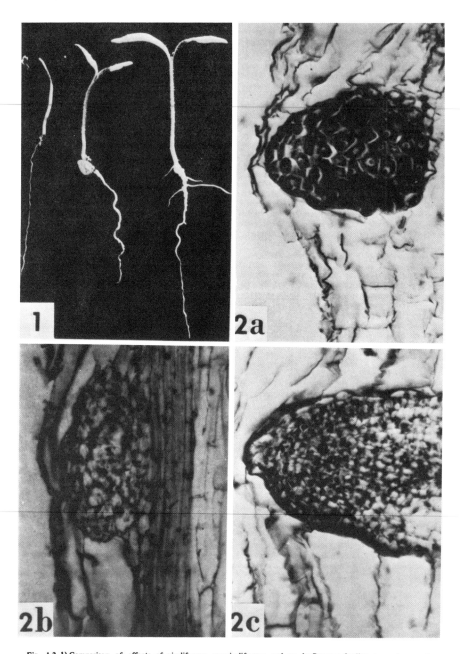

Fig. 1-2. 1) Comparison of effects of viruliferous, nonviruliferous, and no leafhopper feeding upon *Lycopersicon esculentum* seedlings 60 hr after initiation of leafhopper feeding. (Left) Exposed to viruliferous leafhoppers, exhibiting severe wilting and tissue collapse. (Center) Exposed to nonviruliferous leafhoppers, exhibiting stunting and inhibition of branch root initiation. (Right) Healthy control (not exposed to leafhoppers), exhibiting normal growth and branch root development. 2) Comparison of effects of viruliferous, nonviruliferous, and no leafhopper feeding upon nonemerged secondary root tips of *L. esculentum* seedlings 60 hr after initiation of feeding by leafhoppers. a) Healthy control (not exposed to leafhoppers); consisting of normal, functional cells. b) Nonviruliferous; consisting of dead, degenerate cells. c) Viruliferous; consisting of dead, degenerate cells.

cell disorganization and collapse with accompanying cytoplasm degeneration. These abnormalities often involved the entire meristematic region, and possibly extended into the region of maturation. Although a great deal of deterioration was evident, neither hypertrophy nor hyperplasia appeared characteristic of this condition. Secondary root tips which had not yet emerged from primary root cortical tissue at the time of collection exhibited similar effects. In the latter case, the degeneration of embryonic root cells did not extend to immediately adjacent pericyclic and vascular tissues of the primary roots. These effects appeared qualitatively similar in root tips of both viruliferous and nonviruliferous treated seedlings. In contrast, both emerged root tips of control seedlings were comprised of organized, nucleated cells which were obviously functional at the time of collection (Fig. 2).

Some degree of cortical tissue collapse was also evident. This condition appeared more severe in viruliferous-exposed than in nonviruliferous-exposed seedlings. This abnormality occurred mainly in mature regions of primary roots, and may have disrupted vascular tissue, although primary effects were not observed in vascular tissue itself. The cortical collapse appeared distinct from the effects upon root tip cells. Stem tissue appeared normal in plants of all treatments.

DISCUSSION.—A degree of limitation was inherent in these tests, because it was not possible to exclusively observe the effects of the virus upon seedlings as it was to observe the effects of leafhopper feeding alone. Therefore, it was not possible to definitely determine whether the curly top virus itself was capable of causing symptoms similar to those of leafhopper feeding. The absence of qualitatively distinct symptoms between seedlings exposed to feeding by viruliferous and nonviruliferous leafhoppers indicates that subsequent wilting may have been caused primarily by leafhopper feeding. The virus definitely contributed to the severity of feeding symptoms quantitatively, however. Rapid death of young root tips, inability to absorb moisture, and arrested root development were assumed to be the major cause of the observed seedling wilting and death. The occasional collapse of cortical tissue and possible resulting disruption of vascular tissue also may have contributed secondarily to wilting.

The leafhopper-feeding effect upon developing root tips did not appear to result from general removal of photosynthates from the shoots, although this conceivably may have been the origin of cortical

137

collapse in mature roots. A specific leafhopper-secreted toxin is therefore implicated as the cause of sudden death of root tip cells. If the virus alone is not capable of causing wilting, establishment of viral infection in plant tissue may have predisposed the seedlings to a more severe reaction to leafhopper feeding. An alternative possibility would involve the stimulation of increased toxin production by viruliferous leafhoppers as compared with nonviruliferous leafhoppers. This explanation may better account for the short interval (within 12 hr) between the start of feeding and wilting.

The older seedlings apparently acquired considerable resistance to such a phytotoxemia, possibly a result of dilution of the secretion by the larger amount of plant tissue. The distinction between resistance to leafhopper feeding and to curly top itself became discernible in older inoculated plants. As many *L. peruvianum* var. *dentatum* seedlings as *L. esculentum* seedlings wilted and died shortly after exposure to feeding by viruliferous and nonviruliferous leafhoppers. This number was substantially lower, however, among both plant types as compared with that of younger seedlings. Whereas *L. peruvianum* var. *dentatum* seedlings surviving viruliferous leafhopper feeding became stunted but were often able to resume normal growth, *L. esculentum* seedlings that survived the feeding effects later developed typical curly top disease symptoms and died.

Further work using isolation procedures is necessary to definitely establish the presence and nature of the proposed leafhopper-secreted toxin.

LITERATURE CITED

1. BLOOD, H. L. 1942. Curly top, the most serious menace to tomato production in Utah. Utah Farm and Home Science 3:8-11.
2. CANNON, O. S. 1960. Curly top in tomatoes. Utah Agr. Exp. Sta. Tech. Bull. 424. 12 p.
3. CARTER, W. 1962. Insects in relation to plant disease. John Wiley & Sons, Inc., N.Y. 705 p.
4. PRICHARD, D. W. 1969. Comparative response of some tomato and sugar beet varieties to curly top virus infection. M.S. Thesis, Utah State Univ., Logan. 66 p.
5. RANDALL, T. E. 1966. The utility of the reactions of selected host plants to known isolates of the curly-top virus in developing a different approach to breeding problems in tomatoes. Washington Agr. Exp. Sta. Tech. Bull. 49. 18 p.
6. SASS, J. E. 1958. Botanical microtechnique. [3rd ed.] The Iowa State Univ. Press, Ames, Iowa. 228 p.

PSYLLID YELLOWS OF THE POTATO[1]

By B. L. Richards, *Botanist and Plant Pathologist, Utah Agricultural Experiment Station;* and H. L. Blood, *Plant Pathologist, Utah Agricultural Experiment Station, and Agent, Division of Horticultural Crops and Diseases, Bureau of Plant Industry, United States Department of Agriculture* [2]

INTRODUCTION

In August, 1927, Richards, Blood, and Linford [3] reported for the first time what appeared to be a new disease of the potato. Although it resembled current-year symptoms of witches' broom, as described by Hungerford and Dana (8),[4] subsequent studies clearly differentiated between the two disorders. In December, 1927, Richards (14) ascribed this new disease to the feeding process of the tomato psyllid (*Paratrioza cockerelli* Sule). He further reported the disease, as it appeared in Utah, as new to science and proposed the name "yellows."[5]

Subsequent statements have been made concerning the occurrence and the destructive nature of the disease by Linford,[6] Richards (15),[7] Metzger and Binkley,[8] and Binkley (1). Binkley (1) reported the disease, as it appears in the tomato, to be due to a definite virus transmitted by the psyllid nymphs. To the writers' knowledge no further report as to the nature of the disease and its relation to the tomato psyllid has appeared. It is the purpose of this paper to bring together the facts known to date regarding psyllid yellows and to report some additional experimental findings regarding the nature and cause of the trouble. The information regarding the disease is recognized definitely as being incomplete.

OCCURRENCE OF PSYLLID YELLOWS

Psyllid yellows has scarcely a parallel in the history of phytopathology in the uniformity and rate with which it spread. The disease was first noticed by the junior author on June 12, 1927, in experimental plots at Farmington, Utah. In a preliminary survey on June 15

[1] Contribution from Department of Botany and Plant Pathology, Utah Agricultural Experiment Station.
[2] The writers wish to express appreciation for the helpful cooperation of Kathleen L. Hull, formerly of the station staff, and of William Stuart and Melvin Anderson, research students in the Department of Botany and Plant Pathology.
[3] Richards, B. L., Blood, H. L., and Linford, M. B. DESTRUCTIVE OUTBREAK OF UNKNOWN POTATO DISEASES IN UTAH. U. S. Dept. Agr., Bur. Plant Indus. Plant Disease Rptr. 11:93-94. 1927. [Mimeographed.]
[4] Reference is made by number (italic) to Literature Cited, p. 216.
[5] Since the early proposal of "yellows," the name "psyllid yellows" has been employed generally by the authors and their coworkers in both correspondence and in general discussions and by the senior author in recent publications (14, 15). Binkley in 1930 also used the term "psyllid yellows" to designate the disease on tomatoes (1, *Proc. 26, pp. 249-254*). The name "psyllid yellows" seems justifiable as it is both specific and descriptive.
[6] Linford, M. B. FURTHER OBSERVATIONS ON UNKNOWN POTATO DISEASE IN UTAH. U. S. Dept. Agr., Bur. Plant Indus. Plant Disease Rptr. 11:110-111. 1927. [Mimeographed.]
——— PLANT DISEASES IN UTAH IN 1927. U. S. Dept. Agr. Bur. Plant Indus. Plant Disease Rptr. Sup. 59:95-99. 1928. [Mimeographed.]
[7] Richards, B. L. PSYLLID YELLOWS (CAUSE UNDETERMINED). U. S. Dept. Agr., Bur. Plant Indus. Plant Disease Rptr. Sup. 68:28-29. 1929. [Mimeographed.]
[8] Metzger, C. H., and Binkley, A. M. PSYLLID YELLOWS (CAUSE UNDETERMINED). U. S. Dept. Agr., Bur. Plant Indus. Plant Disease Rptr. 68:29. 1929. [Mimeographed.]

JOURNAL OF AGRICULTURAL RESEARCH, 1933, Vol. 46, pp. 189-216.

and 16, the disease was found generally distributed in early potato fields of the Bountiful district of Davis County. Most of the fields at this early date showed 100 per cent infection, and not a single field was found which did not show the trouble to some degree. By June 29, at which time Linford commenced a more detailed survey of the disease, the early potatoes in Davis and Weber Counties were generally infested. Before the survey was concluded on September 15, Linford reported that the "disease had been found in every county of Utah where potatoes had been examined, ranging from Washington County on the south to Cache County on the north"

Table 1, copied from Linford's report,[9] shows the occurrence of the disease in 23 counties visited. No reports were obtained from the other six counties.

TABLE 1.—*Occurrence of psyllid yellows in Utah, by counties, 1927* [a]

County	Fields examined	Fields infested		Heaviest infestation	Average infestation
	Number	Number	Per cent	Per cent	Per cent
Cache	16	9	56.2	100	53.1
Carbon	16	15	100	100	61.1
Beaver	5	5	100		84
Boxelder	5	5	100	100	53.2
Davis	32	32	100	100	56.6
Duchesne	5	5	100	100	91
Emery [b]					
Garfield	4	4	100	100	61.2
Grand	1	1	100	100	100
Iron	21	21	100	100	83.8
Juab	1	1	100	10	10
Kane	4	4	100	100	70
Millard	17	9	52.9	97	24.2
Morgan [c]					
Piute	11	11	100	100	38.2
Salt Lake	24	13	54.2	100	21.7
Sanpete	12	12	100	100	95.8
Sevier	10	10	100	100	80.8
Uinta	6	6	100	100	68
Utah	9	9	100	100	44
Weber	11	11	100	100	74.9
Wasatch [d]					
Washington [e]					

[a] The figures in this table include data from many fields examined before the disease had reached its maximum spread. From the following publication: LINFORD, M. B. Op. cit., p. 98.
[b] Disease said to be present throughout.
[c] Disease reported prevalent late in season.
[d] Disease present.
[e] Crop a total failure from this disease.

Early in 1927 the malady was reported from the western slope of Colorado and was severe especially in the Fruita district of Mesa County, where 100 per cent infection occurred. According to Metzger and Binkley,[10] the ailment was found also in the Gunnison Valley in Delta County, in the Uncompahgre district in Montrose County, and in the Rifle district of Garfield County.

On August 1, the senior author located psyllid yellows in southern Idaho, 3.5 miles north of Pocatello. Two weeks later M. B. McKay reported the disease by letter from Idaho Falls and Twin Falls, Idaho, and from Bozeman, Mont., and H. G. McMillan in personal conference reported it from Wyoming. L. F. Nuffer by correspondence later in the summer reported a general spread of the disease in the

[9] LINFORD, M. B. Op. cit. See footnote 6, second reference.
[10] METZGER, C. H., and BINKLEY, A. M. Op. cit.

140

Idaho Falls district. Shapovalov[11] has also called attention to its presence in California.

Although the tomato psyllid (*Paratrioza cockerelli*) has been known since 1914 to be generally distributed in the Southwestern States, the writers have been unable to find any mention in literature, prior to 1927, of a disease of the potato caused by the insect; neither has reference been found to a disease of the potato similar to psyllid yellows. Comperé (*2, p. 189*), in 1915, states: "In Golden Gate Park, San Francisco, the solanums that were infested with psyllid were rendered worthless." He makes no further reference to the disease phase.

It appears evident from a number of authentic reports that the disease occurred previous to 1927. In 1929 Metzger and Binkley[12] stated:

> The disease was destructive in the Fruita district of Mesa County, Colo., in 1926, and by June 18, 33 per cent of the plants were showing symptoms of a disease, evidently psyllid yellows as described by Richards in 1927.

It is quite possible also that the disease was present in the Fruita district prior to 1926. Linford[13] submits data which show rather conclusively that psyllid yellows was a factor in potato production in the Green River district of Utah, at least as far back as 1925. The senior author has obtained information which indicates that psyllids have figured in potato culture in Washington County, Utah, at least since 1921.

ECONOMIC IMPORTANCE OF PSYLLID YELLOWS

Psyllid yellows in its effect upon the plant must be ranked among the most destructive of known potato diseases. If the plant is attacked when young, prior to tuber formation, no crop results, and early death of the plant frequently ensues. When the plant is attacked during early stages of tuber formation and prior to maturation, serious injury follows, and the resulting crop is of little value. If the plant is attacked after the tubers are well formed, the tubers may sprout, giving rise to new vines (fig. 1, A, B, C), or to sprouted, knobbed, or otherwise malformed tubers, of greatly reduced market value. (Fig. 1, B, C.)

Total crop failures from this disease in individual plantings are not uncommon. In 1927 experimental plots at the Davis County Experimental Farm yielded 40 pounds of marketable tubers from an area estimated to produce from 40 to 50 bushels under normal conditions. In Bountiful, Utah, 250 pounds of marketable tubers were obtained from a 1-acre field, and many of the most successful growers in this same district lost their entire crop, leaving their fields unharvested.

During this same year the disease was so severe that total crop failures resulted in entire valleys. Linford states that in Washington County the entire crop was destroyed. This county was surveyed late in August, long after potatoes are normally harvested, but there was no harvest in 1927, so complete was the destruction.

[11] Shapovalov, M. psyllid yellows (cause undetermined). U. S. Dept. Agr., Bur. Plant Indus. Plant Disease Rptr. Sup. 68: 29–30. 1929. [Mimeographed.].
[12] Metzger, C. H., and Binkley, A. M. Op. cit.
[13] Linford, M. B. Op. cit. See footnote 6, second reference.

Duchesne and Uintah Counties had approximately 50 per cent of a crop at the time the survey was made.

Davis and Weber County growers, who produce early potatoes chiefly, suffered the heaviest financial losses. Based on the acreage planted, it was estimated that 740 cars would have been shipped from Weber County; 110 cars were actually shipped, thus involving a loss of approximately 630 cars. Valued at $420 a car, this amounts to $264,600. Sixty-four cars of seed were shipped into the county at an average of 4.5 cents a pound, making a total outlay of $92,000,

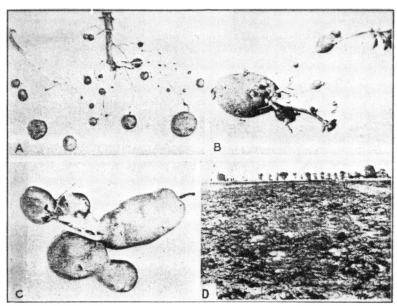

FIGURE 1.—A, Bliss Triumph affected with psyllids showing excess tuberization. One stolon has failed to terminate in tubers and has given rise to new shoots. Several shoots of this type may arise around a single infected mother plant. Note large number of secondary stolons terminating in tubers of various sizes. B, Sprouting of immature Russet Burbank tuber induced by psyllid feeding on parent plant. Practically all buds, both on the mother and the secondary tubers, have become active and have given rise either to new shoots or to a third crop of tubers. C, Sprouting of Russet Burbank tuber characteristic of this variety when parent plant is affected by psyllid nymph late in the season. Such sprouts may develop directly into tubers or may grow through the soil and give rise to second growth in the late-potato districts as in 1927. D, Five-acre field of large, vigorous, and apparently healthy Bliss Triumphs photographed October 4, 1927. These plants grew from small tubers left in the soil during the harvest of the early crop. The first crop was planted April 15 and yielded but 20 sacks per acre; on August 10 it showed 100 per cent psyllid yellows. With the exception of about 15, all plants of this 5-acre field were healthy and apparently free from psyllid yellows at the date the photograph was taken. Psyllid nymphs were present on the 15 plants showing symptons. Seed selected from this late crop gave progeny which were entirely free from any psyllid-yellows symptoms

or $46,000 more than the total value of potatoes actually shipped out. While exact figures are not available, observational data indicate that Davis County suffered even more acutely than Weber County owing to more complete destruction of the crop and to the higher early market prices of potatoes. These two counties lost fully 75 per cent of their crop.

The season of 1927 was especially favorable for potato production in Utah. An average annual acre yield of 185 bushels or more might have been expected, whereas only 135 bushels were realized, entailing a loss of from 25 to 30 per cent of the crop, or approximately

$750,000. The early crop in the State was practically a total failure. The late crop was less severely damaged although greatly reduced in market value. In certain areas little, if any, decrease in yield resulted, while in others isolated fields were seriously damaged. The malformation of the tubers of the late-maturing varieties, the Russet Burbank and the Rural, was of serious consequence. Linford estimated that from certain Russet Burbank fields in Cache Valley not more than 25 per cent of the tubers would pass as United States No. 1, and a local buyer reported that he was unable to find a single car of suitable Russet Burbank potatoes in the entire county.

Metzger and Binkley [14] state that in the Fruita district of Mesa County, Colo., which ships annually about 600 carloads, but 2 carloads were shipped as a result of the heavy infestation in 1927.

Losses from psyllid yellows in Utah during 1928 were greatly reduced as compared with those in 1927. Richards and his coworkers reported for 1928 that while the potato psyllid was almost coextensive with potato culture in the State, the damage was light as compared with the losses in the same areas in 1927, and that the total loss for 1928 would probably not exceed 7 per cent.

Damage to the potato crop during the year varied greatly in the different districts within the State. In Washington County, as in 1927, the destruction was again complete, and the entire crop planted between February 15 and March 10 was plowed under by June 10, except for two experimental plots. Davis and Weber Counties suffered losses between 10 and 12 per cent during the season. In a survey of the Hunter and Pleasant Green districts of Salt Lake County made during August, 1928, 72 per cent of the fields showed psyllid yellows. An average of 9.5 per cent of plants in all the fields visited showed the malady.

The disease occurred in other potato-growing areas, although there exists but little data to indicate the degree of loss. In Cache County the early garden crop was largely destroyed, and material damage was done in many of the late plantings. Sanpete and Sevier Counties were reported to have suffered severely.

Metzger and Binkley [14] report that psyllid yellows was not so serious in 1928 as in either of the previous seasons and that possibly 10 per cent of the acreage was infested so severely that it was plowed under and planted to other crops. The remaining acreage showed a degree of infestation varying from 0 to approximately 10 per cent.

Psyllid yellows was found in a number of areas in Utah in 1929; however, serious loss, so far as is known, was confined almost entirely to Washington County where upwards of 75 per cent of the crop was destroyed.

Psyllid yellows appeared generally throughout Utah in 1930. Reports of damage were obtained from every potato district in the State, although the damage in most areas was relatively light as compared with that of 1927. Washington County, as was the case for the last six years, again lost the major portion of its potato crop, and Utah, Davis, Weber, and Boxelder Counties sustained heavy losses to the early crop. It is significant that the early crop in these four counties, which comprises 85 per cent of the plantings, has been

---

[14] Metzger, C. H., and Binkley, A. M. Op. cit.

143

seriously reduced in yield for three of the seasons since 1927. Psyllid yellows was reported from the Twin Falls and the Idaho Falls districts in Idaho.

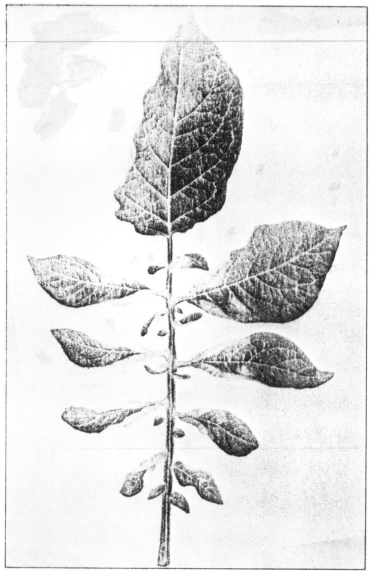

FIGURE 2.—Irish Cobbler potato leaf showing characteristic leaf symptoms of psyllid yellows. Notice the basal rolling and cupping of leaflets. These are accompanied by a characteristic yellowing and purpling, which is a typical expression of the disease on all varieties of potatoes. (Results of insect feeding under natural conditions in field)

During May and early June, 1931, psyllids appeared in great numbers in all early potato-growing areas in Utah, producing psyllid yellows in such quantities as to indicate possibilities of a general

144

epidemic. With the extreme heat and drought of middle and late June, however, the insects disappeared, and recovery from the disease was general. But little damage to either the early or late crop resulted. Psyllid yellows was reported severe, however, throughout the western slope of Colorado.

SYMPTOMS OF PSYLLID YELLOWS

SYMPTOMS UNDER CONDITIONS ACCOMPANIED BY SUMMER-LIGHT RELATIONS

Psyllid yellows is systemic and affects the form and physiology of the entire plant. A marginal yellowing and an upward rolling or cupping of the basal portion of the smaller leaflets on the younger leaves comprise the first symptoms of diagnostic value in the field.

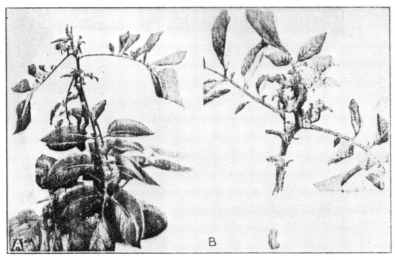

FIGURE 3.—A, Psyllid yellows on Irish Cobbler potato showing characteristic symptoms of the disease induced by the feeding of 200 nymphs from eggs hatched in Petri dishes: nymphs had not fed on diseased plants before transfer to the plant. Note the typical leaf cupping and particularly the peculiar upright and rigid position of young leaflets, also apical hypertrophy and axillary growth. B, Apical hypertrophy of Irish Cobbler shoot induced by confining nymphs to older leaves by means of cloth bags. Note extreme cupping of leaflets and yellowing of cupped portions

(Figs. 2 and 3, A, B.) When diseased plants are exposed to intense sunlight, this basal cupping becomes pronounced. Leaflets affected in this manner tend to curve upward over the petiole and to assume an erect position quite distinct from the normal. (Fig. 3, A.) In the Bliss Triumph and the Irish Cobbler, and to a certain extent in all varieties, the rolled portions, and frequently other aerial portions of the plant, assume a distinct reddish or purplish color which may become so pronounced in cases of severe infection as to give a purplish tint to the entire field. In the more advanced stages of the disease the older primary leaves roll upward over the midrib, become yellow, develop necrotic areas, and degenerate rapidly (fig. 4, B), and as a result a plant is produced which consists principally of secondary leaves and branches supported by the primary stems.

Promptly on the inception of the disease, the aerial shoots usually suffer a sharp delimitation in stem elongation. The nodes enlarge, and the lateral buds are stimulated into activity and may develop

145

into axillary tubers (fig. 3, A, B, 5) or into stocky shoots capped with a rosette of small malformed leaves, which when fully developed give the plant a compact pyramidal shape, scarcely to be recognized as that of a potato plant. (Fig. 5, A, B.) With the enlargement of the nodes and subsequent growth of the axillary buds, the subtending leaves assume a position approximately at right angles to the stem instead of the acute angle characteristic of a normal plant. (Fig. 4, D.) The apical portion of the stems, including the terminal bud

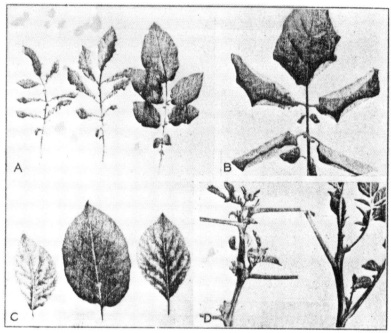

FIGURE 4.—A, Rolling and cupping of young leaflets of Russet Burbank potato very characteristic of the advanced stage of the psyllid yellows on this variety (left and center); normal leaf to the right. B, Effect of psyllid yellows on leaves which were mature at the time of the psyllid infestation. The leaves are somewhat papery and brittle in texture. Under field conditions necrosis sets in rapidly, and death soon results. This is characteristic of all varieties when affected by psyllids. C, Leaf chlorosis characteristic of psyllid yellows when affected plants are grown in the shade or during the short days of late autumn and winter. Affected leaves at left and right show distinct interveinal yellowing, also a distinct change in shape owing to an inhibition of the growth of the basal portion of leaflets, due apparently to the early destruction of chlorophyll in this region. Normal leaf in center. D, Irish Cobbler shoots showing modification of angle of leaf axis, also nodal enlargement characteristic of psyllid yellows. Left, diseased shoot (natural infection); right, healthy shoot

and frequently the first nodes and adjacent internodes, often become involved in a pronounced hypertrophy. (Fig. 3, A, B.)

If plants are attacked when young, stolon formation and tuberization are definitely suppressed, with the result that few, if any, tubers are set. When older plants are affected, the result is quite the reverse, and stolon development and tuberization are stimulated. The terminal buds of the stimulated stolons may fail to produce tubers and instead may grow directly through the soil, giving rise to a second crop of shoots adjacent to the mother plant. (Fig. 1, A.) The lateral buds along the primary stolon may develop directly into tubers (fig. 1, A), or they may give rise to secondary stolon branches which

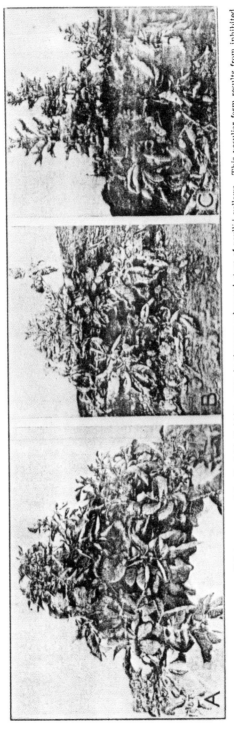

FIGURE 5.—A, Characteristic pyramidal shape assumed by the Irish Cobbler potato in the more advanced stage of psyllid yellows. This peculiar form results from inhibited linear growth and concomitant extension of the lateral secondary shoots that arise from the axis of the old primary leaves. B, Advanced stage of psyllid yellows on the Irish Cobbler. A few primary leaves in advanced stage of deterioration are shown still attached to the primary stem. The apical portion of the plant is shown to consist essentially of secondary leaves and shoots grown from the axis of the primary leaves which have died. In the more advanced stage of the disease, the plants consist primarily of secondary leaves and shoots attached to the primary stem. C, Effect of psyllid yellows on the Early Ohio potato. Primary shoots elongate rapidly, resulting in small, badly curled leaves and axillary growth which is much distorted and usually of yellowish and reddish color. Note position and peculiar curling of the older leaves matured prior to psyllid infestation. This abnormal elongation is peculiar to the Early Ohio variety

in turn may provide opportunity for tuber formation, thereby resulting in development of numerous small potatoes. (Fig. 1, A, B, D.) Such tubers seldom reach a marketable size and may sprout directly without going into a rest period. (Fig. 1, B, C.) Such sprouting may give rise to new stolons, to leafy and apparently normal shoots, or to a variety of malformed tubers. (Fig. 1, B, C.) Discarded tubers from early harvest often produce a second crop of healthy vigorous vines. (Fig. 1, D.)

Plants affected after tubers have entered the early stages of dormancy may resume growth and produce stolons and many small tubers. The more mature tubers, if still attached to the parent plant when it is attacked, may also commence growth and develop into tubers of undesirable shape and low market value. (Fig. 1, C.) This breaking of the rest period in tubers after dormancy has been established and the inhibition of its establishment in developing tubers provides one of the constant and outstanding features of psyllid yellows.

SYMPTOMS UNDER CONDITIONS OF REDUCED LIGHT INTENSITY

The types, vigor, and sequence of symptomatological expression vary so greatly under both the intensity and the duration of light that symptoms characteristic of the open field are of little value in judging results under protected conditions in the greenhouse or under conditions of relatively dense shade. This fact was first suggested from observations made during the winter of 1927. Subsequent study, however, has provided a basic symptomatology for the study of psyllid yellows under shaded conditions and during the late fall, winter, and early spring months, and under cloth cages during the summer months. In fact, this symptomatology appears quite as reliable as that under natural conditions in the field and has been used as a criterion of judgment for all work conducted under cloth or under winter greenhouse conditions.

With decreased light intensity and duration, basal cupping and coloration do not occur uniformly. Instead, the basal lobes of the young leaflets turn distinctly yellow and are inhibited in growth, giving rise to linear leaflets quite distinct from those of the normal leaf. (Figs. 3, A; 4, C.) Yellowing finally appears in the interveinal portions of the affected leaflet, giving a general leaf chlorosis, seldom seen under field conditions. (Fig. 4, C.) A similar type of interveinal yellowing develops progressively from the younger to the older leaves, advancing slowly in later stages and showing a typical interveinal chlorosis in the most advanced stages of the trouble. The necrotic areas characteristic of the late stages of leaf deterioration in the open field have not as yet been observed under the more protected conditions. On the whole, the rate at which the plant succumbs to the disease under conditions of reduced light intensity and duration is much slower than that found in the open field; diseased plants under such conditions may survive quite as long as and sometimes longer than the healthy individuals.

The degree and type of bud activity both below and above the ground appear to be affected but little with varying light conditions.

148

RELATION OF THE PSYLLID TO THE DISEASE

During the early survey studies in June, 1927, Linford[15] first noted a small scalelike insect on plants showing symptoms of psyllid yellows. Subsequent studies showed a high correlation between the occurrence of the insect, which was later determined to be *Paratrioza cockerelli* by the Bureau of Entomology (fig. 6, A, B), and the characteristic symptoms of the disease. Survey studies throughout 19 counties in Utah showed this parallelism to be complete. Even in the most remote and isolated fields the disease and the insect were found constantly associated. In August, 1927, M. B. McKay, in a personal letter, reported the disease from Montana and southern Idaho, and in all cases the disease was associated with the insect. A

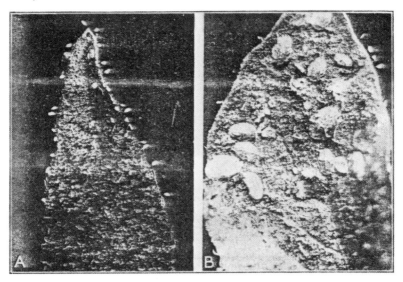

FIGURE 6.—A. Eggs of *Paratrioza cockerelli* Sulc on young potato leaflet. ✕ 9. B, Nymphs of *P. cockerelli* feeding on young potato leaflet. Note eggs on leaf margin and scattered irregularly over the surface of the leaf. ✕ 9

similar report was obtained from H. G. McMillan for Wyoming and Colorado. Such observations indicated rather clearly that the tomato psyllid was definitely concerned in the etiology of the disease.

On July 15, psyllids were taken from Davis County and placed on 50 plants in the pathological garden at Logan and covered with gauze insect cages. All plants developed the disease. Later, however, the disease spread throughout the ⅛-acre experimental plot, finally involving 100 per cent of the exposed plants. Forty plants in this plot, however, had been grown under insect cages and were kept covered until October 15, and 39 of the 40 remained entirely free from the disease. During the season a triangular rent was made in one of the cages, through which parts of the covered plant protruded. This plant became infested with insects and developed a clear case of psyllid yellows.

---

[15] LINFORD, M. B. Op. cit. (See footnote 6, first reference.)

Five experiments to test the etiological relation of *Paratrioza cockerelli* were made during September and October, 1927. On September 5, 40 psyllids were confined on each of three plants grown in the greenhouse under celluloid cages. Similarly, caged plants free from insects were held as controls. By September 9, one of the plants with insects had developed definite basal leaf rolling, a second plant had developed symptoms by September 18, and a third by October 2.

On September 9, 30 nymphs were transferred to each of 8 plants grown under celluloid cages. Three plants covered with cages but free from the insects were used as controls. By September 28, all plants on which the insects fed had developed advanced stages of the psyllid yellows disease. The controls remained normal.

On September 20, 30 nymphs were placed on each of 3 plants under celluloid cages; 2 plants were kept for controls. By September 30, 10 days later, 2 of the plants had exhibited marginal yellowing and basal rolling, and the third had developed the disease by October 10. The 2 control plants remained disease-free until discarded on November 1. Another series was started September 21 in which 30 insects were transferred to each of 7 plants. Four plants were held as controls. By October 10, the 7 insect-infested plants had developed clear-cut symptoms of the disease. The controls at this date were free from symptoms and insects. Later 1 of the check plants was found infested with nymphs and subsequently developed the disease.

In the fifth series plants were started in the greenhouse without cages. These plants were grown in 8 inches of soil on the greenhouse bench. All plants were in a vigorous growing condition on September 23, at which time the transfer of insects was made. Twenty plants distributed uniformly throughout the bed were employed and nymphs were carefully placed on 1, 2, or 3 leaves of each of the plants. The nymphs were confined to the leaves with gauze bags in such a way as to maintain complete isolation of other parts of the inoculated plant and of the control plants. Thirty insects were used to each plant; 51 plants were left as controls. Of the 20 to which insects were transferred, 3 showed marginal yellowing and basal leaf rolling within nine days. On October 10, 15 plants exhibited basal rolling as well as the characteristic yellowing and reddening. By November 1, when the experiment was terminated the plants had developed the disease and exhibited the various symptoms characterizing psyllid yellows in the field. The 51 controls remained disease-free. Nineteen diseased and nineteen healthy hills were selected and the tubers dug and weighed to determine the effect of the disease on tuberization. The data are summarized in Table 2.

TABLE 2.—*Effect of psyllid feeding on tuberization of Irish Cobbler potatoes in preliminary experiments*

Condition of plant	Hills	Tubers	Average tubers per hill	Average total weight per hill	Average weight per tuber
	Number	*Number*	*Number*	*Grams*	*Grams*
Diseased	19	317	16.6	75.5	4.5
Healthy	19	79	4.2	92.5	22.0

150

In these preliminary tests all phases of the disease as found in the field were produced under controlled experimental conditions, following an incubation period of six to nine days. The results justify the conclusion that the disease in some way is induced during the feeding process of nymphs of *Paratrioza cockerelli*.

RELATION OF NYMPHAL FEEDING TO THE DISEASE

Relation of the Number of Nymphs to Symptom Expression

In the preliminary tests typical symptoms of psyllid yellows were produced consistently with as few as 30 active nymphs. In late autumn what were considered characteristic symptoms of the disease failed to develop in the greenhouse on plants carrying as many as 60 to 75 nymphs. The following March, however, the progeny of these insects which had failed in the winter to induce psyllid yellows again consistently induced the disease. At first the cause for this apparent lack of potency on the part of the insect was not clear. In the course of the experiments, however, it became apparent that both the intensity and the duration of sunlight in some way either influenced the insect in its feeding or determined the type of symptom expression.

During 1928 and 1929 attempts were made to determine more accurately the quantitative relation between nymphal feeding and the disease. On August 11, three series of experiments were started in the field under gauze cages, using 10, 15, and 30 nymphs per plant. The time of feeding varied from 3 to 15 days, after which time the insects were killed by fumigation. The results are given in Table 3. All plants on which psyllids fed showed the early symptoms within 9 to 15 days after the insects commenced feeding. A study of the subsequent development of the disease on these plants was rendered valueless because of the general psyllid infestation of the field.

TABLE 3.—*Relation between number of psyllid nymphs and the length of feeding period and the first symptoms of psyllid yellows under cages in open field*

[Period of feeding, 3 to 15 days, commenced August 11, 1928]

Series No.	Plants	Nymphs per plant	Length of feeding period	Plants diseased	Series No.	Plants	Nymphs per plant	Length of feeding period	Plants diseased
	Number	Number	Days	Number		Number	Number	Days	Number
1	4	30	3	4	3	2	10	5	2
	4	30	3	4		2	10	7	2
	4	30	7	4		4	10	10	4
	4	30	10	4		2	10	15	2
	4	30	15	4					
2	4	15	5	4					
	4	15	10	4					

Between April 22 and July 25, 1929, four separate series of tests were completed, using from 1 to 9 nymphs per plant. In these tests nymphs failed to produce psyllid yellows, although comparable numbers during the past three years have occasionally been noted to induce the disease.

151

Additional data were obtained in four sets of experiments conducted under greenhouse conditions between March 19 and June 25, 1929. The numbers and the distribution of the nymphs, together with a summary of results, are given in Table 4.

TABLE 4.—*Summary of four series of experiments, showing relation between numbers and distribution of psyllid nymphs and the symptom expression of psyllid yellows on the Irish Cobbler potato*

[Feeding period, March 19 to April 12, 1929; data taken 41 days after insect transfer, 12 plants used in each experiment]

Distribution of nymphs	Psyllids per plant	Plants diseased	Plants remaining healthy	Distribution of nymphs	Psyllids per plant	Plants diseased	Plants remaining healthy
Nymphs placed on one leaf	300	11	1	Nymphs distributed equally on three leaves—Continued.	30	4	8
	150	11	1		15	0	12
	75	7	5		6	1	11
	30	3	9	Nymphs distributed equally on six leaves	300	12	0
	15	3	9		150	12	0
	6	0	12		75	10	2
Nymphs distributed equally on three leaves	300	12	0		30	7	5
	150	10	2		15	1	11
	75	9	3		6	0	12

Results of all the various experiments indicate that under greenhouse conditions and during the shorter days of late fall or early spring the number of nymphs feeding, and possibly the distribution of the insect on the plant, are vital factors in the production of psyllid-yellows symptoms. Much additional work under controlled environmental conditions must be done to determine more accurately this quantitative relation of nymphs to the occurrence of the disease.

RELATION OF NYMPHAL FEEDING PERIOD TO THE PRODUCTION OF EARLY SYMPTOMS OF THE DISEASE

Experiments were started on March 6, 1930, to determine the shortest period of insect feeding necessary to produce psyllid yellows. In the experiment, 200 nymphs (100 on each of two leaves) were confined on each of 20 healthy plants. Insects were removed at intervals as follows: Plants 1–5, after 2 days; plants 6–10, after 3 days; plants 11–15, after 4 days. Insects on plants 16–20 were allowed to feed for the entire period of 36 days. Ten plants, Nos. 21–30, were kept free from insects and remained free from the disease throughout the entire experiment. This experiment was repeated with essentially the same results. The results are recorded in Table 5.

Results indicate that at least three days' feeding is necessary to produce the first definite symptoms of psyllid yellows. Four days' feeding gave a more vigorous expression of the early symptoms and resulted in a more permanent effect, although with a 4-day period the disease did not progress far beyond the early manifestation.

This failure of symptoms to appear as a result of fewer than three days' feeding was not occasioned by any peculiar masking effect of the environment, as the early appearance of the disease resulted when the same number of insects fed for longer periods, and a complete expression of symptoms was produced by nymphs feeding continuously for a period of 36 days.

TABLE 5.—*Relation between short periods of nymph feeding and the production of early or first symptoms of psyllid yellows in the Irish cobbler potato*

[Feeding time 2, 3, 4, and 36 days; 200 insects used on each plant]

Plant No.	Feeding period	Condition of plant at removal of nymphs	Condition of plant 10 days after feeding commenced	Condition of plant 36 days after the beginning of nymph feeding
	Days			
1	2	No symptoms.	Normal	Large plant apparently normal.
2	2	do	do	Very slight marginal yellowing, otherwise normal.
3	2	do	do	Do.
4	2	do	Mere trace of marginal yellowing.	Slight basal yellowing and restriction, otherwise normal.
5	2	do	Normal	Slight basal yellowing, otherwise normal.
6	3	do	Slight interveinal yellowing.	Basal, marginal, and interveinal yellowing distinct early symptoms.
7	3	do	Normal	Normal except slight yellowing of young leaves.
8	3	do	Slight trace of yellowing on young leaflets.	Slight yellowing of 3 leaves, otherwise normal.
9	3	do	Normal	Young leaflets yellow and some interveinal yellowing could be considered type of early symptoms.
10	3	do	Slight marginal yellowing.	Distinct basal yellowing on a number of younger leaves.
11	4	do	Normal	Do.
12, 13, 14	4	Symptoms	Early symptoms of disease; basal, marginal, and interveinal yellowing.	Distinct basal, marginal, and interveinal yellowing on younger and older leaves, showing that feeding had some effect on subsequent growth.
15	4	do	Marginal, basal, and interveinal yellowing.	
16, 17, 18, 19, 20	36	do	Marginal, basal, and interveinal yellowing; all symptoms exhibited.	Full expression of symptoms of disease above and below ground.
20-30	0	Healthy	Healthy	Healthy, with occasional plants showing slight yellowing of younger leaflets.

RELATION OF NYMPHAL FEEDING PERIOD TO THE SEQUENCE AND DEGREE OF SYMPTOM EXPRESSION

During the earlier greenhouse and field studies instances were observed frequently which indicated the existence of a definite relation between the length of the feeding period and the final degree of disease expression. In many cases, especially under greenhouse conditions, apparent recovery was noted, and in general the accumulated evidence suggested that continued feeding of nymphs was necessary to produce the full expression of psyllid yellows.

On February 23, 1930, two series of experiments were started to determine more accurately the relation of the feeding period to the early appearance and to the continued development of symptoms of psyllid yellows. Twenty plants, exclusive of controls, were used in each of the two series. In series 1, 200 nymphs (100 on each of two leaves) were confined by means of gauze bags to each of 20 healthy plants. The insects were then removed from the plant by clipping off the infested leaf as follows: Plants 6–10, after 12 days' feeding; plants 11–15, after 16 days, and plants 16–20, after 26 days' feeding. Plants 1–5, inclusive, were fed upon for 48 days.

Series 2 was set up in the same manner as series 1. Plants 1–5, inclusive, were fed upon for a period of 50 days, or during the entire time the experiments were run. Insects were removed as follows:

Plants 6–15, after 9 days; plants 16–20, after 14 days. Eight insect-free plants were used as controls for series 1 and nine plants for series 2. All plants in both series were grown openly in the greenhouse bench in 8 inches of soil. A summarized statement of series 1 and 2 is recorded in Table 6. (Fig. 7, A, 1–5.)

TABLE 6.—*Summary of results of experimental series 1 and 2 in which 200 psyllid nymphs were fed on Irish Cobbler potato plants for various periods longer than the incubation period*

[See text for details and also Figure 6A, 1–5

SERIES 1

Length of feeding	Plants involved	Average height	Average number of leaves per plant	Average length of leaves	Average tubers per hill	Average weight of tubers per hill	Average weight per tuber	General expression of symptoms at the end of the experiments, which lasted 50 days
Days	*Number*	*Inches*	*Number*	*Inches*	*Number*	*Ounces*	*Grams*	
0	5	16.0	10.3	10.3	4.5	6.7	42.2	Normal.
12	5	15.2	11.6	11	8.8	5.8	18.7	Some apparently normal; others slightly yellowed; some axillary growth.
16	5	14.2	13	9.9	8.8	4.05	13.0	Distinct interveinal yellowing; abundant axillary growth.
26	5	13.1	12	9.9	11.4	4.02	10.4	Clearly diseased; yellowing of younger and older leaves.
50	5	11.3	12	8.7	14.0	1.6	3.2	Severe disease of all plants; yellowing, reddening, and cupping of apical leaves; apical and axillary hypertrophy.

SERIES 2

Length of feeding	Plants involved	Average height	Average number of leaves per plant	Average length of leaves	Average tubers per hill	Average weight of tubers per hill	Average weight per tuber	General expression of symptoms at the end of the experiments, which lasted 50 days
0	8	14.3	....	9.8	4.8	5.6	23.1	Normal.
9	10	13.7	....	9.08	9.0	5.4	17.0	Some apparently normal; others slightly yellowed; some axillary growth.
14	5	13.3	....	8.3	8.4	4.6	15.5	Distinct interveinal yellowing; abundant axillary growth.
50	5	12.8	....	9.5	13.4	2.3	4.8	Severe disease of all plants; yellowing, reddening, and cupping of apical leaves; apical and axillary hypertrophy.

Most of the infested plants in the two series showed slight marginal and interveinal yellowing by the sixth day. All plants showed unmistakable symptoms at the end of the tenth day. Many plants exhibited marked rolling and cupping of the smaller and younger leaflets. Basal, marginal, and interveinal yellowing was pronounced on all plants from which insects were removed on the twelfth day in series 1 and by the ninth day in series 2. A number of these plants also showed basal leaf cupping and reddening of younger leaves. More advanced symptoms, such as leaf rolling, pronounced interveinal yellowing, slight nodal enlargements, and beginning axillary growth, were evident at the end of the sixteenth and twenty-sixth days.

In all cases, on the removal of the insects, the progress of development of the symptoms appeared to cease rather abruptly. All red and purple coloring that had developed during the feeding period on affected leaves completely disappeared. Leaf rolling or cupping ceased, and the rolled leaves uniformly unrolled and assumed normal

154

position and shape. A definite tendency toward recovery was noted also in both marginal and interveinal yellowing. Where but slight yellowing occurred prior to insect removal, recovery was apparently complete; however, when the yellowing was well advanced, the

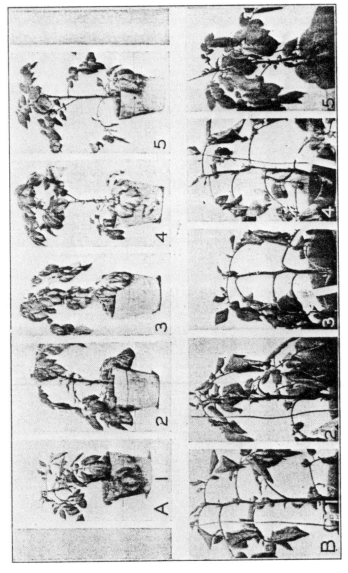

FIGURE 7.—A, Irish Cobbler potatoes on which psyllid nymphs have fed for varying periods. For data see page 200 and Tables 10 and 11. The feeding periods were as follows: Plant No. 1, 50 days; plant No. 2, 26 days; plant No. 3, 16 days; plant No. 4, 12 days; plant No. 5, no feeding (control). B, Psyllid yellows induced in Irish Cobbler plants by nymphs from eggs hatched in Petri dishes on normal potato leaves. Plants Nos. 1, 2, and 3 are representative of separate series on which nymphs from different broods, kept free from all diseased plants, fed. Plant No. 4, injured by nymphs from diseased potato plants. Plant No. 5, control, kept free from all sources of infection

normal green color was seldom regained. Plants fed upon for fewer than 16 days assumed practically normal linear growth and in many cases equaled the unaffected plants. Subsequently, axillary and apical growth was of a normal green color and of apparently normal texture. Certain physiological processes, however, were so disturbed during the feeding that the plants did not completely recover from the effects of the disease. This is clearly shown in the relative height of plants (fig. 7, A), number of tubers per hill, average weight of tubers per hill, and average weight per tuber. (Table 6.) In all cases, a greater number of tubers with a decreased total hill yield and decrease in tuber weight resulted with increased length of feeding. All symptoms characteristic of the disease developed prominently in plants on which the insects were fed for the total 50 days. (Fig. 7 A, 1.)

Results indicate clearly that the symptom complex characteristic of psyllid yellows is entirely contingent upon the feeding process of nymphs of *Paratrioza cockerelli* and further that a complete expression of symptoms in their characteristic sequence and intensity, under greenhouse conditions, is entirely dependent on the continued feeding of the nymphs.

RELATION OF ADULT FEEDING TO THE DISEASE

Studies with nymphs have given no clue as to the exact effect of adult feeding on symptom expression. Two sets of experiments were set up July 16, 1929, in which adult psyllids were allowed to feed for a period of 28 days on healthy Irish Cobbler plants in the open field. In the first series, 50 adults were fed on each of 10 plants. These were confined in groups of 10 on each of 5 different leaves of the plant, by means of small spring cages. In the second series, 75 insects were fed on each of 10 plants, 15 in each spring cage on each of the 5 separate leaves. Five of the insect-infested plants of each series were then placed under insect-proof cages and kept covered for the entire time of the experiment. The other five plants of each series were left uncovered and exposed to the natural weather conditions in the field. Cages with insects were shifted to new feeding areas on the leaf every third day and the eggs laid during the period destroyed. All insects lost through death or escape were promptly replaced by additional insects from the insectary. No indication of the disease developed from adult feeding either during or subsequent to the 28-day period.

Five additional series of experiments were started on August 22 in the greenhouse to determine whether adults in numbers greater than those used in the earlier field studies could induce yellows. In these experiments the insects were confined to the plants in large celluloid cages under which the plants had been grown, thus allowing feeding over the entire plant surface. To insure against nymph feeding, the adults were removed at intervals of four days and all eggs destroyed. In this process, adults were removed from the cages by suction guns and placed in small vials. The eggs were then crushed and the original number of insects replaced. All adults used in the experiment were obtained from diseased plants in the insectary.

In series 1, 100 adults were placed on each of 10 plants on August 22 and allowed to feed until September 16, a total of 25 days. At the end of the feeding period, none of the plants showed symptoms of psyllid yellows. Eggs laid during the last 4-day period of insect feeding, September 12 to 16, were allowed to hatch on 6 of the 10 plants used in the experiment. All 6 of these plants showed typical symptoms within 9 to 12 days after the hatching of the eggs. The other 4 plants, kept free from nymphs, did not develop psyllid yellows after the removal of the adults.

156

Series 2 was a duplication of series 1 except that 150 instead of 100 adults were used. Eight of the ten plants remained free from symptoms for 28 days, at which time the experiment was terminated. Two plants showed unmistakable symptoms of disease. When examined, however, both diseased plants were found to carry a number of psyllid nymphs, hatched from eggs which were overlooked in the experiment. All adults were removed from the 10 plants at the end of 28 days. As in series 1, the eggs laid during the last 4 days of the experiment were allowed to hatch on 6 plants, all of which developed psyllid yellows within 8 to 12 days after the nymphs commenced feeding.

Series 3, 4, and 5 differed from 1 and 2 only in the number of adults used. In series 3, 200 adults were allowed to feed on each of 5 plants; in series 4 and 5, 500 and 1,000 adult insects, respectively, were placed on each of 3 plants. After 28 days' feeding, none of the 11 plants in the three series showed the slightest symptom of disease. Plants fed upon by these larger numbers, however, were evidently stunted in growth, and when the numerous nymphs from eggs laid during the last four days of the experiment were allowed to feed, 7 of the plants were killed.

The five experiments on adult feeding were carefully checked, (1) by placing 50 nymphs on 10 healthy plants and allowing them to feed during the 28 days, all of them developing psyllid yellows, and (2) by placing 7 plants under cages not exposed to insect feeding but treated as if eggs were being crushed at the same period as eggs were crushed in the experiments. Except for apparent stunting and occasional leaf mutilation, these latter plants showed no indication of treatment. A final check was provided by growing 10 plants under cages free from insects and untouched. The check plants remained free from disease during the 28 days of the experiment and grew somewhat larger than did those exposed to insects.

Results of the five series on adult feeding are given in Table 7.

TABLE 7.—*Results of five series of experiments in which various numbers of adult psyllids were fed for 25 days on healthy Irish Cobbler potato plants*

Experiment No.	Insects used per plant	Stage of insect	Plants used	Diseased plants	Healthy plants
1	100	Adult	10	0	10
2	150	do	10	[a] 2	8
3	200	do	5	0	5
4	500	do	3	0	3
5	1,000	do	3	0	3
Control	60	Nymph	20	20	0

[a] As explained in the text, these 2 plants showing unmistakable symptoms were found to have a number of nymphs feeding on them.

RELATION OF NYMPHS TO INFECTIVE PRINCIPLE

The failure of adult psyllids to induce the disease at once raises the question as to the origin or source of the substance injected by nymphs which produces the pathological symptoms characteristic of psyllid yellows in the potato. An attempt was made to separate the nymphs from this substance by removing eggs from the leaves of potato plants to healthy disease-free leaves in Petri dishes where they were allowed to hatch. The resulting nymphs were then transferred to healthy plants on which they were allowed to develop into adults and finally to lay eggs. From these eggs three separate broods of nymphs (A, B, and C) were obtained and were placed on healthy potato plants in the greenhouse. Two hundred nymphs were placed on each plant used in the experiment. Two plants were used for insects from brood A, 3 for brood B, 4 for brood C. Nymphs were allowed to feed for 27 days. Eight plants were held free from insects as controls, and additional plants were inoculated, each with 200 nymphs from diseased potato plants. All nine plants fed on by the nymphs from broods A, B, and C developed uniformly symptoms entirely characteristic of psyllid yellows and in a more severe form than that produced by nymphs from diseased potato plants. The results are recorded in Table 8.

TABLE 8.—*Results from the feeding of psyllid nymphs which were obtained from eggs hatched in Petri dishes on disease-free potato leaves*

[Feeding period, 27 days, March 25 to April 22, 1929]

Source of insects	Plants employed	Insects per plant	Diseased plants	Healthy plants	Incubation period	Degree of severity of disease
	Number	Number	Number	Number	Days	
Brood A	2	200	2	0	6	Severe expression.
Brood B	3	200	3	0	6	Do.
Brood C	4	200	4	0	6–8	Do.
From diseased plants	8	200	8	0	6–8	Mild to severe; only 2 plants equalled in severity the plants fed upon by insects, broods A, B, and C.
Insect-free (control)	8	0	0	8		

TRANSMISSION STUDIES

During 1928 and 1929 various standard methods used for the artificial transfer of virus diseases were employed in attempts to transmit psyllid yellows from diseased to healthy potato and tomato plants. Large numbers of plants in different stages of development were used as sources of inoculum and for inoculation. All these attempts gave negative results. Binkley (*1, r. 26*) also reports negative results in his attempts to transmit artificially the disease in the tomato. In preliminary experiments grafting has also proved ineffective as a means of transmission. To date, the nymph of *Paratrioza cockerelli* appears to be the only known means by which psyllid yellows can be transmitted from diseased to healthy plants, if such transfer actually takes place, or by which the disease is induced directly into healthy plants. Further work is now in progress to test all known methods of artificial transmission.

Observational and experimental evidence further indicates that psyllid yellows is not transmitted through the tuber from diseased parents to the progeny under field or greenhouse conditions in Utah. Young plants from attached tubers produced by diseased plants or from tubers detached from the mother plants show no symptoms of the disease; however, both may develop the disease with equal readiness when fed upon by psyllid nymphs. It is also quite possible that young attached shoots may in time develop the disease through the mother plant, when the latter is fed upon continually by nymphs, although this relation has not been clearly established. In the field shown in Figure 1, D, only 18 plants were found to exhibit distinct psyllid symptoms on October 4, 1927, when the photograph was taken. Nymphs were found actively feeding on all of these. Three bushels of tubers selected from this same crop and planted in 1928 produced vigorous plants entirely free from any signs of the disease.

Because of the vigor of the plants, the owner selected seed from this same stock for his 1929 planting. Although in 1928 the plants were infested with the psyllids later in the season, the plants in 1929 again appeared entirely free from the disease and remained so throughout the season. Other observations similar to the foregoing were made during 1927 to 1930, inclusive, and plantings made for the purpose of determining this relation gave similar results. In 1929, 15 fields of second-crop potatoes from discarded infested tubers were observed to show no symptoms of psyllid yellows until fed upon by psyllid nymphs later in the season. Under no observed conditions have plants, grown from tubers produced by infected parents and kept free from insects, shown symptoms of psyllid yellows either in the greenhouse or in the field.

EPIDEMIOLOGY OF PSYLLID YELLOWS

GENERAL NATURE

The sudden appearance of psyllid yellows in 1927 provides an interesting problem for analysis. According to data already presented, the disease appeared rather suddenly in the early crop throughout Utah, the western slope of Colorado, southern Idaho, and local areas in Montana and Wyoming. This apparently sudden and extensive distribution was no less startling than the degree of uniformity with which the disease occurred. In Utah few, if any, fields in the infected areas escaped the disease, and in certain localities, particularly those growing early potatoes, infection was so complete that scarcely an unaffected plant could be found. Isolated fields in canyons many miles removed from the main valley centers of potato culture became infected before the end of the season. A similar situation existed throughout the western slope of Colorado where the disease almost completely destroyed the potato crop in many districts.

FACTORS INVOLVED

The sudden appearance and widespread and uniform distribution of psyllid yellows in 1927 are explainable only by the presence of some prolific and rapidly disseminated etiological factor, such as is found in the tomato psyllid. The distribution of *Paratrioza cockerelli* prior to 1927, the nature of the insect, that is, its natural means of dissemination, rate of development, longevity and degree of fecundity, insect parasitology, and the number and distribution of host plants are, therefore, vital factors. The various environmental factors, such as temperature, humidity, and air movement enter into the problem chiefly as a result of their influence on the fecundity and dissemination of the insect.

159

The suddenness with which psyllid yellows occurred and the novelty of the disease in the infested areas during 1927 suggests an early migration of *Paratrioza cockerelli* from a few local areas in which the insect normally survived into the various parts of Utah, Idaho, Montana, Wyoming, and parts of Colorado. On the other hand, it is quite possible that the insect had previously occupied these infected areas but had occurred in such small numbers as to entirely escape notice, especially as an etiological factor; thus, with a disturbance of some peculiar balance, the involvement of the entire region of the 1927 epidemic was made possible.

Survey studies subsequent to 1927 have established the fact that *Paratrioza cockerelli* had been present and responsible for psyllid yellows during 1925 and 1926 in the Green River and Washington County districts in Utah and in certain districts in Colorado. It is conceivable that the insect might have spread from these various areas throughout the range occupied in 1927. The more general distributions of the insect reported by Crawford (4) in 1914 appears to furnish the more plausible explanation for the 1927 epidemic of the disease. This writer gives the distribution of the species of *Paratrioza cockerelli* as covering the entire southwestern part of the United States and reports the specific localities in which the insect has been found as follows: Boulder, Rocky Ford, and Canon City, Colo.; Milford and Park City, Utah; Tucson and Fort Yuma, Ariz.; Madagascar Mountains, N. Mex.; Claremont, El Centro, San Luis Obispo, Argus Mountains, Alameda, and Death Valley, Calif. The occurrence in Milford and Park City, Utah, is especially interesting, and the further fact that the Utah station entomologists have observed *Paratrioza cockerelli* in the infested areas in previous years suggests the distinct possibility that the insect might have been more generally distributed than had been supposed. The ability of the insect to overwinter in those areas to which it spread in 1927 and its early appearance in Davis County, Utah, apparently bear out this possibility.

NATURE OF THE INSECT

Crawford (3, 4), Ferris (7), and Lehman (10) describe *Paratrioza cockerelli* as a small homopterous insect of the family Cheridae with a small, active clear-winged adult stage, varying in size from 1.3 to 1.8 mm in length and from 0.39 to 1 mm in width. This small adult is extremely active; when disturbed, it springs quickly into the air by means of its powerful hind legs. The springing habit of the insect, assisted by flight and by the wind, undoubtedly functions effectively in the distribution of the species and consequently in the spread of the disease at least within relatively localized areas. The insect is so minute that when once in the air it might readily be transported considerable distances by the air currents. It is conceivable that the combination of these factors may result in the transportation of the insect over long distances.

Observations as to the longevity of the adult vary. Compere (2) noted that *Paratrioza cockerelli* adults lived for three months in captivity. Knowlton and Janes (9) gave 64 days as the longest life period for an adult male and 189 days for an adult female, with an average life of 25.22 days for males and 34.4 days for females. The writers found the life of the female to vary from a few hours to 60 days, with an average longevity under greenhouse conditions of 45 days. The long life of the insect may result in overlapping of broods, which fact, coupled with a long oviposition period, aids greatly in increasing the number of affected individuals.

Compere (2) observed that egg laying commenced three days after copulation, although he did not state the length of the preoviposition period. Knowlton and Janes (9) reported a preoviposition period varying from 5 to 25 days, with an average of 10.1 days from emergence of adult female until the first eggs were produced. Similar results to those of Knowlton were obtained by the writers. It will be noted from Table 9 that the preoviposition period for the 10 females varied from 4 to 20 days, with an average of 9.7 days between emergence and the production of the first eggs. Compere (2) stated that three adults in captivity laid eggs for a period of 3 days. Knowlton and Janes (9), on the other hand, gave a much longer period of egg laying, varying from a few days to a maximum of 179 days. They found the average oviposition period of 58 females to be 21.45 days. For 10 insects observed under greenhouse conditions, the writers found the oviposition period to vary from 20 to 53 days, with an average of 35.2 days. (Table 9.)

TABLE 9.—*Egg-laying history of 10 adult females of Paratrioza cockerelli (Sulc) under greenhouse conditions*

[One pair of adults was confined to leaves of potatoes by means of spring cages; at the end of each 24 hours the cages with insects were removed to a new leaf area and eggs laid during the 24 hours counted]

Adult No.	Pre-egg-laying period of adult	Length of egg-laying period	Total eggs laid	Adult No.	Pre-egg-laying period of adult	Length of egg-laying period	Total eggs laid
	Days	Days	Number		Days	Days	Number
1	5	20	430	8	20	35	553
2	6	21	458	9	17	31	497
3	11	33	851	10	5	36	641
4	16	28	504				
5	4	53	1,460	Minimum	4	20	430
6	6	46	979	Maximum	20	53	1,460
7	5	49	829	Average	9.7	35.2	720

In the shortest oviposition period of 20 days, as shown in Table 9, the insect laid 430 eggs, while the female with an oviposition period of 53 days deposited 1,460 eggs. Also, as shown in Table 9, the 10 insects averaged 720 eggs. Knowlton and Janes (9) report a total of 19,833 eggs from 60 females, with an average of 330.55 eggs for each of the 60 females. These writers also record a maximum of 1,352 eggs for a single female, laid during a period of 179 days.

Knowlton and Janes (9, p. 285) record a high percentage hatchability of psyllid eggs. Of 9,615 eggs observed, 7,989, or approximately 83 [16] per cent, hatched, giving rise to living nymphs. The large number of eggs, their hatchability, and the extended period during which the female psyllid may lay eggs undoubtedly plays an important part in the epidemiology of psyllid yellows.

Paratrioza cockerelli passes through an incomplete metamorphosis with the usual stages of adult, egg, and nymph. The time required

---

[16] This should be 83 per cent.

for completion of the life cycle has been variously estimated and has been shown to depend to quite an extent upon the influence of environment on the development of the insect during the various stages of growth. Compere (2) reports that approximately 45 days were evidently required to complete the life cycle under the conditions imposed in his experiments. He further states that the broods "are continuous throughout the year." Lehman (10) gives 25 days as the time necessary for the life cycle of the insect. Knowlton and Janes (9, p. 286), in laboratory studies with a much larger number of insects than observed by Compere, give the time for development of the various instars shown in Table 10.

TABLE 10.—*Time of development of various instars of Paratrioza cockerelli as given by Knowlton and Janes*

Instar	Nymphs observed	Average days required	Instar	Nymphs observed	Average days required
First	252	2.76	Fourth	151	2.72
Second	186	2.44	Fifth	133	4.87
Third	158	2.49			

Knowlton and Janes (9) state that the total time for nymphal development for some 800 nymphs observed varied with conditions from 12 to 21 days, with an average of 16 days. These data correspond essentially with the observations of the present writers. Judging from the data supplied by Knowlton, the life cycle of *Paratrioza cockerelli* from egg laying to adult emergence may be completed within from 25 to 37 days, depending on the conditions to which the insect is exposed. These data are significant in view of the fact that nymphs have been observed under the rather vigorous climate at Logan, Utah, as early as May 4, and in an active state as late as November 2. In view of these data, it appears possible that from three to five broods may develop during a single season. Consequently, the progeny from a single female adult under favorable conditions may number into the millions in a single season. In view of such fecundity and length of life favorable ecological conditions for overwintering and propagation may initiate an epidemic any season.

PARASITOLOGY OF INSECT

Little is known of the parasites of *Paratrioza cockerelli*, although the writers have observed that such do occur and undoubtedly play an important part in the survival of the species. Whether the absence of psyllid parasites played a significant part in the epidemic of 1927 and in the persistence of the insect during 1928–29 and 1930–31, there is no way of determining. However, as the variation in the physical environment appears inadequate to explain the epidemic of 1927, it would seem that the abundance and sudden appearance of the insect during the particular year might be adequately explained by a serious disturbance of the biological balance which ordinarily keeps the insect in check. The parasitology of *Paratrioza cockerelli* remains as a problem for further study.

162

The food plants of *Paratrioza cockerelli* are undoubtedly important in facilitating the distribution of the insect. The degree of influence which these food plants exert, however, is still problematic, although the number of plants on which the insects have been found is significant. Crawford (*4, p. 72*) lists food plants as follows: "Pepper (*Capsicum annum*), tomato (*Solanum nigrum*), potato (*Solanum tuberosum*), * * * spruce (*Picea* sp.) pine (*Pinus monophylla*), alfalfa (*Medicago sativa*). List (*11, 12*) reports psyllids as being abundant on the cultivated tomato in Colorado.

Ferris (*7*) observed adults and nymphs from California on tobacco (*Nicotiana tabacum*), and Compere (*2*) stated that the insects on which he made observation in the Golden Gate district of California were found on the Jerusalem cherry (*Solanum capsicastrum*). Van Duzee (*17*) listed the insects on members of the following genera: Capsicum, Solanum, Purshia, Picea, Pinus, and Medicago. Essig (*5, p. 438*) in 1917 added *Datura* sp. and *Solanum nigrum* to the list of host plants. The writers have found *Paratrioza cockerelli* nymphs and adults feeding abundantly on tomato (*Lycopersicum esculentum*), groundcherry (*Physalis longifolia*), matrimony-vine (*Lycium vulgare*), and on all varieties of the potato (*Solanum tuberosum*) grown in Utah during the past three years. In the greenhouse the nymphs have been found to feed on tobacco.

The common groundcherry appears to be a most favorable host of *Paratrioza cockerelli* in Utah, second possibly only to the potato in importance. In 1927, this plant was universally infested with psyllids throughout the State, and even in isolated areas miles from potato fields it was found to support large numbers of both nymphs and adult psyllids. The general distribution of this Physalis species in Utah undoubtedly facilitated the dissemination of *P. cockerelli* in 1927 and figured as an important factor in the epidemic of psyllid yellows in that year, as well as in the general epidemiology of the disease.

DISCUSSION

Accumulated evidence clearly indicates that *Paratrioza cockerelli* in some definite way is involved in the etiological complex of psyllid yellows. Exactly in what manner the insect produces the disease, however, has not been revealed, although some facts are sufficiently suggestive as to merit definite consideration. The total absence of visible disturbances at the point of insect feeding, together with the systemic nature of psyllid yellows and the few insects necessary to induce the disease, precludes mechanical injury or food extraction as possible elements in disease production. On the other hand, these basic relations considered in connection with other features of the disease suggest more definitely that the disease is produced either by a virus, transferred from plant to plant, or by some toxic substance injected into the plant tissue during the feeding process of *P. cockerelli* nymphs. Facts have been obtained which support both possibilities.

The more critical studies have revealed facts which are difficult to fit into the virus theory. The abrupt cessation of symptom development with the removal of the insect followed by an apparent uniform tendency to recover from the disease, is especially pertinent in this connection. These facts, when taken together with the development of apparently healthy organs from axillary buds and the absence of tuber transmission of the disease, renders acceptance of the virus concept particularly difficult. In this connection it is also necessary to recall that the adult psyllid is incapable of producing psyllid yellows after feeding on diseased plants, and that the infective principle, whatever its nature, is probably inseparable from the psyllid nymphs, which alone are capable of producing the disease. The foregoing, however, must be considered in view of the fact that Shapovalov (*16*) reports tuber transmission of psyllid yellows and that Binkley (*1*) claims to have separated that which he considers as a virus from the nymph and has unhesitatingly designated the disease as of virus origin. On these two points the meager data presented by these workers raise a serious question as to the justification for their conclusion. Whether or not the substance injected into the potato plant by *Paratrioza cockerelli* is a virus remains a question for future research.

To the writers the explanations that appear most plausible, especially in view of a number of the foregoing facts, is that *Paratrioza cockerelli* during its feeding processes injects into the plant tissues some toxic substance which quickly becomes systemic and possibly produces the exaggerated responses characteristic of the disease by its interference in some way with the carbohydrate metabolism of the plant.

It is interesting in this connection to note that Monteith and Hallowell (*13*) report a condition involving the feeding of leaf hoppers on legumes which resemble closely the etiological complex and symptomatological responses involved in psyllid yellows. They suggest that the pathological symptoms involved are probably the result of some "chemical or enzymatic toxin," secreted by the leaf hoppers.

Should the toxin theory of psyllid yellows prove correct, it would appear that this disease, also the whitetop of alfalfa and other legumes, the hopperburn of potatoes, and possibly other diseases, constitute a group of plant maladies that may truly be designated, based on their peculiar etiology, as insect diseases.

SUMMARY

Psyllid yellows as a disease of the potato first came to the attention of plant pathologists in 1927, although there is evidence that the trouble has existed in certain isolated areas in Utah for a number of years prior to this date.

The disease may develop suddenly over a vast area in any one season and is capable of extensive and frequently complete destruction in both the early and the late potato crop.

Studies since 1927 have shown the dangerous nature of psyllid yellows and indicate that in certain districts it is a perennial menace even to the extent of eliminating the potato as a crop. This condition exists particularly in Washington County in southern Utah, and also in the early potato-growing areas of Davis and Weber Counties in the northern part of the State. A similar condition is reported also for the Fruita section in the Grand Junction district of Colorado (western slope).

In survey studies the tomato psyllid (*Paratrioza cockerelli* Sulc) has been found constantly associated with psyllid yellows of the potato, and experiments have shown that the disease is in some way induced during the feeding processes of the nymphs of this insect.

Under conditions especially favorable for symptom expression as few as three to five nymphs might occasionally produce psyllid yellows, although uniformity of appearance and full expression of symptoms seldom result with fewer than 15 to 30 actively feeding nymphs.

The adult form of *Paratrioza cockerelli* in numbers up to 1,000 per potato plant appear incapable of producing psyllid yellows symptoms on the plant in the field or in the greenhouse.

The symptomatology of psyllid yellows varies greatly with the number of insects feeding, the length of feeding period, and the intensity and duration of light exposure during the time of feeding.

Psyllid-yellows symptoms under conditions of unmodified sunlight consist of yellowing, basal leaf rolling and purpling of the younger leaves, yellowing and rolling of older leaves, nodal enlargement, increased axillary angle, aerial tubers and shoots, frequent rosetting, various apical growths, and distortion, excess tuberization, and inhibition of rest period. Under conditions of decreased exposure and intensity of light, basal, marginal, and interveinal yellowing becomes a constant feature of the disease.

Progress in symptomatological expression is stopped abruptly when insects are removed at intervals of 12, 16, and 26 days after feeding has commenced, indicating that the full expression of symptoms of psyllid yellows results only when nymphs of *Paratrioza cockerelli* are allowed to feed continuously on the tissues of the infested plant. A tendency toward recovery results when time of feeding in the greenhouse is less than 16 days. Recovery in the field has also been observed. So far as is known, *P. cockerelli* is the only factor capable of producing psyllid yellows in the potato and in related plants.

Attempts to transmit psyllid yellows from diseased to healthy plants have failed. Under Utah conditions the disease does not appear to be transmitted from diseased plants to the following generation through the tuber.

The size, motility, prolific fecundity, longevity, and long oviposition period of the female are important factors in the rate of dissemination of the insect. These factors, when considered in connection with the apparent general distribution of the insect, provide, in part, at least, an explanation of the sudden widespread epidemic of psyllid yellows in 1927.

In preliminary tests nymphs of *Paratrioza cockerelli* were not separated from the infective principle by hatching eggs on healthy potato leaves in Petri dishes. In fact, nymphs so hatched produce a more vigorous symptom response on healthy Irish Cobblers than psyllid nymphs of the same age grown on infected potato plants.

The true nature of the infective principle injected into potato plants by *Paratrioza cockerelli* at present remains unknown. Available facts, however, question somewhat the virus theory of the disease and suggest the possible existence of some toxic substance which is produced in some way during the feeding process of the psyllid nymphs. Additional facts will be necessary before final conclusions can be drawn as to the true etiology of psyllid yellows.

LITERATURE CITED

(1) BINKLEY, A. M.
   1929–30. TRANSMISSION STUDIES WITH THE NEW PSYLLID-YELLOWS DISEASE OF SOLANACEOUS PLANTS. Science (n. s.) 70:615, 1929. Also Amer. Soc. Hort. Sci. Proc. (1929) 26:249–254, 1930.

(2) COMPERE, H.
   1916. NOTES ON THE TOMATO PSYLLA. Calif. Comn. Hort. Mo. Bul. 5:189–191, illus.

(3) CRAWFORD, D. L.
   1911. AMERICAN PSYLLIDAE. III TRIOZINÆ. Pomona Col. Jour. Ent. 3:[421]–453, illus.

(4) ———
   1914. A MONOGRAPH OF THE JUMPING PLANT-LICE OR PSYLLIDAE OF THE NEW WORLD. U. S. Natl. Mus. Bul. 85, 186 p., illus.

(5) ESSIG, E. O.
   1917. THE TOMATO AND LAUREL PSYLLIDS. Jour. Econ. Ent. 10:433–444, illus.

(6) ———
   1926. INSECTS OF WESTERN NORTH AMERICA, A MANUAL AND TEXTBOOK FOR STUDENTS IN COLLEGES AND UNIVERSITIES AND A HANDBOOK FOR COUNTY, STATE, AND FEDERAL ENTOMOLOGISTS AND AGRICULTURISTS AS WELL AS FOR FORESTERS, FARMERS, GARDENERS, TRAVELERS, AND LOVERS OF NATURE. 1035 p., illus. New York.

(7) FERRIS, G. F.
   1925. OBSERVATIONS ON THE CHERMIDAE (HEMIPTERA: HOMOPTERA) PART II. Canad. Ent. 57:46–50, illus.

(8) HUNGERFORD, C. W., and DANA, B. F.
   1924. WITCHES' BROOM OF POTATOES IN THE NORTHWEST. Phytopathology 14:[372]–383, illus.

(9) KNOWLTON, G. F., and JANES, M. J.
   1931. STUDIES ON THE BIOLOGY OF PARATRIOZA COCKERELLI SULC. Ann. Ent. Soc. Amer. 24:283–290, illus.

(10) LEHMAN, R. S.
   1930. OBSERVATIONS ON THE LIFE HISTORY OF THE TOMATO PSYLLID (PARATRIOZA COCKERELLI SULC.) (HOMOPTERA). Jour. N. Y. Ent. Soc. 38:307–312.

(11) LIST, G. M.
   1918. TESTS OF INSECTICIDES. Colo. State Ent. Circ. 26:36–45.

(12) ———
   1925. THE TOMATO PSYLLID, PARATRIOZA COCKERELLI SULC. Colo. State Ent. Circ. 45:16.

(13) MONTEITH, J., JR., and HOLLOWELL, E. A.
   1929. PATHOLOGICAL SYMPTOMS OF LEGUMES CAUSED BY THE POTATO LEAF HOPPER. Jour. Agr. Research 38:649–677, illus.

(14) RICHARDS, B. L.
   1927–28. A NEW AND DESTRUCTIVE DISEASE OF THE POTATO IN UTAH AND ITS RELATION TO THE POTATO PSYLLA. Potato Assoc. Amer. Proc. 14:94, 1927. Also (Abstract) Phytopathology 18:140–141, 1928.

(15) ———
   1931. FURTHER STUDIES WITH PSYLLID YELLOWS OF THE POTATO. (Abstract) Phytopathology 21:103.

(16) SHAPOVALOV, M.
   1929. TUBER TRANSMISSION OF PSYLLID YELLOWS IN CALIFORNIA. (Abstract) Phytopathology 19:1140.

(17) VAN DUZEE, E. P.
   1917. CATALOGUE OF THE HEMIPTERA OF AMERICA NORTH OF MEXICO, EXCEPTING THE APHIDIDAE, COCCIDAE AND ALEURODIDAE. 902 p. Berkeley, Calif. (Calif. Univ. Pubs., Ent. v. 2.)

INTRODUCTION TO SECTION III:
INSECT-BACTERIA RELATIONSHIPS

With only a few exceptions, bacterial plant pathogens are not dependent on insects. In most cases where
insects and bacteria are associated, the relationship is
a general one with each member capable of surviving
entirely without the other. Such a generalized relationship is described in the paper on fire blight transmission by Keitt and Ivanoff (1941) and the paper by
Allen, Pinchard and Riker (1934) on bacterial transmission by the apple maggot.

Sometimes a closer relationship is found whereby
specialized transmission of a bacterial pathogen is
provided by an insect. Leach's paper on cucurbit wilt
and its association with cucumber beetles is presented as
an example of such a relationship.

Rarely, a much more intimate association exists
whereby both the insect and the bacterial pathogen
benefit from the relationship, a type of mutualism.
Petri's classic paper on the intestinal bacteria of the
olive fly (1910) presents such a relationship.

TRANSMISSION OF FIRE BLIGHT BY BEES AND ITS RELATION TO NECTAR CONCENTRATION OF APPLE AND PEAR BLOSSOMS

By G. W. Keitt, *professor of plant pathology*, and S. S. Ivanoff, formerly *research associate in plant pathology, Wisconsin Agricultural Experiment Station* [2]

INTRODUCTION

The pioneer investigations of Waite (*17, 18, 19*)[3] and later experiments and observations by many others have established beyond doubt that the honeybee and some other insects are capable of transmitting the blossom blight of apple (*Malus sylvestris* Mill.) and pear (*Pyrus communis* L.) incited by *Erwinia amylovora* (Burr.) Winslow et al. For many years after this discovery insects were generally thought to be the only important agents for transmission of blossom blight. Later investigations (e. g., *2, 3, 4, 7, 10, 16*), however, have shown that meteoric water is an important factor in its spread and that under some conditions minute aerial strands of bacterial exudate may be disseminated by wind. The relative importance of insect and water transmission, which seems to vary greatly with conditions, is subject to considerable difference of opinion. Since blossom blight is one of the most important phases of the fire blight problem, a better understanding of its epidemiology is highly desirable.

Though it is generally accepted that bees can transmit blossom blight, comparatively little experimental work has been done on the details of this transmission or on the factors that favor or limit it. It has been the purpose of the present work to contribute to a reexamination of these aspects of the problem in the light of recent information, especially in their relation to nectar concentration. These studies, which were pursued in the spring of 1936 and 1937, were unavoidably interrupted when one of the authors was called to another post. The available results are reported herein. A companion study on nectar concentration in relation to the growth of *Erwinia amylovora* and infection of blossoms following artificial inoculation is reported elsewhere in this Journal (*8*).

Literature on the transmission of fire blight has been reviewed by Parker (*11*) and others. Consequently, only papers that seem especially pertinent to the present work are cited herein.

DIRECT TRANSMISSION FROM CONTAMINATED TO UNCONTAMINATED BLOSSOMS

An objective of the following experiments was development of methods whereby transmission of fire blight from one blossom to another by honeybees (*Apis mellifera* L.) could be studied experimentally under adequate control. Some needs for specific information

---

[2] Grateful acknowledgments are made to Dr. Erwin C. Alfonsus, formerly instructor in beekeeping, University of Wisconsin, for assistance in handling the bees and advice on some phases of this problem.
[3] Italic numbers in parentheses refer to Literature Cited, p. 752.

JOURNAL OF AGRICULTURAL RESEARCH, 1941,
Vol. 62, pp. 745-753.

168

concerning such transmission in relation to the epidemiology of blossom blight have been discussed elsewhere (8).

Experiments were performed in three ways: (1) Individual marked bees of an uncontaminated nucleus hive in a large cloth cage in the greenhouse successively visited inoculated [4] and uncontaminated blossoms of potted trees; (2) bees of an uncontaminated nucleus hive in a large cloth cage in the greenhouse freely visited two potted trees, one with inoculated blossoms and the other with uncontaminated ones; and (3) an uncontaminated bee, handled in a specially designed wire cage, visited inoculated blossoms and then uncontaminated ones in the greenhouse or the orchard.

Evidence that the bees were not contaminated with the fire blight bacteria at the beginning of the experiments is based on the following precautions and tests. The bees of the nucleus hives were brought from Louisiana in early spring before they had opportunity to leave the hive. If the hive had been contaminated in the preceding year, the evidence is strongly against the possibility that the bacteria would have overwintered in it (6, 11, 12, 14, 15). When the hives had been placed in the cloth cages, the bees were allowed on 2 successive days to visit uncontaminated blossoms of potted apple and pear trees that had been held in a moist chamber to bring the nectar to a dilution favorable for infection. Each individual bee used in experiments with the small wire cage was allowed to work on a few uncontaminated blossoms before it was employed in the subsequent transmission experiments. In all these control experiments the bees were seen to introduce the glossa into the receptacle cup and remain in position long enough to indicate that they were sipping nectar. Throughout all the experiments on transmission, no indication was found that the bees were contaminated before they were permitted to visit the inoculated or diseased blossoms.

Some typical experiments on transmission are described below as illustrative of the methods and results.

About 50 blossoms of a 3-year-old dwarf Bartlett pear tree in the greenhouse were inoculated in the nectar by means of a small camel's hair inoculator at about 6 p. m. The tree had previously been held for a few hours in a moist chamber (9) with the curtains wet but spray not running, in order to bring the nectar to a concentration low enough to favor infection.[5] After inoculation it was kept overnight in another moist chamber. On the following morning measurements of nectar by means of an Abbé refractometer showed that the sugar concentration varied from 3 to 5 percent, whether the blossoms had been inoculated or not. Platings were made from inoculated and uninoculated blossoms at 3 time intervals that day. Fire blight bacteria, which subsequently caused typical infection in inoculation tests, were isolated in all trials from inoculated blossoms, but in no case from uninoculated ones. On the morning after inoculation, this tree, with a like one that had received similar moist treatment but no inoculation, was placed in a cloth cage. Each tree was protected by mosquito netting, so that

[4] Unless otherwise stated all inoculations were made on the preceding day by introducing a drop of about 1/100 cc. of bacterial suspension into the receptacle cup by means of a camel's hair inoculator, with care not to wound the host tissue.

[5] Unless otherwise stated all potted trees, before and after being used in the transmission experiments, were placed overnight in the moist chamber at about 20° C., with the curtains wet but the water not running. The inoculated and the uncontaminated trees were kept in separate chambers. At the end of a moist treatment, the nectar in the blossoms was usually abundant, and contained 3 to 5 percent of sugars. On keeping the trees in the greenhouse for 1 hour at about 24°, the concentration of nectar sugars usually rose to 10 or 12 percent.

individual blossom clusters could be exposed to visitation by bees or covered at will. An uncontaminated nucleus hive of bees was then placed in the cage. An inoculated cluster was exposed, with the aim of having one bee sip nectar from the blossoms.[6] Most of the bees flew about above the trees but only a few actually approached the exposed cluster. As soon as one alighted on an exposed blossom it was marked on the thorax with a droplet of specially prepared aniline dye and no other bees were permitted to touch this cluster. This bee was allowed to work on the inoculated blossoms until it had a good chance to become contaminated but not long enough to get its fill of nectar. The inoculated cluster was then covered and one on the uninoculated tree was exposed. The marked bee, without returning to the hive, alighted on the blossoms and worked on each of them, at times returning to a blossom it had already sipped from before going to another it had not yet visited. Each blossom the bee touched was marked, and the order of visitation was recorded. After the bee had visited all the blossoms, it was caught and the cluster was covered. The glossa was cut off with sterile instruments and its apical part dipped successively into the nectar of 10 blossoms of a third available tree having abundant nectar of a concentration favorable for infection. The glossa and the honey stomach were crushed and plated. The three trees were then incubated overnight in the moist chamber at about 20° C., with the curtains wet but the water shut off. On the following morning the blossoms of all the trees were found to contain abundant nectar. The trees were then further incubated in the greenhouse for 7 days at about 22° to 24°, after which the results were taken. The trees were kept under observation for another month.

The results of this experiment show that the bee transmitted the disease from the inoculated blossoms to 2 of the 4 uncontaminated blossoms it visited. No disease developed in the 10 blossoms that were touched with the bee's glossa. The glossa, however, yielded a few fire blight colonies that were subsequently shown by inoculation to be pathogenic. The honey stomach yielded a great number of micro-organisms, none of which resembled the fire blight pathogen. Most of the blossoms inoculated with the camel's hair inoculator showed macroscopic symptoms of blight within 4 days. Blossoms that were not inoculated did not show any disease. The experiment just described was performed four more times under similar conditions. Only one of these trials gave positive results.[7]

Transmission was also accomplished in two trials of another type, in which an inoculated and an uninoculated tree were kept together in a cloth cage for 5 hours, the bees of an uncontaminated hive freely visiting the blossoms of both trees. In the first trial 32 of the 61 blossoms of a dwarf Bartlett pear tree (uninoculated when placed in the cage) became diseased within a week after the bees' visitation, and in the second 46 of the 87 blossoms on a Seckel pear tree (likewise uninoculated when placed in the cage) blighted. The disease was therefore transmitted to 52 percent of the blossoms of these two trees.

[6] Bees may visit blossoms to collect pollen or reconnoiter without sipping nectar. In these experiments they were regarded as sipping nectar when they extended the glossa into the receptacle cup and remained in position for a distinctly longer period than would be required for reconnoitering.

[7] The amount and concentration of nectar changed rapidly after the trees were taken out of the moist chamber. For instance, in one case the concentration of nectar sugars rose from 3.5 percent to 11 percent in 50 minutes. In a few hours the volume of nectar was so diminished that measurable samples were not obtainable. These changes in the amount and concentration of nectar during the course of an experiment may have influenced the amount of infection (8), notwithstanding the fact that the moist treatment of the plants after visitation by the bees induced nectar concentrations favorable for infection.

Most of the tests on direct transmission of blossom blight by selected individual bees were made with the use of a small wire bee cage or trap (fig. 1). The chief advantage of this cage is that it permits keeping a particular bee with known history through several operations in association with any selected clusters as long as the bee remains alive and active. The cage, made of 16-mesh galvanized wire screen, is about 10 inches long and 4½ inches in width and height. It consists of two detachable halves connected with hinges on one side and with a hook on the opposite side. Two sliding doors, each placed near the outer end of one of the hinged sections, cut off small compartments (fig. 1, *a* and *c*). A bee is easily caught with this cage and confined in the central large compartment (fig. 1, *b*). Then

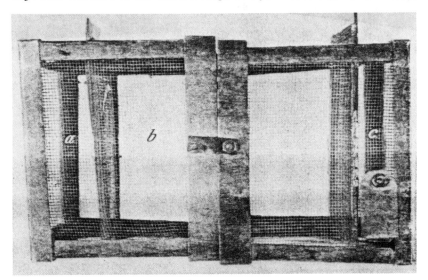

FIGURE 1.—Wire bee cage used in the inoculation experiments: *a* and *c*, Small outer compartments; *b*, large central compartment.

one of the trap doors is lifted and the insect is confined in the small outer compartment. Later the central compartment is opened, placed about a blossom cluster, then closed and hooked. The trap door is lifted, and the bee is allowed to visit the blossom cluster. After it has worked on the blossoms sufficiently, it is driven back into the small compartment and the sliding door is closed. The same bee is then used again on other blossom clusters, carried safely from one orchard to another, kept overnight, or handled otherwise according to the requirements of the experiment.

Transmission experiments with the wire bee cage included the following steps:

1. In an orchard in which no naturally occurring fire blight had been found, 10 blossom clusters of apple or pear were bagged separately, 2 of which were inoculated with the fire blight organism suspended in pure water or in artificial nectar[8] of various concentrations, as desired.

[8] The artificial nectar used contained invert sugars and sucrose in the proportions reported by Beutler for apple nectar—6.4 parts by weight of dextrose, 6.4 of levulose, and 8.5 of sucrose being dissolved in the following weak nutrient solution: Asparagine, 0.1 percent; sodium chloride, 0.01 percent; dibasic potassium phosphate, 0.05 percent; magnesium sulfate, 0.02 percent; calcium chloride, a trace. The solution was adjusted to approximately pH 7.0. The details of preparation are reported elsewhere (8).

2. About 1 to 3 days later, a bee was caught in the sterilized cage and allowed to sip nectar from two of the uninoculated clusters. The total number of blossoms worked on was noted.

3. As soon as the cage could be shifted into position, the same bee was allowed to sip nectar from an inoculated cluster.

4. After a similar brief interval, the same bee was allowed to work on four of the uninoculated blossom clusters.

5. The bee then was decapitated, its glossa and honey stomach plated, and the pathogenicity of the recovered bacteria tested.

In some special trials the concentration of the nectar in the blossoms was measured just before or just after the bee's visit.

By using the technique just described, in some cases omitting steps 1 and 5, 32 transmission tests were made in the greenhouse or the orchard at Madison in 1936. Ten of these gave positive results; i. e., the bee transmitted the disease from an inoculated to an uncontaminated blossom.

The transmission tests were continued during the same season at Sturgeon Bay, Wis., where the blooming season is later than at Madison. In all cases the transmission was attempted with single bees, trapped in the wire cage. Of the 26 individual tests, 7 gave positive results, 13 negative, and 6 doubtful. Of the tests that gave positive results, 5 were made when the receptacle cups were moist or wetted and only 2 when they were apparently dry. None of the 13 tests that gave negative results were made when the receptacle cups were moist or wetted.

LENGTH OF TIME AFTER INOCULATION THAT BLOSSOMS ATTRACT BEES

One experiment was performed to gain evidence on the length of time after inoculation that blossoms will attract bees and serve as sources of contamination. It consisted in placing with an uncontaminated hive in the cloth cage two different Bartlett pear trees each day, one inoculated and the other not. The inoculated tree introduced on the first day had been inoculated 5 days; that on the second, 4; the third, 3; the fourth 2. The results showed that under the conditions of the experiment the bees could transmit the disease to healthy blossoms from diseased blossoms that had been inoculated for 5 days. The diseased blossoms on the tree introduced 5 days after inoculation were already wilted and light brown in color. Three bees on more than 5 occasions touched these diseased blossoms with the glossa, then moved to the healthy blossoms. It was evident, however, that the healthy blossoms attracted more bees than the diseased ones and that the bees lingered longer on healthy than on diseased blossoms. The tree that was uninoculated when placed in the cage with the tree inoculated for 5 days had 46 blossoms, 29 of which were found diseased 10 days after the bees' visit.

CONCENTRATION OF NECTAR IN BLOSSOMS AT THE TIME OF THE BEE'S VISIT IN RELATION TO TRANSMISSION

In a greenhouse trial (table 1) some potted Bartlett pear trees were given a treatment in the moist chamber that brought the sugar concentration of their nectar within a range of 3 to 8 percent. They were then placed in a cloth cage and subjected to visitation by contaminated bees with similar trees that, having received no moist treatment, had

172

nectar with a sugar concentration of 45 percent. After removal from the cage the trees with low nectar concentration received a second moist treatment, whereas the others did not. Thirty-eight percent of the visited blossoms with the lower nectar concentration and none of those with the higher blighted.

TABLE 1.—*Nectar concentration in blossoms of 2-year-old Bartlett pear trees in relation to transmission of fire blight by contaminated honeybees* [1]

Bee No.	Moist treatment of blossoms before or after bee's visit [2]	Concentration of sugars in nectar before bee's visit [3]	Blossoms visited by bee	Blossoms diseased	
				Number	Percent
		Percent	*Number*		
1	Treated before and after	3, 4, 8	3	2	
1	___do___	3, 4, 8	5	2	
2	___do___	3, 4, 8	3	0	38
2	___do___	2, 3	4	1	
2	___do___	2, 3	2	2	
3	___do___	4, 5	4	1	
4	No moist treatment	45 or higher	4	0	
1	___do___	45 or higher	5	0	
4	___do___	45 or higher	5	0	0
5	___do___	(4)	3	0	
6	___do___	(4)	4	0	

[1] The bees had just been contaminated by sipping nectar from blossoms artificially inoculated on the preceding day. The experiments were performed in the greenhouse at 20° to 21° C.
[2] A bee visited from 2 to 5 blossoms of a cluster.
[3] Values are for individual samples. The concentration of nectar rose in some of the blossoms to 15 percent during the time the bee worked and before the tree was put back into the moist chamber.
[4] Receptacle cups dry.

In a field trial it was aimed to control in part the nectar concentration of the blossoms from which the bees obtained inoculum, as well as of those to which they were to carry it. In a pear orchard in which no naturally occurring blight had been found, blossoms were inoculated on various days with fire blight bacteria suspended in artificial nectar solutions with sugar concentrations varying from a trace to 40 percent. At the same time small drops of artificial nectar of the same range of concentration, but containing no bacteria, were placed in the receptacle cups of uncontaminated blossoms. Some of the treated blossoms were bagged in an attempt to check the rapid increase of nectar concentration. On the following day individual uncontaminated bees were allowed to sip nectar, first from some of the inoculated blossoms, then from uninoculated ones containing the artificial nectar drops. Shortly before or after the bees visited the blossoms, the concentration of the nectar in these and other blossoms was measured. It was found in most cases that the concentration had undergone changes. Some of the drops that originally had contained a trace or 1 percent of nectar sugars were later found to contain as high as 10 or 12 percent. Likewise, blossoms that originally contained 40 percent of nectar sugars were found to have 70 or 75 percent. The results of these trials, which are summarized in table 2, show that when a bee worked on inoculated blossoms with nectar containing 2 to 12 percent sugars and then on uncontaminated ones with nectar containing 0 to 35 percent sugars, 49 percent of the latter group blighted. A higher percentage of infection might have resulted if the concentration of nectar in some of the blossoms had not risen so high. On the other hand, no infection resulted when the bees first worked on blossoms with nectar containing, respectively, 10–14, 42–56, and 48–75 percent sugars and then on others with nectar containing, respectively, 10–18, 44–47, and 46–70 percent. Likewise, bees that worked on inoculated blossoms with apparently dry receptacle cups and then on uncontaminated ones with dry receptacle cups did not transmit the disease

TABLE 2.— *Concentration of pear nectar in relation to transmission of blossom blight by honeybees, Sturgeon Bay, Wis., 1937* [1]

Range of concentration of sugars in nectar of inoculated blossoms from which bees sipped	Range of concentration of sugars in nectar of healthy blossoms from which contaminated bees sipped	Bagging of blossoms after bees' visit	Bees used	Blossoms	
				Used	Diseased
Percent	*Percent*		*Number*	*Number*	*Percent*
2–8	0–10	Bagged	12	50	56
3–12	0–35	Not bagged	8	42	40
10–14	10–18	Bagged	6	22	0
42–56	41–47	....do	10	34	0
48–75	46–70	Not bagged	9	36	0
([2])	([2])	....do	18	52	0

[1] Wire cages were used for controlling the bees and the experiments were performed on orchard trees.
[2] Receptacle cups dry.

DISCUSSION

It is recognized that some degree of artificiality may attend all experiments with bees handled in captivity, and that results from such work are reliable only in proportion to the adequacy with which they are observed and controlled.

Transmission of the disease from one blossom to another was demonstrated by each of the three methods tried, and each method may be useful. However, work with individual bees greatly facilitates adequate observations and controls. Use of the bee cage substantially increases the range and flexibility of experimentation with individual bees.

The large number of instances in which blossoms did not blight after visitation by a contaminated bee indicates that there are important limitations on the efficiency of this insect in transmitting the disease. Indeed, if this were not the case, it would be very difficult to understand how our apple and pear culture could continue, in view of the great number and activity of bees.

The results of these experiments on transmission of blossom blight by bees indicate that nectar concentration is a very important factor limiting this mode of transmission. They are in general accord with the results of studies (5, 8, 13, 14) of nectar concentration in relation to fire blight infection initiated by artificial inoculation. However, in many cases in which the nectar was at a favorable concentration, little or no infection occurred after contaminated bees had sipped from it. It is, therefore, apparent that other factors besides nectar concentration are important in limiting blossom-blight transmission by bees. An experimental study of such factors lies beyond the scope of the present paper.

The need for information on factors favoring or limiting blossom-blight infection under conditions of natural transmission has been discussed elsewhere (8). The present investigation was interrupted soon after experimental methods for such work had been developed. Further studies under various conditions are needed. It would seem especially desirable to perform additional greenhouse and orchard experiments in which contaminated bees visit uncontaminated blossoms containing nectar too concentrated to permit infection. The time during which bacteria thus deposited will live and the range of conditions they will tolerate without losing the capability to infect when favorable conditions occur are vitally important considerations in relation to the epidemiology and control of the disease. While work with artificial inoculation is very valuable in helping to define and interpret problems relating to blossom-blight transmission by bees and other insects, further experimental work on transmission by the insects themselves seems essential to an adequate understanding of their role in disseminating the disease.

SUMMARY

Transmission by honeybees of fire blight of apple (*Malus sylvestris*) and pear (*Pyrus communis*), incited by *Erwinia amylovora*, was studied by three experimental methods. The most flexible and convenient one employed individual bees handled in a specially designed wire cage.

Bees were attracted to blighting blossoms that had been inoculated 5 days before, and transmitted the disease to healthy blossoms.

In greenhouse and orchard experiments contaminated bees freely transmitted blight to healthy blossoms when the sugar concentration of the nectar was in the lower range encountered in nature, but not when it was in the medium or higher range.

In the experiments reported herein, nectar concentration was an important factor in limiting blossom-blight transmission by bees. However, in many cases in which the nectar was at a favorable concentration, little or no infection occurred after contaminated bees had sipped from it. It is apparent that other factors in addition to nectar concentration are important in limiting blossom-blight transmission by bees.

LITERATURE CITED

(1) BEUTLER, RUTH.
    1930. BIOLOGISCH-CHEMISCHE UNTERSUCHUNGEN AM NEKTAR VON IMMEN-BLUMEN. Ztschr. f. Vergleich. Physiol. 12: [72]-176, illus.
(2) BROOKS, A. N.
    1926. STUDIES OF THE EPIDEMIOLOGY AND CONTROL OF FIRE BLIGHT OF APPLE. Phytopathology 16: 665-696, illus.
(3) GOSSARD, H. A., and WALTON, R. C.
    1917. FIRE-BLIGHT INFECTION: RAIN PROVES AN IMPORTANT CARRIER OF DISEASE IN OPEN ORCHARDS. Ohio Agr. Expt. Sta. Monthly Bul. 2: 357-364, illus.
(4) ———— and WALTON, R. C.
    1922. DISSEMINATION OF FIRE BLIGHT. Ohio Agr. Expt. Sta. Bul. 357: [79]-126, illus.
(5) HILDEBRAND, E. M.
    1937. THE BLOSSOM-BLIGHT PHASE OF FIRE BLIGHT, AND METHODS OF CONTROL. N. Y. (Cornell) Agr. Expt. Sta. Mem. 207, 40 pp., illus.
(6) ———— and PHILLIPS, E. F.
    1936. THE HONEYBEE AND THE BEEHIVE IN RELATION TO FIRE BLIGHT. Jour. Agr. Res. 52: 789-810, illus.
(7) IVANOFF, S. S., and KEITT, G. W.
    1937. THE OCCURRENCE OF AERIAL BACTERIAL STRANDS ON BLOSSOMS, FRUITS, AND SHOOTS BLIGHTED BY ERWINIA AMYLOVORA. Phytopathology 27: 702-709, illus.
(8) ———— and KEITT, G. W.
    RELATIONS OF NECTAR CONCENTRATION TO GROWTH OF ERWINIA AMYLOVORA AND FIRE BLIGHT INFECTION OF APPLE AND PEAR BLOSSOMS. Jour. Agr. Res. 62: 732-743.

175

(9) KEITT, G. W., BLODGETT, E. C., WILSON, E. E., and MAGIE, R. O.
    1937. THE EPIDEMIOLOGY AND CONTROL OF CHERRY LEAF SPOT. Wis. Agr. Expt. Sta. Res. Bul. 132, 117 pp., illus.
(10) MILLER, P. W.
    1929. STUDIES OF FIRE BLIGHT OF APPLE IN WISCONSIN. Jour. Agr. Res. 39: 579–621, illus.
(11) PARKER, K. G.
    1936. FIRE BLIGHT: OVERWINTERING, DISSEMINATION, AND CONTROL OF THE PATHOGENE. N. Y. (Cornell) Agr. Expt. Sta. Mem. 193, 42 pp., illus.
(12) PIERSTORFF, A. L., and LAMB, HOWARD.
    1934. THE HONEYBEE IN RELATION TO THE OVERWINTERING AND PRIMARY SPREAD OF THE FIRE-BLIGHT ORGANISM. Phytopathology 24: 1347–1357.
(13) THOMAS, H. EARL, and ARK, P. A.
    1934. NECTAR AND RAIN IN RELATION TO FIRE BLIGHT. Phytopathology 24: 682–685.
(14) —— and ARK, P. A.
    1934. FIRE BLIGHT OF PEARS AND RELATED PLANTS. Calif. Agr. Expt. Sta. Bul. 586, 43 pp., illus.
(15) —— and VANSELL, GEORGE H.
    1934. RELATION OF BEES TO FIRE BLIGHT. Amer. Bee Jour. 74: 160.
(16) TULLIS, E. C.
    1929. STUDIES ON THE OVERWINTERING AND MODES OF INFECTION OF THE FIRE BLIGHT ORGANISM. Mich. Agr. Expt. Sta. Tech. Bul. 97, 32 pp., illus.
(17) WAITE, M. B.
    1892. RESULTS FROM RECENT INVESTIGATIONS IN PEAR BLIGHT. (Abstract) Amer. Assoc. Adv. Sci. Proc. (1891) 40: 315.
(18) ——
    1902. THE RELATION OF BEES TO THE ORCHARD. Calif. Cult. 18: 390–391.
(19) ——
    1906. PEAR-BLIGHT WORK AND ITS CONTROL IN CALIFORNIA. Calif. Fruit Growers' Conv. Off. Rpt. (1905) 31: 137–155.

FREQUENT ASSOCIATION OF PHYTOMONAS MELOPHTHORA, WITH VARIOUS STAGES IN THE LIFE CYCLE OF THE APPLE MAGGOT, RHAGOLETIS POMONELLA[1]

T. C. ALLEN, J. A. PINCKARD AND A. J. RIKER

INTRODUCTION

Phytomonas melophthora A. and R., which causes rot of ripe apples, has been studied in relation to various stages in the life cycle of the apple maggot, *Rhagoletis pomonella* Walsh. This work was undertaken because of the various indications (reviewed by Allen and Riker (2)), of a frequent relation between the larvae of this insect and the rot organism. It seemed desirable to determine, if possible, how the larvae and the bacteria became associated and the frequency of this association throughout the life cycle of the insect.

The economic importance of the combination of *Phytomonas melophthora* with the apple maggot is manifest both in the orchard and in storage. Under natural conditions in the orchard the dissemination of the bacteria and the mode of their entry into the fruit are apparently dependent upon the insect. Under storage conditions subsequent development of rot in the fruit seems associated with the presence of maggot infestation. Consequently, further study of this relation appeared desirable.

The problem has been studied primarily by means of certain bacteriological methods applied to various stages of the insects and to their immediate environment. This type of study has already shown its value in the excellent work by Leach (6) and Johnson (4) on the relation of certain insects to the spread of soft-rot bacteria. The technic employed by the writers is reviewed briefly.

MATERIALS AND METHODS

The materials used in these studies included (1) the various available stages in the life cycle of the insect and (2) the accompanying decay in apple tissue, as listed in table 1. Infested fruits were obtained in 1931 and 1932 from Gays Mills, Madison, Sparta, and Winneconne, Wisconsin. Adult flies and the fruits that contained both eggs and the ovipositor punctures were collected at Gays Mills. Several varieties of maggot-infested apples were used in the studies: viz., Dudley, McMahon, Snow, Wealthy and Yellow Transparent.

[1] Published with the approval of the Director of the Wisconsin Agricultural Experiment Station. These studies have been made in cooperation between the Departments of Economic Entomology and Plant Pathology.

PHYTOPATHOLOGY, 1934, Vol. 24, pp. 228-238.

Isolations from apple tissue were made in accordance with the usual laboratory technique as employed by Allen and Riker (2), except as noted. Isolation studies from the various stages of the insect involved variations in procedure. Adult flies, eggs, egg-shells, and larvae were placed in broth and removed after 20 minutes. The broth was incubated 48 hours at room temperature before dilution plates were poured. Suspensions from the broth were transferred into healthy apples. When bacterial decay developed in the apple tissue, poured-plate isolations were made on nutrient glucose agar. Flies were killed with chloroform or ether before crushing in tubes of nutrient glucose broth.

Methods for treatment of flies, eggs, and larvae with surface disinfectants were as follows: The material was placed in 70 per cent alcohol for 3 minutes to remove air, washed in sterile water and transferred to bichloride of mercury, 1 to 1000. After 5 minutes it was washed in sterile water and placed in a tube of broth for 20 minutes. Then it was transferred to another tube of broth and crushed. The bacteria on the surface, reached by this method, were certainly killed, but the possibility remains that those embedded in slowly soluble material upon the surface may have escaped injury. The natural openings make it difficult to differentiate between surface and partial internal sterilization. However, in the data that are presented later, the interpretation is made that, when the tubes of broth in which the material remained for 20 minutes remained sterile, any bacteria subsequently recovered came from inside. The development of growth in a check broth tube was interpreted to mean that microorganisms occurred on the surface of the material and no further isolations were attempted. When growth appeared in the tube where the insect was crushed, inoculations with the broth were made into apples and reisolations were made as previously described (2).

Eggs, which were nontreated and incubated to obtain developing larvae, were removed from apple tissue and transferred aseptically to dark moistened blotting paper within small sterilized vials. These vials were kept slightly above room temperature. As larvae hatched, they were transferred aseptically to needle pricks in surface-sterilized fruits. As decay developed in the apples, isolation studies were made of the rot that developed adjacent to the larval burrows. Certain difficulties of technique remain to be overcome with eggs treated with a surface disinfectant, for only 2 out of 25 trials were successful. In these 2 successful attempts, the larvae from treated eggs died a couple of days after being placed in apple tissue. No rot developed in the surrounding fruit tissue.

Several methods were tried before successful isolation of the organism was obtained from the pupal stage. The following method gave the most satisfactory result. Puparia were removed from soil and placed in 5 cc.

of physiological salt solution for 20 minutes with frequent agitation. This salt solution was diluted approximately 1 to 6, 1 to 35, and 1 to 200. One cc. from each dilution was placed into each of 3 Petri dishes with glucose yeast-infusion mineral-salt agar. This medium was similar to that employed by Wright (7). Its composition was glucose, 10 grams; magnesium sulphate (MgSO$_4$ · 7 H$_2$O), 0.2 grams; sodium chloride (NaCl), 0.2 grams; dipotassium phosphate (K$_2$HPO$_4$ · 3 H$_2$O), 0.1 gram; calcium chloride (CaCl$_2$), 0.1 gram; 10 per cent yeast infusion, 100 cc. and distilled water 900 cc. The reaction was adjusted to pH 6.8.

Puparia were also treated in disinfectant as described earlier, except that they were previously washed 3 times in tubes of sterile salt solution. Instead of 3 dilutions as used earlier, 8 successive dilutions were made to approximately 1 to 1,000,000. Three plates were poured from each dilution, making a total of 24 plates from each puparium. This relatively large amount of work was performed because it increased the chances for success.

The pathogenicity of the cultures isolated was determined in each case on one of several varieties that included Delicious, McIntosh, Wagner, and Yellow Transparent.

The results secured with these methods are given briefly in the following pages.

RESULTS

Phytomonas melophthora, the cause of bacterial storage rot of apples in Wisconsin, has been found associated with all stages examined in the life cycle of the insect, *Rhagoletis pomonella*. The life cycle of this insect, with its accompanying plant pathogen, has been followed in material from the orchards at Gays Mills. Certain parts of the cycle were studied with material from other sections of the State. The results of isolation studies from the various stages of the insect and from corresponding decay in apples are reported in detail in the following pages and are summarized in table 1. The same sequence of the work on different forms of the insect and associated apple tissue is followed both in the text and in this table.

ADULT FLIES

The adult flies used in these experiments were commonly found harboring *Phytomonos melophthora* in such quantities that they were readily isolated by methods outlined above. The reasons for suspecting the adult fly as a vector in the production of this disease were (1) the rot that sometimes followed the wound produced during oviposition in relatively ripe fruit (Fig. 1, C), and (2) the association of the apple maggot with rot, as considered earlier (2).

The flies examined were secured, 13 from the orchard and 12 from a series of emergence cages previously placed over piles of infested fruit.

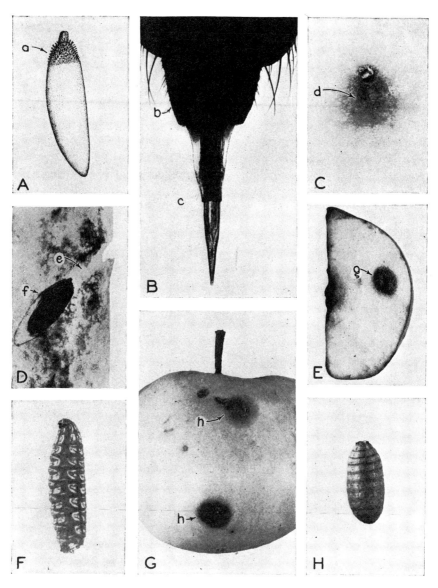

Fig. 1. A. Egg of the apple maggot and reticulation, *a*, at posterior end. ×51.
B. The posterior of a female fly, showing the end of the abdomen, *b*, and the partially
extended ovipositor, *c*. ×23. C. Egg puncture viewed from the surface of a ripe
apple. Decayed tissue, *d*, appears about the puncture. ×15. D. The egg, *f*, at normal
position in apple tissue, showing ovipositor or egg puncture, *e*. ×31. E. Rot, *g*, about
larval burrow in apple. ×1½. F. Mature larva. ×6. G. Rot, *h*, about larval exit
holes in apple. ×1½. H. Puparium. ×4.

Two broods of flies, some of which were obtained from 2-year-old puparia, were involved in the collection as explained by Allen and Fluke (1). The age of the flies collected in the orchard was uncertain, but only 1-day-old flies were used from the emergence cages.

Isolations were made to determine whether the flies were actually carrying the bacteria. The flies were subjected to the fumes of either chloroform or ether before the isolations. Both male and female flies were used for dilution plates either with or without surface treatment with a disinfectant as follows: Eight of 10 trials with nontreated female flies were positive for *Phytomonas melophthora*. Three trials with treated females were all positive. Four of 6 trials with nontreated male flies were positive. All of 6 trials with treated males were positive. These results are summarized in table 1. The larger percentage of positive results from the treated flies was perhaps the result of freedom from troublesome contaminations. Since about half of the males and females were only a day old and were from emergence cages it is suggested that they carried the bacteria either from the puparia or perhaps from the surrounding material. This question is considered further in the next paragraph and in connection with studies of the puparia. From these studies it appears that *Phytomonas melophthora* may be carried both internally and externally by the mature fly in quantities sufficiently large to account for the observed dissemination of the bacteria in Wisconsin orchards. This raises the question concerning how the association occurred.

Soil isolations were attempted in an effort to learn whether the flies became contaminated as they emerged. Four soil samples obtained within emergence cages were examined. Each soil sample was collected from the surface 2 inches in a sterile glass vial, mixed and divided into approximately 2 equal portions. One portion was plated in nutrient dextrose agar in triplicate from 6 dilutions that ranged up to 1 in 2,000,000. Part of the other portion of each sample was introduced into apple according to the method of Ark (3) with the exception that ripe Yellow Transparent apples were substituted for green pears. The negative results secured, perhaps because of inadequate technique, are not interpreted to mean that the soil does not harbor *Phytomonas melophthora*, but that, under the conditions of the above experiment, this organism was probably not present in the soil in relatively large quantities. Since more than three-fourths of the flies emerging from this soil carried the pathogenic bacterium, it appears more probable that the insects carried the bacteria from the puparia. How the flies transmitted the bacteria to the eggs was next considered.

Ovipositor Punctures

The ovipositor puncture was studied to determine the frequency of its inoculation. Five different varieties of apples were collected from 4 sources in the State, as mentioned earlier. The wounds made during oviposition, (Fig. 1, C) were located with binoculars. With sterile instruments the tissue of the fruit was cut away exposing the ovipositor puncture, e, and egg, f (Fig. 1, D). Isolations were made from the wound according to methods previously discussed. Results of isolations from 22 ovipositor punctures revealed that 10 of these contained *Phytomonas melophthora*. In connection with these results one should recall that relatively green apple tissue is not a favorable medium for the rot bacteria (2). These results suggest that bacteria may be transferred by means of the ovipositor (Fig. 1, B) and that, when conditions are favorable, rot may develop in the fruit following injuries made by the fly. Only a small percentage of the punctures were found devoid of eggs or egg-shells. The rate at which rot developed about the wound appeared to be influenced by the maturity of the fruit.

The inoculation of the ovipositor puncture might be accounted for by the habit of the adult fly. The ovipositor is extended and forced through the epidermis by several up and down movements. Any bacteria present on the ovipositor may therefore be smeared over the surrounding apple tissue. Following egg deposition, the ovipositor is generally cleaned by the rear legs of the insect before it is withdrawn into the abdomen. This cleaning habit also is performed in the same manner following defecation and can perhaps explain the distribution of rot bacteria over the ovipositor. Knight (5) has suggested that 2 pathogenic fungi were carried on the ovipositor of the apple maggot.

Eggs

Eggs of the insect (Fig. 1, A and D, f) were deposited a short distance under the epidermis of the apple fruit. Fifteen eggs were dissected from the apple parenchyma and isolations made from surface washings, according to the above-described technic. The results of these isolations showed that eight of the eggs were contaminated with *Phytomonas melophthora*. The projections on the proximal end of the egg (Fig. 1, A, a) apparently serve both to prevent any reverse movement of the egg and perhaps to harbor bacteria.

Eggs from captive flies were obtained by placing pairs of flies in a glass rearing cage together with a ripe apple, and a little yeast-water honey mixture. After the adult had been observed to deposit the egg, the fruit was removed from the cage, the egg dissected from the host tissue and, examined as earlier described. Three eggs were successfully extracted and isolations made from their surfaces without injury to the egg. In each attempt *Phytomonas melophthora* was recovered. In addition, 2 others were successfully obtained and treated with disinfectants without killing the contained embryos. The larvae were subsequently hatched and were found to be free from *Phytomonas melophthora* as described later. While the number is too small for conclusions, this evidence suggests that the bacteria do not occur inside the egg. The number of eggs employed is small because of the difficulty already mentioned that was experienced in removing them from the apple tissue and in handling them without injury.

Egg Shells

Egg shells found in apple tissue were treated in the same manner as the eggs. Larvae had emerged from the eggs after 4 to 6 days. Results of isolations from 24 egg shells showed that one-third of them carried the rot bacteria. It appears from the evidence available that as the larva emerges from its shell, it may frequently make contact with the apple-rot bacteria.

Larvae from Orchard

Young larvae were collected in apples taken from the orchard. Isolations made from 13 such larvae, not treated with surface disinfectants, showed that 3 of them were carrying the bacteria. It is probable that when the bacteria were present they were unable to increase in number much, if any, because of the relatively unfavorable condition in the green fruit. Similar larvae treated with surface disinfectants gave the same results from the same number of trials as those not treated. This indicated that the bacteria were present inside as well as on the surface of the larvae. Since the early life of the larvae is usually spent in relatively green fruit, decay rarely develops about the wounds made during oviposition or about the egg. The larvae hatch, but development is retarded until the fruit reaches a relatively mature condition. The number of bacteria available for isolation from such larvae as have hatched within 2 or 3 days, therefore, is quite small. If the parasitized fruit is removed from the tree while still in a "green" condition, further progress of both the larvae and rot seems to be dependent on the physiological processes of ripening and can be hastened or retarded by manipulation of the storage conditions. Larvae developed rapidly in ripe stored fruit usually amid conspicuous infection of the host parenchyma (Fig. 1, E, *g*). The above observations correspond to those following artificial inoculations on fruits in various stages of maturity (2).

Mature larvae (Fig. 1, F) from fallen fruit in the orchard were examined. Isolations from 13 of this group revealed that all contained *Phytomonas melophthora*. Thirteen similar larvae, which were treated with disinfectants, also revealed that all carried the plant pathogen. These trials showed that the mature larvae of this insect carried the rot-producing pathogen in relatively large numbers. While it was noted that the larvae apparently preferred the decayed portion of the fruit, no investigations were undertaken on the relation of the products of decay to the nutrition of the insect.

Larvae from captive flies were obtained from the eggs laid in insect cages. Nontreated larvae from this source were allowed to develop normally in the apple tissue until they neared maturity. Six of them were then crushed in broth. In each trial *Phytomonas melophthora* was recovered from the larvae in large quantities. Larvae from nontreated eggs of captive flies also were hatched on sterile blotting paper. The larvae were placed in broth for 20 minutes and then transferred to sterile apple tissue. Rot was produced in each of these trials and the bacteria were recovered from both the apple tissue and the tubes of broth. These larvae pupated in the usual manner. Larvae from treated eggs of captive flies were hatched as above and placed in broth for 20 minutes and then into healthy apple tissue. No cloudiness appeared in the broth after 2 weeks' incubation and the larvae were assumed to be free from bacteria. After 3 days both of the insects used in this experiment had burrowed in the apple tissue for a few centimeters and had died. There was no apparent increase in size of the larvae. No signs of decay were detected in the apple tissue.

The rot that developed about the larvae from captive flies also showed the presence of the typical rot bacteria in each of 3 trials. No difference was observed in the character of the rot observed in the insect cages from that found in the orchard.

Larval Burrows

Larval burrows (Fig. 1, E, *g*) in a variety of stages of decay and development were tested for the presence of *Phytomonas melophthora* during the course of these studies. Nineteen attempted isolations showed that 12 of them were infected with the bacteria. A greater portion could have been obtained had the writers rejected the burrows made by very young larvae in unripe apple tissue.

Exit Holes

Exit holes in the fruit were commonly observed to show progressive decay in nature (Fig. 1, G, *h*). At this period the larvae had matured and worked out of the fruit to pupate in the soil. Spread of the rot about the exit holes progressed until the whole apple was decayed by *Phytomonas melophthora* or until other bacteria or fungi entered and completed this process in advance. Twenty-three apples were collected showing various stages of rot developing about exit holes. Positive cultures of the bacteria were secured from 11 of these fruits. Although all the exit holes showed decay, considerable difficulty was experienced in a number of cases owing to other bacteria and fungi. An unidentified fungus resembling Mucor was particularly troublesome and was probably responsible for much of the failure to recover the apple-rot bacteria. The above experiments indicate that the larvae commonly enter the pupal stage carrying a considerable quantity of the plant pathogen.

Puparia

Puparia (Fig. 1, H) were collected and stored in sand in the ice box for approximately 7 months. The purpose of storage was to try to determine

TABLE 1.—*Summary of isolation studies made on the association of apple-rot bacteria with different stages in the life cycle of the apple maggot and on the decay of apple tissue*

Source of isolation	Specimens employed	Specimens yielding pathogenic cultures	Isolations successful
	No.	*No.*	*Per cent*
Adult flies treated[a]	9	9	100
" " nontreated	16	12	75
Ovipositor puncture	22	10	45
Surface of eggs	15	8	53
Eggs from captive flies			
Treated[a]	2	0	0
Nontreated	3	3	100
Egg shells	24	8	33
Larvae from orchard			
Young larvae treated[a]	13	3	23
" " nontreated	13	3	23
Mature larvae treated[a]	12	13	100
" " nontreated	13	13	100
Larvae from captive flies			
Nontreated	6	6	100
From nontreated eggs[b]	3	3	100
From treated eggs[ab]	2	0	0
Rot about larvae of captive flies	3	3	100
Larval burrows	19	12	63
Exit holes in fruit	23	11[c]	48
Puparial surface washings	25	16	64
Puparia treated[a]	20	0	0

[a] The treatment was with a disinfectant, as described in the text.
[b] The eggs were removed from the apples and hatched in vials.
[c] The low number of positive results was probably because of secondary organisms, as explained in the text.

if time had a bearing on mode of overwintering of the bacteria. Twenty-five healthy puparia were chosen from the group and isolations made from surface washings. Ordinary methods of isolation failed in studies of the puparia, so certain modifications were employed as described earlier. Sixty-four per cent of these puparia were found to carry *Phytomonas melophthora* on that portion of the puparia that can be wet by water. These results indicate that overwintering in the field is likely to occur on the surface of the puparia.

Puparia, treated with disinfectants before crushing, gave no evidence of internal transmission of *Phytomonas melophthora*. Twenty puparia were used in these attempts, all of which gave negative results. Considerable difficulty was experienced with other bacteria and fungi that appeared in large numbers on the dilution plates. Cultures were secured from almost all of the various colonies appearing on these plates, and inoculations made into apple fruits gave negative results. The fact presented earlier that 1-day-old flies often carried the rot bacteria suggests that these bacteria were associated with the fly in the pupal stage. In this and earlier isolation studies it should be borne in mind that the rot bacteria, when present, might easily be missed, especially in badly contaminated material. The results of the above experiments suggest that *Phytomonas melophthora* may overwinter more abundantly on the surface of the puparia than inside.

SUMMARY

Phytomonas melophthora, the apple-rot bacterium, has been studied in relation to the various stages in the life cycle of *Rhagoletis pomonella,* the apple maggot. The bacteria have been found commonly associated with both male and female adult flies, eggs, larvae, and puparia. They have also been found in the ovipositor punctures, larval burrows, and exit holes in apple-fruit tissue. The bacteria were recovered from adult flies, and larvae, following treatment with surface disinfectants.

This work, based on 244 isolations, 54 per cent of which were positive, indicates that these apple-rot bacteria may be frequently associated with various stages in the life-cycle of the apple maggot.

LITERATURE CITED

1. ALLEN, T. C., and C. L. FLUKE. Notes on the life history of the apple maggot in Wisconsin. Jour. Econ. Ent. 26: 1108–1112. 1933.
2. ALLEN, T. C., and A. J. RIKER. A rot of apple fruit caused by *Phytomonas melophthora,* n. sp., following invasion by the apple maggot. Phytopath. 22: 557–571. 1932.

3. ARK, P. A.   The behavior of *Bacillus amylovorus* in the soil.   Phytopath. 22: 657–660.   1932.
4. JOHNSON, DELIA E.   The relation of the cabbage maggot and other insects to the spread and development of soft rot of Cruciferae.   Phytopath. 20: 857–872. 1930.
5. KNIGHT, H. H.   Studies on insects affecting the fruit of the apple.   N. Y. (Cornell) Agr. Exp. Sta. Bul. 410.   1922.
6. LEACH, J. G.   Relation of the seed corn maggot (*Phorbia fusciceps* Zett.) to spread and development of potato black-leg in Minnesota.   Phytopath. 16: 149–177. 1926.
7. WRIGHT, W. H.   The nodule bacteria of soybeans: I. Bacteriology of strains.   Soil Sci. 20: 95–130.   1925.

187

Observations on Cucumber Beetles as Vectors of Cucurbit Wilt

J. G. Leach

According to present concepts, cucumber beetles (*Diabrotica vittata* Fabr. and *D. duodecimpunctata* Oliv.) are the only proved vectors of cucurbit wilt caused by *Erwinia tracheiphila* (E. F. Sm.) Holland, and the only known method of survival of the pathogen over winter is in bodies of hibernating beetles. Absolute proof of the survival of the bacteria in this way has never been presented because of the failure of all efforts to overwinter the beetles experimentally, but Rand and Enlows (7) have offered strong circumstantial evidence by demonstrating survival of the pathogen in beetles held in cold storage for 6 weeks, when all the insects were dead. Also the isolation of the pathogen in early spring from beetles assumed to have over-wintered as adults has been generally accepted as strong supporting evidence for this method of survival.

Carter (2) recently questioned this concept, pointing out that overwintering beetles emerge and feed for some time on nonsusceptible plants before cucurbits are available, and has expressed the opinion that any wilt bacteria that may have survived in the digestive tracts of the beetles would have been lost by the cleansing effect of such feeding. According to Carter, "a more likely occurrence is that the wild cucumbers and perhaps other hosts are first infected, so that when the cultivated cucurbits are attacked, the insects are by then carrying fresh inoculum in their intestines." The absence of perennial or biennial cucurbits or any evidence of seed transmission weakens this hypothesis but does not rule it out completely.

Burkholder (1) called attention to the unique nature of *E. tracheiphila* among plant pathogenic bacteria and to certain facts suggesting that "it is more at home in the beetle than in the plant" and that this may point to the possible origin of the disease. He suggested

188

also that *E. tracheiphila* might be parasitic upon the insect but recognized that the ability of the beetle to remain alive, whereas the plant dies, is one argument against this theory.

The survival of the beetle and the death of the plant would not be inconsistent with the concept of a symbiotic relationship between the beetles and the bacteria. Several bacterial plant pathogens are known to live symbiotically in the bodies of their insect vectors (5, 6), and in some cases special anatomical adaptations in the form of caeca provide a reservoir of bacterial inoculum. Leach (5), in discussing beetles as vectors of cucurbit wilt, pointed out that bacteria in the bodies of insects had not been studied by histological methods and that it was not known whether such a symbiotic relationship is involved.

Because of the anomalous state of our knowledge of this relationship, a histological study of the insects was undertaken. Adult beetles were caught and processed for sectioning in early spring, in midsummer, and in late summer. Specimens of both the striped and spotted beetles with wings removed were embedded in paraffin, sectioned and stained with basic fuchsin and counterstained in picric acid, a method previously shown to be satisfactory for staining gram-negative bacteria and the various insect tissues (4, 5). Some of the specimens were fed on wilted plants for 48 hr or longer before killing, whereas others were killed as soon as caught in the field. Approximately 75 insects were sectioned, stained and examined. Surprisingly few bacteria were found in the intestinal tracts, even in those insects killed after feeding on wilted plants. Those bacteria present were mixed with the ingested food material in a heterogenous arrangement showing no evidence of multiplication in situ. No intestinal caeca were observed in which bacteria could accumulate and serve as reservoirs of inoculum. Most of the bacteria observed were short rods well within the morphological limits for *E. tracheiphila* but, of course, could not be identified. When cultures were made from dissected sections of the intestines, many nonpathogenic bacteria were present and it was difficult to obtain *E. tracheiphila* in pure culture. Isolations from the intestines from 5 beetles of each species yielded only one culture of the pathogen; this was from a beetle that had been experimentally fed upon a wilted plant prior to killing.

The bacteria were more abundant in the midintestine than in the fore- and hind-intestine, and there was no evidence of concentration of living bacteria in the hind intestine and rectum as is found in some dipterous insects. In many sections, a few bacterial cells occurred in chains adhering to the peritrophic membrane suggesting the possibility of multiplication. No significant differences in the presence of bacteria were observed between the two species of insects or between males and females. Of the insects collected in late summer, it was observed that there were more males than females, but in early spring the sexes were about equal in number. Whether or not this has any significance is not known.

Because of the small numbers of bacteria in the intestinal tracts, it was thought possible that some significant concentration of bacteria might have escaped detection. It is evident that there is a normal intestinal flora of facultative-anaerobic bacteria in the intestinal tract and that multiplication is, in some manner, held in check as long as the insect is alive. If the insects could be killed without killing the bacteria, and then incubated, the surviving bacteria should develop without the insect's restraining influence (5). To test this, specimens of freshly caught beetles were placed at $-20°C$ for 24 hr, then incubated at $+25°C$ for 4, 8, and 16 hr before fixation. When these were cut and stained masses of orderly arranged cells of short rods were found in the midintestine but in no other parts of the insect. It was concluded that the relatively few bacterial cells observed in the midintestine before freezing were living cells that multiplied promptly when the restraining influence of the living insects was removed. Isolations indicate that if the wilt pathogen is present in the insect, it probably is there in small numbers along with nonpathogenic species and is subject to the same restraining influence.

Assuming that the pathogen does survive over winter in the intestinal tracts of the beetles and is not lost during the preliminary feeding on nonhost plants, bacteria must find their way into fresh wounds when they become available in order to infect cucurbits. Since the beetles have no salivary glands and apparently do not regurgitate in their feeding process, it is not likely that primary infection results from contaminated mouth parts. Smith (8) recognized this and demonstrated that infection could take place if fecal pellets of experimentally contaminated insects were placed upon fresh feeding wounds.

Secondary infection is easily explained as the mouth parts of beetles, in feeding on infected stems of cucurbit plants, would become contaminated and transfer the bacteria to fresh feeding wounds on susceptible plants.

Because of the apparently small numbers of bacteria found in the intestinal tracts of beetles, and the extensive feeding on nonhost plants before cucurbits are available, there seems to be justification for questioning the present concept of the method of survival over winter and the source of primary inoculum. According to Gould (3), the striped cucumber beetle has been recorded as feeding on 68 species of plants in 20 families; but, for 40-50 days in early spring before cucumber plants are available, the beetles feed extensively on the blossoms of early blooming plants, chiefly in the family Rosaceae. These plants should be given more consideration as possible sources of primary inoculum.

The author has no alternative explanation to offer, but the present concept of survival seems to be a weak one for a pathogen for which no other method of survival is known. The problems of survival over winter and the sources of primary inoculum need to be studied further.

LITERATURE CITED

1. BURKHOLDER, W. H. 1960. Some observations on Erwinia tracheiphila, the causal agent of the cucurbit wilt. Phytopathology 50:179-180.
2. CARTER, W. 1962. Insects in relation to plant diseases. Interscience Publishers. New York. 705 p.
3. GOULD, G. E. 1944. The biology and control of the striped cucumber beetle. Indiana Agr. Expt. Sta. Bull. 490.
4. LEACH, J. G. 1933. The method of survival of bacteria in the puparia of the seed-corn maggot. Zeitschr. für Angewandte Entomologie. 20:150-161.
5. LEACH, J. G. 1940. Insect transmission of plant diseases. McGraw-Hill. New York. 615 p.
6. PETRI, L. 1910. Untersuchungen über die Darmbakterien der Olivenfliege. Zentralbl. für Bakt. II 26:357-367.
7. RAND, F. V., and ELLA M. A. ENLOWS. 1920. Bacterial wilt of cucurbits. U.S. Dept. Agr. Tech. Bull. 828.
8. SMITH, E. F. 1911. Bacteria in relation to plant diseases. Carnegie Inst. Publ. 27, 2.

Ref. Zentralblatt für Bakteriologie II
26:357-367 (1910)

69-1725
Translated from German

Original reports from bacteriological and
zymological institutes, laboratories, etc.

Royal Plant Pathology Station, Rome[1]/

RESEARCH ON THE INTESTINAL BACTERIA OF THE OLIVE FLY

by Dr. L. Petri, Rome
(with seven figures)

The digestive apparatus of the larva of <u>Dacus oleae</u>

(Rossi) Meigen, and to be more particular the four blind

pockets of the midgut, contain a large bacteria colony

from the moment the larva emerges from the egg until it

reaches the stage of pupation (Fig. 1). The position

of this large colony in relation to the chitin coating

of the proventriculus and the peritrophic membrane is

1/ This article summarizes a report published by the
   Royal Experimental Station for Plant Pathology in Rome
   under the title "Research on the Intestinal Bacteria
   of the Olive Fly" (in Italian), qto, 130 pages, 1
   table and 37 figures in the text, Rome (G. Bertaro)
   1909.

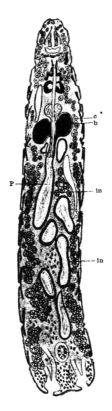

Fig. 1 Half-schematic longitudinal
        section of an adult larva.
        o = blind pockets of the
        midgut, b = bacteria, in =
        midgut, p = peritrophica

such that the bacteria cannot be forced out during moulting (Fig. 2). These micro-organisms multiply continuously and the excess bacteria which have no room in the blind pockets are repeatedly pushed out through the anal opening, following the path of the other ingested substances. In the saliva glands and malpighian vessels there are neither bacteria nor micro-organisms of any other type. In the last instar before pupation, when the larva is still capable of moving, the blind pockets and the rest of the digestive tube are almost completely emptied.

Very few bacteria still remain at the lower opening of the cardia; afterwards they are transferred to the oesophagus, where they lodge between the folds of the intima to remain there throughout the entire histolytic and histogenetic process of the pupa stage. During this time no spore formation has been observed. Before the oesophagus of the imago is completely formed, every trace of bacteria disappears, and the time during which this occurs varies according to the season, being one to two days in summer and early autumn, whilst in

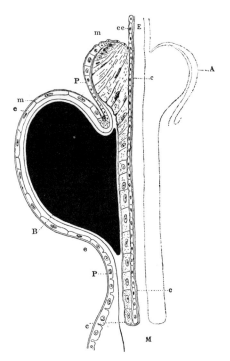

Fig. 2 Schematic longitudinal section of the
upper part of the alimentary tract.
E = oesophagus, oe = oesophagus epithelium, c = cuticula of the proventriculus, P = peritrophica, e = epithelium of the blind pockets, m =
muscle, B = colony of bacteria, M =
midgut

winter it is one, two or even three months. Later, bacteria can be detected in an unpaired glandular dorsal tube in the pharynx (Fig. 3). The bacteria develop in this gland immediately after the birth of the adult insect as a result of the profuse secretory activity of the epithelial cells covering the inner walls of the gland. From here the bacteria spread in the course of a few hours to the midgut, where within 24-48 hours after birth (in summer or autumn) they form a multiplicity of oval conglomerations linked together by a transparent, mucous substance. In the female, bacteria are also to be found in numerous, minute, finger-like anal glands, which unite to form two paired groups just before the anal opening. This opening is at the end of the ovopositor on the abdominal side and opens along with the vagina into a cloaca (Figs. 4 and 5).

In the adult insect, development of the bacteria is totally independent of the food; it depends more on the physiological activity of the insect, particularly - if only indirectly - on the maturity of the sexual organs.

In the case of females emerging during the winter,

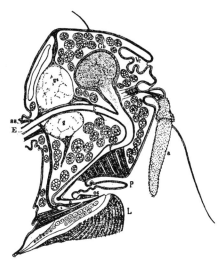

Fig. 3 Schematic longitudinal section (centre) through
head of olive fly.
a = feeler, Gb = pharynx gland filled with
bacteria, F = pharynx (gullet), E = oesophagus,
gs, g = upper, lower pharynx ganglion, P = palp,
O = hypopharynx, os = upper lip, L = labellum,
ss = salivary ducts. The ptillinum (Vo) is
drawn in.

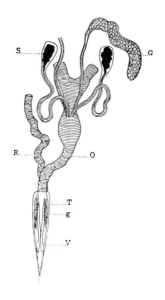

Fig. 4 Part of the female sexual apparatus in <u>Dacus</u>
<u>oleae</u>.
G = ancillary gland (?), g = anal glands, O =
fallopian tubes, R = endgut, S = ovaries, T =
ovipositor, V = cuticular plates limiting the
cloacal furrow

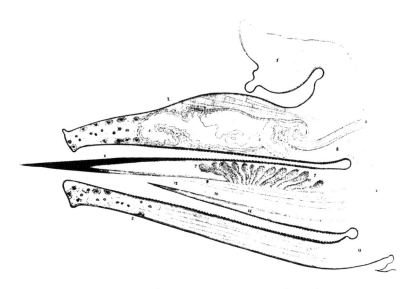

Fig. 5 Longitudinal section of the ovipositor.
1. The 5th abdominal segment
2. The ovipositor opening
3. Opening of the ancillary glands and ovaries
4. Vagina
5. Fallopian tubes
6. Laying duct
7. Anal glands with bacteria
8. Endgut
9. Anus
10. Opening of vagina
11. Paired abdominal plate restricting the cloaca
12. Peritrophica with expelled bacteria

in which the egg forms very slowly, the development of the bacteria in the pharynx gland is considerably delayed. With insects in which this large glandular space is completely empty, the pharynx along with the rest of the intestinal tract is very often subject to infection by parasitic or saprophytic organisms. The transfer of bacteria from the mother to the egg takes place when the egg is laid in the olive, through the separation of a small number of bacteria from the anal glands. Since these glands open near the anus, which is almost in contact with the vagina, micro-organisms can spread over the surface of the egg at the moment it passes through the ovopositor.

During the development of the embryo the bacteria multiply very rapidly around the micropyle owing to a small amount of mucous substance which surrounds the egg, being thicker at the micropyle end (Fig. 6). The bacteria can penetrate to the inside of the egg through the chorion via the numerous air tubes which open around the micropylar thickening (Fig. 7). In the egg yolk and in the developing embryo no bacteria have been found; they are to be found

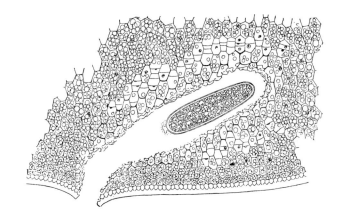

Fig. 6   Section through olive with egg of
         Dacus oleae. The bacteria at the
         micropyle end are proliferating.

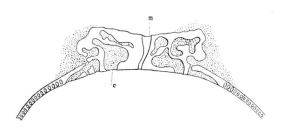

Fig. 7   Section through the micropyle end of
         the chorion.
         m = micropyle, o = airtubes filled
         with bacteria

in the proventriculus, however, in the section corresponding to the beginning of the four blind pockets, at the
time when the larva is still enclosed in the chorion.

In this stage of development the mouth parts are
already fully armed and the larva can cut through part
of the chorion with its hooks. Very probably infection
of the digestive tube in the young larva is attributable
to these punctures; since the bacteria are already present
in the air tubes of the micropyle and have already penetrated the chorion, infection could also have taken place
even if the punctures had been confined to the yolk sac.
Before the larva is born, its midgut bacteria live on
yolk particles.

After a first moulting, which always takes place in
the egg, the larva frees itself from the now unnecessary
cast skin and starts to bore a passage through the soft
parts of the olive whilst the blind pockets of the mid-
gut are almost entirely filled with bacteria. Attempts
to develop an embryo without the presence of bacteria
have all failed completely. All experiments lead to the
hypothesis that the development of the bacteria in the

egg micropyle is quite independent of the development of the embryo itself. Usually the bacteria in the blind sacs do not form a homogeneous colony, and the specific micro-organism which is present in each stage of the insect's development is often joined by Ascobacterium luteum[1]. Its development in the blind sacs of the mid-gut increases with the age of the larva; during the first instars this bacterium is totally absent, but in the later stages it can nearly always be found, often in such large numbers that it alone constitutes a significant part of the bacteria colony. Within limits, the development of Ascobacterium in the digestive tube of the larva is not harmful to the host, and in fact it can even be assumed that the lipolytic effect of this micro-organism is beneficial to the larva: it improves the digestive action of the stomach juices, since the food is mainly

---

[1] Cf. Cornil and Babes, Les Bacteries (Bacteria) 3rd ed., Vol. 1, 1890, pp. 155-158, Figs. 54, 55;
Mace, Traite pratique de bacteriologie (Practical Treatise on Bacteriology), 4th ed., 1901, p. 1018, Pl. XXI;
Petri, Rendiconti d.R. Accad. Lincei. Vol. 14, 1905, p. 400, Vol. 15, 1906- p. 648.

fatty, especially with ripe olives.

This latter effect may be responsible for the fact that Ascobacterium is found in larger numbers in the larval digestive tube during November and December. Or perhaps we should assume that this micro-organism develops and multiplies better because the larval intestine is more susceptible to infection in olives which are often already rotting.

It can indeed be shown in many cases that the Ascobacteria pass through the anal opening into the body of the larva where they may remain in the hindgut, at least to start with, infecting the blind sacs of the mid-gut only later. It is also to be noted that these micro-organisms are much more widely distributed on the olive trees towards the end of the autumn, owing to the fact that the larvae spread out over an extensive area when pupation takes place.

For pathological reasons, this micro-organism can only rarely constitute the entire bacterial content of the intestine. The Ascobacterium can be transferred from the larva to the adult insect; transference from the

the insect to the egg occurs only in rare cases.

It is my opinion that the bacterium normally living symbiotically with Dacus oleae is the same micro-organism that causes rot in olive trees, namely Bacterium savastanoi Smith[1].

This micro-organism is not normally culturable with the olive fly, especially during its development around the egg micropyles in the first instars and in the midgut of the winged insect.

The only way of proving that it is identical with the rot bacillus is to inoculate the olive branches with pharynx gland bacteria from a fly recently born in a sterile medium. Typical rot tuberoles can usually be obtained in this way and by normal processes an organism which is identical with the Bacillus savastanoi can be isolated from them. I was only rarely successful in

---

[1] Cf. United States Department of Agriculture, Bureau of Plant Industry, Bull. No. 131, Washington, 1908; Petri, L., Untersuchungen Uber die Identität des Rotzbacillus des Ölbaumes (Research on Identity of Rot in the Olive Tree) (Central bl. f. Bakt. Abt. II Bd. 19. 1907. p. 531).

isolating it directly from the blind pockets of the larva
and from the alimentary canal of adult insects. In these
cases it is never found alone, but always together with
Ascobacterium luteum, in mixed colonies. These results
are completely analogous with those from previous culture
experiments on the micro-organisms of olive tree rot.
It should be noted, however, that as long as it is not
possible to produce a food substrate on which bacteria
isolated directly from the insect's intestine can be
cultured, the question whether Bacillus savastanoi or
Ascobacterium luteum are both contaminants cannot be
settled once and for all. The other results I have obtained lead me to believe that the rot micro-organism
is the only inhabitant of the Dacus intestine. During
the entire development cycle of the olive fly, therefore,
there is a constant symbiotic relationship with a micro-
organism whose multiplication inside the host depends on
the physiological activity and the anatomic structure of
the host in such a manner that, once separated from it, the
organism can only rarely live saprophytically on artificial
culture plates.

It should not be forgotten that we are dealing here with an hereditary union, which results, in the course of subsequent generations of the micro-organism in question, in the weakening or complete disappearance of certain special characteristics of the primary metabolism of the free original species. A too rapid transition from the symbiotic to the autotrophic, saprophytic state kills it.

When removed from the insect's alimentary tract, the micro-organism can develop again in an artificial medium if it is able to exercise its parasitic properties on some living organism, even a plant (olive tree). It seems to have become a biological necessity for this bacterium to act on living organisms to produce a reaction which modifies the substrate in such a way as to have a beneficial nutritional effect. What then is the significance of this symbiosis?

Is it really a case of two symbionts, with mutually useful complementary properties? Above all we must recognize the parasitic nature of the relationship between the micro-organism and its host. The former certainly finds the most favourable conditions for development in the diverticles of the alimentary tract, both in the larva and in the adult, living on the substances processed by the epithelial cells. B. savastanoi indeed finds its nourishment exclusively in the secretions of the blind pockets of the larva, or in the secretions of the pharynx gland and anal glands in adults, and probably also in the secretions of the vaginal or saliva glands when it develops about the egg micropyle. If these secretions are not present, no proliferation takes place; the death of the insect hinders further development. The parasitic nature of the relationship between this micro-organism and its host is also indicated by the accessibility of the Dacus digestive apparatus to widely differing parasitic organisms.

It has in fact been shown that in adults whose pharynx gland is completely empty owing to delay in the development of B. savastanoi, bacterial or mould infections frequently occur.

The cause of the original infection of the fly's intestine by the rot bacteria is therefore clear, and so is the advantage which this bacterium derives from its parasitic life; but what is the value to the fly which carries this micro-organism? I have already postulated the hypothesis that the secretion of the blind pockets is modified by the metabolic products which B. savastanoi has to eliminate for its further development. In a living larva of Dacus oleae the alimentary tract should in fact present a markedly different picture, as regards the chemical composition of the stomach juices, depending on whether it contains bacteria or not. So far, it has not been possible to demonstrate this fact, and in my opinion every attempt to do so would be fruitless. However, this can clearly be regarded as a possible consequence of an enormous multiplication of this bacterium in a section of the intestines having an exceptional digestive capacity. Whether such qualitative or quantitative changes in the stomach juices are beneficial to the larvae is an un-resolved question. From my investigations it appears that there is never any digestion of bacterial cells in the blind pockets. In this respect, however, I am in some doubt as regards the bacterial cells which, as a result of superfluous proliferation, are continuously eliminated by the blind pockets.

It is my belief, therefore, that one cannot entirely reject the hypothesis that the larva gradually digests the micro-organisms taken up.

In ripe olives the larva is forced to take in a large amount of oil in order to get the necessary nitrogenous substances. An insufficient amount of these substances could be compensated somewhat by digestion of the bacteria which have penetrated into the mesenteron and which under certain conditions are capable of assimilating nitrogen from the air. The oil that finds its way through into the alimentary tract remains for the most part unchanged and is eliminated with the excreta, converted to a fine emulsion and separated into glycerine and fatty acids. The emulsion can be directly observed if the intestinal tract is removed from a feeding larva and is perhaps due to the alkaline salts dissolved in the stomach juice.

In invertebrates it has not yet been possible to demonstrate the presence of gall salts, but it must nevertheless be assumed that the digestive secretions contain alkaline salts like those contained in the gall of the higher animals (phosphates?). According to the old investigations of Plateau, and the more recent ones of Cuenot and Blatta, the fats are broken down in the midgut and its diverticles.[1/] . Insects are thus capable of digesting fats without the help of special micro-organisms, but using the emulsive, lipolytic secretion which is peculiar to the intestinal epithelium.

Many larvae existing on oily endosperm in fact have no intestinal bacteria.

The larvae of the wool moth, which derive their nourishment from a substance which is hardly attacked by the stomach juices, have an alimentary tract completely free of micro-organisms. In the larva of _Dacus oleae_, which requires special nourishment, symbiosis with bacteria capable of processing large quantities of lipase may be very useful, through the accelerated breakdown of triglyceride, especially in larvae living in very ripe olives, where oil forms the main part of the material sucked

_____

[1/] Furth, O. von, Comparative chemical physiology of the lower animals (in German), Jena (G. Fischer) 1903.

up by the larva. It is precisely at this time that a relatively great proliferation of <u>Ascobacterium</u> <u>luteum</u> takes place in the intestine.[1]

The present results of our work force us to be content with such suppositions regarding the biological significance of symbiosis during the larval life of the olive fly. With the completely developed insect the significance is clearer and more important: Janet[2] has observed in certain ants the presence of two-paired, branched, actinie-like pharynx glands which correspond in every respect to the pharynx gland of <u>Dacus</u> <u>oleae.</u> In these diverticles there is usually a nematode (<u>Pelodera</u> <u>janeti</u> Lac. Duthier), which can be

---

[1] At this same time a large amount of alkaline salts is required in the alimentary tract in order to saponify and neutralize the free fatty acids which are present in ripe olives in high proportion. The reaction of the midgut is a proof that this neutralization of fatty acids really takes place. So far we do not know to what extent the presence of the bacteria enhances the processing of these substances required for digesting the ingested food.

[2] Janet, Nematodes in the pharynx glands of ants (in French), Compt. Rend. Acad. Sc., Vol. 117, 1893, p. 700.

regarded as a harmless and hence tolerated parasite. It is frequently but not always present, and other parasites or saprophytes can inhabit the pharynx glands. The saliva glands of _Limax cinereus_, too, are usually inhabited by a worm (_Leptodera flexilis_ Duj.).

These organisms, in which some gland cavities may house harmless parasites, lead us to certain views regarding the biological significance of symbiosis in the life of the olive fly and regarding the possible origin of this union.

The facts observed by Janet with ants[1] show that often certain gland cavities can accommodate different

---

[1] In his work on _Cyclostoma elegans_, Garnault has observed the presence of symbiotic bacilli together with urine products in a closed organ (Claparedas concretion gland) (Anatomic and histological research on _Cyclostoma elegans_ (in French), 1887). Giard has also observed similar symbiosis phenomena in the completely closed kidney organs of ascidia (molgulid group). The kidney parasite _Nephromyces_ Gd. apparently renders the host a great service by freeing the kidneys of excretion products; these products would otherwise very quickly clog the kidneys as the latter have no outlets (_Nephromyces_, a new kind of parasitic fungus in the kidney of molgulids (in French), Compt. Rend. Acad. Sc. 1888).

micro-organisms as a result of their special position.

These micro-organisms may be either harmful or harmless; in the first case they are difficult to detect because of the rapid disappearance of the hosts. Cases, however, where the antagonism between the two symbiotic organisms is practically zero and the parasite is tolerated without harmful effects are much easier to find.

Under certain conditions of life the olive fly shows a surprising similarity to the ants investigated by Janet. In insects emerging in the water or at the beginning of spring the intestinal bacteria develop late and slowly so that the pharynx gland remains quite empty even though it may be completely formed and its epithelium secreting. As a result, it can be very easily attacked by the parasitic or saprophytic micro-organisms taken in with the food.

Among these micro-organisms, one species of Torula has a fatal effect on the fly: it multiplies enormously in the alimentary tract, causing the insect's death within a few hours. Even Ascobacterium luteum, which under normal conditions of life is harmless for the summer generations, may cause the death of flies emerging in the winter or at the beginning of spring.

If the pharynx gland is completely filled with proliferating B. savastanoi, no other micro-organism except Ascobacterium seems able to develop there; as I have already proved, however, the latter can never be harmful to the fly if its proliferation is restricted by the opposing effect of the rot bacillus. In this way B. savastanoi protects Dacus oleae against the penetration of micro-organisms into the digestive apparatus from outside and against their harmful consequences. The large pharynx gland with its special secretions would always be susceptible to dangerous infections without the presence of its specific bacillus. The mortality of flies emerging in the winter or at the beginning of spring is often very high, owing to the failure of B. savastanoi to develop (or to develop as fast as it should) during the first moments of life when the search for food and its uptake are particularly intensive. This delay in the reappearance of the symbiotic micro-organism in the intestine of the adult insect seems to be related to slow egg formation or spermatogenesis in the male. The sexual organs of the females are usually slower to mature. Apart from this indirect factor the low temperature also has an effect on the bacteria. The flies live even during the coldest winters, whereas B. savastanoi can only multiply at moderate temperatures (well above zero). One can even say that at 5°C it does not at all intents and purposes proliferate at all.

The above-mentioned examples of pharynx glands in which harmless parasites can exist, and the irregular nature of this symbiosis, indicate that although there is no pronounced antagonism between host and parasite, one must be very careful in regarding such unions as the result of a deep-rooted and necessary mutualism.

At the same time, however, these instructive examples help to explain a symbiosis in which, as with the olive fly, the two organisms have become inseparable. Although the digestive apparatus of this insect, especially the female, is remarkably suited for the development and reproduction of the micro-organism, we must avoid regarding this as a cause-and-effect relationship. I have already stressed that the formation of the pharynx gland is quite independent of any irritating and modifying effect which the bacteria may have during histogenesis in the reconstruction of the foregut walls. If the bacteria developed earlier and were localized in the pharynx region, we could assume that a blind pocket diverticle was formed at this point through protrusion due to proliferation. During formation of the imago however, the bacteria are in a completely latent state and there is a complete absence of irritant effect. The pharynx gland, like most of the head organs, is produced through the differentiation of a special imaginal disc. Likewise, the characteristic end of the rectum in the female is in no way due to the effect of bacteria.

Although, with Dacus oleae and in many other cases, we must be satisfied with the mere observation of facts since exact explanations cannot be found, we can still assume, on the basis of the processes occurring not only with other insects but also with plant and animal organisms living symbiotically with micro-organisms, that species now serving as hosts have, since their very origin, possessed certain structural characteristics which serve to promote or produce the parasitic action of micro-organisms living as saprophytes in the external medium.

Although we have no explanation at the moment, we could regard these unusual examples of tolerance vis-a-vis harmless parasites as the result of natural selection, since during the alternation of generations the only unions that have persisted to the present day are those in which symbiosis is based not only on tolerance but also on mutually useful properties. The fact that with some animal or plant organisms either the digestive system or the external appearance is quite different from what is typical of related species in the same systematic group may point to a secondary change. With the olive fly, however, the alimentary tract has anatomical characteristics differing greatly from the other Muscids, and it is difficult to believe that such pronounced changes are only secondary and have taken place only to promote the symbiotic conditions between the intestinal bacteria.

In nature we find all stages between symbiotic mutualism and true parasitism; the examples mentioned above and the facts we have presented regarding <u>Dacus</u> <u>oleae</u> show that in this case symbiosis must be based on parasitism coupled with special host properties of the insect. It is my opinion that with the olive fly the basic reason for the symbiosis is to be found in the special structure of the digestive apparatus. The type of micro-organism taken up can perhaps be regarded as having a secondary significance.

If the parasites were really older than the species they attack, we would have to regard the olive fly as the initial cause of olive-tree rot. This would mean that the insect constituted a double menace to the plant, since the latter serves to accommodate, and make possible the proliferation of, the micro-organism which is the fly's doughtiest ally in its fight for existence.

As regards methods of combatting olive fly in the agricultural sector, the results produced by the present research on the biology of these insects are of no help; nevertheless, I should like to point out that my results explain a number of aspects of the life of <u>Dacus</u> <u>oleae</u> which have so far been rather obscure, for instance the

fact that in certain years the flies are reduced in
numbers even though this cannot be attributed entirely to
the direct effect of cold or to other influences on the
winter pupae. It is my opinion that this irregularity
in the development period from one year to another is due
to the fact that, as a result of the cold delaying the
opening of the pupae, the vitality of the micro-organisms,
always diminished during pupation, is reduced still
further so that the flies are without the specific micro-
organisms immediately after emergence and even for a period
of several days. Even if the micro-organisms had been
transferred alive to the adult insect, their development
in the pharynx diverticle would be delayed through the
cold.

I think it is highly likely, or even almost certain,
that under such circumstances real epidemic infections
take place, and that in a given zone the number of insects
emerging in the winter or at the beginning of spring is
greatly reduced. These winter insects of course play
an important part in preserving the species from one year
to the next. Future research on the digestive apparatus

of the olive fly, especially in the spring generations, will thus be of practical, as well as theoretical, interest.

Another important question is whether with all _Dacus_ species the digestive apparatus is formed like that of _Dacus oleae_, and if so whether it is inhabited by the same or by other micro-organisms.

Research in this direction has also indicated the presence of bacteria in the larval intestine of _Dacus longistilus_, a parasite of _Olea chrysophylla_.

INTRODUCTION TO SECTION IV:
INSECT-FUNGUS RELATIONSHIPS

Fungi are the most numerous plant pathogens with which man must contend. Most fungi have effective means of dissemination and few depend upon insect vectors for their spread. Insects do, however, play a significant role as vectors of fungus pathogens. In some cases insects act as accidental vectors acquiring and disseminating fungus spores during pollinating or nectar collecting activities. The classical paper by Sturgis (1898) describes such a relationship. In other instances a closer relationship exists between fungi and their insect vectors. The two biological entities live in close contact for prolonged periods and sometimes the relationship appears to be mutually beneficial. The paper by Leach et al. (1938) describes such a relationship between bark beetles and blue stain fungi. A similar relationship may exist between the Dutch elm disease fungus and its bark beetle vectors. Parke et al. (1941) discuss the important aspects of _Ceratocystis ulmi_ transmission by bark beetles.

Some fungi, such as the Dutch elm disease-pathogen, are vectored by one or two specific insect species. Others may be vectored by numerous insects. The recent paper by Hinds (1972) illustrates the latter case in which numerous insect species vector a fungal pathogen.

Whether insect transmission of pathogenic fungi is strictly accidental or a closer biological relationship exists, insects do increase the efficiency of fungal pathogens. They may increase the effective range of a pathogen, deposit inoculum in infection courts protected from adverse environmental conditions, provide wounds which serve as avenues of infection, or protect inoculum from adverse conditions in transit. Insects also conserve fungal inoculum by carrying it in a positive manner from susceptible host to susceptible host. When wind or water serves as the agent of dissemination the process is random and much inoculum is wasted when it falls on non susceptible hosts. We have attempted to include papers in this section which describe most of these vector-fungus relationships.

ON SOME ASPECTS OF VEGETABLE PATHOLOGY AND THE CONDITIONS WHICH INFLUENCE THE DISSEMINATION OF PLANT DISEASES

W. C. Sturgis.

The modern vegetable pathologist finds himself confronted at the very outset of his investigations by many preliminary questions which he is obliged to answer more or less satisfactorily before he can recommend with any degree of certainty a definite line of preventive or curative treatment.

He must be familiar with the main principles of vegetable physiology in general and the normal anatomy and histology of the special plant under consideration, in order that he may decide when and how the general course of the physiological activities of the plant is disturbed, and whether the structure which he observes is normal or otherwise. In case the anatomy is evidently morbid, he must be prepared to diagnose the case with as great a degree of accuracy as possible. Let us suppose that, as a result of extended observations upon one plant or a series of plants showing similar symptoms of disease, he finds that a particular organism is generally or constantly associated with the disease. I pass over the large class of cases in which no such organism is observed, and in which therefore the pathologist must put all his knowledge to the test, examine the environment with the utmost attention to detail, exhaust all his resources, and test every possible theory in his search for operative causes.

But, having found a possible connection between the diseased condition under observation and a living organism, the arduous portion of his work begins, viz., the determination of the parasitism or the mere saprophytism of the organism in question. For it is not enough merely to observe the associa-

BOTANICAL GAZETTE, 1898, Vol. 25, pp. 187-194.

tion of a living organism of fungous or bacterial nature with the diseased condition, no matter how intimate or constant such association may be. Of course, there may be cases, such as the "black-knot" of plum trees, in which the effect of the fungus is so apparent and its parasitic nature so manifest that the evidence of the unaided eye is almost conclusive (though even in this case it will be remembered that for years the knots were supposed to be caused by insects), but in the vast majority of cases a far more searching proof is necessary. The organism whose parasitic nature is in question must be isolated from its host and grown in a pure culture; thence it must be transferred with due care to the uninjured tissues of a healthy plant of the same species as that from which it was derived, growing under normal conditions; in this plant it must produce symptoms of disease identical with those originally observed; and, finally, from this plant the same organism must again be isolated. Only under the fulfillment of such conditions can an organism be stamped as an absolute parasite.

These are rules made familiar to us by the methods of modern bacteriology, but they too seldom enter into the practice of the vegetable pathologist. It may be said in passing that their fulfillment cannot always be attained. It is more than probable that only an extremely small proportion of the diseases of plants which are commonly attributed to fungous parasites are absolutely parasitic in their nature — that is, due to organisms which can attack and penetrate the uninjured tissues of healthy plants growing under normal conditions, and live therein at the expense and to the detriment of the host. In most cases the pathologist must be prepared to search for injured tissues offering an opportunity for saprophytic, followed possibly by parasitic attacks, or for unfavorable surroundings weakening the plant or rendering it peculiarly susceptible to the attacks of semiparasitic organisms. Such conditions are easily induced, and great care has to be exercised in drawing conclusions from results obtained in the laboratory or greenhouse from inoculations of wounded tissues of plants kept under conditions of warmth and moisture which seldom, if ever, obtain in the field. The pathologist must be prepared to ascertain and to correct the predisposing as well as the apparent causes of disease, and among such causes he may even be forced to include the long process of artificial selection which has had as its almost exclusive aim the development of plants along lines of fruitage only, with too little regard to those factors which tend to produce hardy stock resistant to unfavorable conditions.

I make these statements with some hesitation, yet I believe them to be borne out by facts. It is becoming more and more apparent that in combating the host of fungi which invade our orchards and truck farms in these days of intensive farming, due regard must be paid to what we may call the hygiene of plant life. The proper regulation of the water supply by drainage and tillage; the securing of the free access of air and sunlight by pruning, thinning, and training; care in the selection of healthy, resistant stock; the intelligent use of fertilizers and their adaptation to the needs of the plant—these are some of the sanitary measures which, duly considered and acted upon, will do more than the mere use of fungicides to insure success in dealing with fungous diseases.

To take individual proofs of these general statements: Experiments recently conducted at the Rhode Island Experiment Station have gone far to show that the two most serious diseases of celery are due, not primarily to the attacks of the fungi associated with them, though both of them might properly be placed among Sorauer's "Schwäche-Parasiten," but to a weakening of the plants attributable to the purely artificial level method of culture whereby the roots are exposed to all the temperature-changes of the surface soil. A mulch, consisting even of the leaves of diseased celery teeming with the spores of the fungi in question, served to prevent the spread of the disease. That proper attention to purely cultural conditions will very largely decrease the prevalence of apple "scab" is a matter of common observation, and I have myself seen a peach orchard, showing the first symptons of a serious attack of *Cercospora Persica*, completely restored to health by tillage and a judicious application of nitrate of soda. I would direct the attention of every vegetable pathologist to the words in which Professor Bailey summarizes one of his bulletins on the care of orchards, and to the order of the terms which he uses, " Till, feed, prune, spray." I have outlined the steps which the vegetable pathologist must take in order to secure a trustworthy diagnosis. Having learned to distinguish a morbid condition through a working acquaintanceship with normal physiology and anatomy, he must determine the final cause of disease; by careful investigation he must decide whether it is parasitic or otherwise, and, if so, in what degree; and he must determine whether the attack of the parasite is immediate, or superinduced by the local destruction of tissues or by the general debility of the plant.

One very important question remains to be considered, viz., When and how the parasite, if such it be, secures entrance to the host and is thence disseminated. Upon the answer to this question depends in great measure the whole philosophy of preventive treatment. One method of determining the matter is, of course, the careful study of the life history of the fungus in question. If it be known, with a reasonable degree of certainty, that a certain pathogenic fungus depends largely upon aerial summer-spores for its dissemination, we naturally recommend preventive treatment with fungicides; if it is a perennial mycelium to which the fungus owes its continuous vitality, we are prepared to advise pruning. If it is ascertained that certain spores, seemingly delicate, are enabled to pass uninjured through an animal's digestive tract, the manure heap demands our first attention; and if careful research in the field and the laboratory is at length rewarded by the discovery of resistant spores produced during the winter in or upon the refuse of a diseased crop, we very properly lay the utmost stress upon a thorough cleaning up and destruction of all such refuse. A knowledge of such facts connected with parasitic fungi is absolutely essential to any intelligent application of preventive measures, and we cannot value too highly such researches as those of Thaxter upon "potato-scab," or of Aderhold upon the ascosporic forms of *Fusi-*

cladium dendriticum, and *F. pyrinum*.   But fruitful results are also to be obtained by observations upon the direct means by which the reproductive bodies of parasitic fungi are borne hither and thither and become fresh sources of contagion.

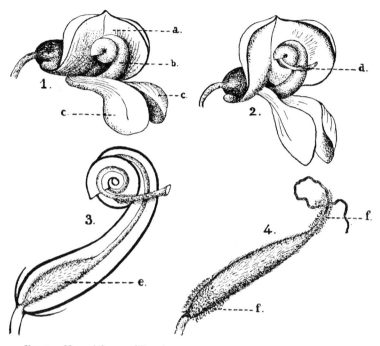

FIG. 1.—Normal flower of lima bean.
FIG. 2.—The same, with wing-petals depressed and style protruded.
FIG. 3.—Section of keel, showing the ovary and protruded style.
FIG. 4.—Young pod, showing mildew at the two extremities.

This leads me to speak of a rather striking case which came under my observation during the past summer.   For several years the growers of lima beans in southern Connecticut have suffered great losses through the destructive attacks of the mildew, *Phytophthora Phaseoli* Thaxter. This fungus attacks the pods, sometimes covering them with its white, felt-like mycelium ; it also occurs upon the leaves, though rarely and inconspicuously, and upon the fruiting branches where it does extensive injury by destroying the tissues below the flowers, thus causing the death of all the young pods above the point of attack. Before proceeding farther let us recall the structure of the bean flower. It will be remembered that the pistil and the stamens are completely enclosed in the spirally coiled keel (*fig. 1*). No portion of them is exposed to view except the very base of the ovary, and that only when the surrounding petals are forced apart. Under these conditions not only would close-fertilization seem to be assured, but it would appear certain that, however the mildew gained access to the host, it certainly could not be by infection of any part of the pistil before the fall of the flower. Yet, continuous observation convinced me that the mildew failed to appear to any serious degree before the flowers began to expand, that fairly mature pods seldom showed areas of fresh infection, that the young pods often showed a copious growth of fruiting hyphæ and spores indicative of infection before the fall of the blossom, and that the points of infection were always at the extreme base or tip of the young pods. These observations led to the supposition that insects were mainly responsible for the dissemination of the mildew.

Further investigation confirmed this view. I have called attention to the enclosed and protected position occupied by the pistil; this obtains until the flower is visited by an insect of considerable size, generally a honeybee. The projecting wing-petals offer a convenient landing place, and, as the bee alights on them, his weight deflects both wings and keel, the style is protruded from the keel, the bee's abdomen brushes over it, and in his efforts to reach the bottom of the flower the petals are forced apart, the base of the ovary exposed and the bee's head comes in contact with it (*figs. 2, 3*). Thus cross-fertilization is secured, but if the bee has, by chance, touched a mildewed pod with either head or abdomen, fungous infection no less surely occurs. It will be noted that the only portions of the pistil touched by the bee are the base of the ovary and the style. An examination of scores of flowers showed that in the majority of cases they were infected, and in these cases, without exception, the points of infection were identical with the spots touched by the bees (*fig. 4*). One additional point might be mentioned. On a very badly diseased plantation it was noticeable that the spread of the mildew practically ceased about September 10, although the vines continued to flower and produce pods until October. I am at a loss to account for this sudden cessation of fungous activity, but it is worthy of notice in this connection that after the date above mentioned hardly any bees were seen in the plantation.

It seems almost certain then, that in the case of this mildew at least, insects are the principal agents in the dissemination of the fungus.

But I have already stated that the fungus sometimes appears elsewhere than upon the young pods. In some cases it is apparent from the respective positions of old and fresh points of infection upon the leaves or mature pods that the spores have been carried by the rain or dripping dew from one portion of the vine to a subjacent one, but certain facts led me to think that the wind played a considerable part in the infection of older tissues. In order to test this matter I pursued the following course. The mildew is usually confined to comparatively low, damp situations. The grounds of the Connecticut Experiment Station occupy an elevated position, the land is well drained, the soil light and sandy, and so far as I know, lima beans on this land have never mildewed. During the past summer they occupied two rows running east and west. Directly south of them, at a distance of about 100 feet, were two rows of bush limas running north and south (*fig. 5*). On August 14, when the mildew had been abundant for a month or more on a farm at a distance of about a mile in a straight line from the Station, the Station vines were carefully examined and found to be perfectly free from mildew. The following day two mildewed pods were brought from the farm above mentioned, and the mildewed surface of one of them was rubbed upon a single healthy and almost mature pod at the east end of each row of pole limas. The prevailing winds at the time and for the ten succeeding days varied from northwest to northeast. Within a week the mildew appeared abundantly upon the two infected pods and from this point swept down both rows from east to west, and in two weeks the crop was practically ruined. Meantime the two rows of bush limas were examined daily. About ten days after the first infection of the pole limas, mildewed pods were found upon the bush limas, but only at the north end of the

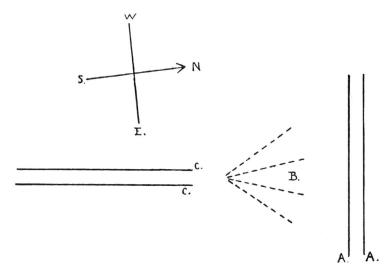

Fig. 5.— *A, A,* points of primary artificial infection on pole beans; *B,* course of prevailing winds; *C, C,* points of secondary natural infection on bush beans.

rows nearest to the source of infection. From this point it spread rapidly southward until both rows were completely involved.

The conclusion seems inevitable that not only do insects play an important part in the dissemination of fungous diseases, but that the wind certainly does its share.

How this particular fungus is propagated from season to season is a question of great importance, but it is apart from the object of the present paper which is to call renewed attention to the divers lines along which the vegetable pathologist is obliged to direct his attention, and the importance and interest which attaches to all observations relative to the dissemination of fungous diseases.

THE INTERRELATIONSHIPS OF BARK BEETLES AND BLUE-STAINING FUNGI IN FELLED NORWAY PINE TIMBER [1]

By J. G. Leach, *associate plant pathologist and botanist*, L. W. Orr, *instructor in forest entomology*, and Clyde Christensen, *assistant forest pathologist, Minnesota Agricultural Experiment Station* [2]

INTRODUCTION

It is a well-known fact that trees injured by fire or heavy defoliation, or those felled by wind or in the course of lumbering operations, are very susceptible to attack by bark beetles, wood borers, and fungi. Such timber deteriorates rapidly and is often rendered almost worthless in one season. This fact is very important in forestry operations where it becomes necessary to leave cut logs in the woods for a season or more before they are taken to a mill.

The rapidity with which such timber may decline has been pointed out by Boyce (*1*),[3] who made a study of the deterioration of western yellow-pine trees felled in connection with control of the western pine beetle. He showed that the sapwood of such trees was completely blue-stained by the end of the first season after felling. Decay was also very rapid, especially in the sapwood, but was more pronounced the second season. However, Boyce did not mention any relationship between the bark beetles and the development of the stains and decay.

Graham (*6*), in a study of the felled tree trunk as an ecological unit, found that there was a definite succession of insects and fungi in the log as the chemical and physical character of the wood changed during the process of disintegration and decay. He pointed out that along with the insects typical of each region and stage of decomposition of the log there also were fungi equally typical of the parts where they occur. He further observed (*6, p. 399*) that "In some cases there is a distinct symbiotic relationship between wood inhabiting insects and fungi, as in the case of the ambrosia beetles; and in many other instances a looser type of symbiosis can be demonstrated." The details of these relationships, however, were not studied. The work reported in the present paper is the result of one phase of a project planned to study in some detail the interrelations of certain insects and fungi attacking felled logs kept under more or less controlled conditions.

PLAN OF EXPERIMENTS

The field experiments, initiated in the spring of 1931, were carried out at the Lake Itasca Forest Forestry Biology Station, Arago, Minn. Because of its long, smooth bole and relative freedom from

Paper no. 1228 of the Journal Series of the Minnesota Agricultural Experiment Station. Cooperative investigations by the Division of Plant Pathology and Botany and the Division of Entomology and Economic Zoology. Supported in part by a grant from the research funds of the Graduate School of the University of Minnesota.

[2] The writers wish to express their appreciation to Dr. Louise Dosdall for assistance in identifying some of the fungi and to Vera Koerper for assistance in the histological studies and for the drawings made from them.

[3] Reference is made by number (italic) to Literature Cited, p. 340.

JOURNAL OF AGRICULTURAL RESEARCH, 1934, Vol. 49, pp. 315-342.

limb scars, Norway pine, *Pinus resinosa* Ait., was chosen for the study. Healthy standing trees of suitable size were selected and felled on May 18 and 19. The trunks were immediately cut into logs 40 inches long and 7 to 12 inches in diameter. These logs, after treatment as indicated below, were placed in position under a slanting roof made of laths spaced so as to provide approximately 50 percent shade. The logs were placed upon wooden supports so that the north end was about 6 to 8 inches and the south end about 4 inches above the ground. The wooden supports had previously been painted with a copper

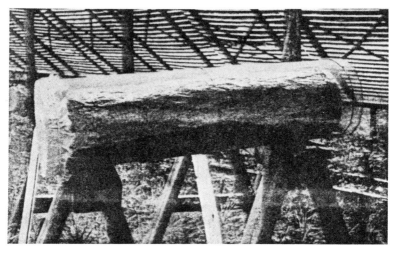

FIGURE 1.—A log from series C, sealed and enclosed in an 18-mesh screen-wire cage.

sulphate and linseed-oil paint as a precaution against spread of decay from the supports to the logs.

The logs were divided into 6 series of 8 logs each, except the check series, in which there were 16 logs. Each series was handled differently, as follows:

A. Not caged; no treatment (check series).

B. Not caged; ends and limb scars disinfected with a 2-percent aqueous solution of ethyl mercury chloride, then sealed with roofing pitch and covered with burlap.

C. Same as series B but enclosed in a cage of 18-mesh aluminum-coated screen wire (fig. 1).

D. No end treatment but enclosed in a cage of 18-mesh screen wire.

E. Not caged; ends and limb scars sprayed at frequent intervals throughout the summer seasons with a 2-percent aqueous solution of ethyl mercury chloride.

F. Same as series E but enclosed in a cage of 18-mesh screen wire.

It was planned that series A should serve as a check series, duplicating as nearly as possible the conditions in nature, being exposed to normal insect attack and any fungus spores disseminated by them as well as to infection by wind-blown spores through the exposed ends and limb scars.

Series B was designed to eliminate infection by wind-blown spores but to leave the logs exposed to normal insect attack. Thus, any fungus infection would be due to inoculum introduced by insects or entering through holes made by the insects.

In series C elimination of both fungus infection and insect attack was attempted.

Series D was planned to eliminate insect attack but to leave the logs exposed to infection by wind-blown spores.

Since logs sealed with pitch and burlap, as in series B and C, would obviously maintain a higher moisture content than unsealed logs and since this treatment might influence the results, the ends of the logs in series E and F were sprayed with a solution of ethyl mercury chloride but not sealed. This treatment, as was determined later, effectively prevented infection through the exposed ends and did not interfere with the normal drying of the logs.

One-fourth of the logs of each series were to be removed for examination at the end of each summer for 4 successive years. In this way the progress of insect attack and fungus infection under the different conditions could be followed and any associations between insect and fungus could be detected.

A record was kept of the particular tree from which each log was cut and the logs were so distributed in each series that any differences in results due to differences in individual trees would be evident. Each log was weighed at frequent intervals throughout the summer in order to determine the variations in weight.

In addition to the experiment outlined above, other experiments were started from time to time in which freshly cut logs were treated and caged, as in series C and F, and into which individual species of insects were introduced. In this way logs sealed against infection by wind-blown spores were subjected to attacks by individual species of insects. Thus the association between a given insect and fungus could be studied without being complicated by the presence of other insects or fungi.

Throughout the course of the investigation the progressive development of the insects and fungi was observed in logs that were barked and cut up at suitable intervals. Cultures of fungi were made from the logs and from the insects in various stages of development. Also insects in various stages of development were killed and embedded in paraffin for histological examination in order to determine the more intimate relationships between the insects and associated fungi. In this way it was hoped to gain a fairly accurate picture of the association of the insects and the fungi involved in the deterioration of the logs.

Two species of bark beetles, *Ips pini* Say and *I. grandicollis* Eich, were among the first insects to attack the exposed logs. This paper presents the results of a study of these two beetles and the fungi associated with them in their development in the logs.

LITERATURE RELATING TO BARK BEETLES AND BLUE STAIN

Apparently the bluing of timber was first described in 1878 by Hartig (8), who recognized its fungal nature and also mentioned the presence of insects in trees affected with blue stain. Münch (12), MacCallum (11), Wilson (20), and others in later years observed the association of blue stain with insect injury, but, apparently, made no study of the nature of the association. Von Schrenk (19), in 1903, investigated more closely the relation of insects to the spread of blue stain. In addition to describing in detail the development of blue stain in and about the tunnels of *Dendroctonus ponderosae* Hopk., in trees of the western yellow pine, *Pinus ponderosa* Lawson, Von Schrenk dissected a number of beetles and attempted to isolate the blue-stain fungus from the intestinal tract and from feces. He failed to obtain the blue-stain fungus but found a characteristic bacterium present. He considered these trials "by no means conclusive for they were not exhaustive" and more work on a larger scale was projected, but the results were never published. The blue-stain fungus described by Von Schrenk was *Ceratostomella pilifera* (Fr.) Wint., and Rumbold (*17, p. 848*) is of the opinion that "possibly *C. pilifera* was a secondary blue stain in the wood that he used for starting his cultures and that the fungus that first stained it had lost its vitality by the time the wood reached the laboratory." This error and his failure to isolate the fungus from the beetles probably are responsible for Von Schrenk's conclusion (*19, p. 18*) that

The spores of the "blue" fungus are probably blown about by the wind in countless thousands, and at the time of the beetle attack in July and August some of the spores lodge in the holes made in the bark of the living pine tree by the bark and wood-boring beetles.

After Von Schrenk's work in 1903 very little attention was given to this insect and fungus association until 1928, when Craighead (*5*) called attention to the constant association between tree-killing bark beetles (*Dendroctonus*) and blue stain. Craighead pointed out that the girdling of the trees by the bark beetles was not sufficient to cause the rapid death of the trees and suggested a symbiotic relation between bark beetle and blue-stain fungus in which the later contributed to the death of the tree. This was soon followed by the experiments of Nelson and Beal (*15*) and the more extensive studies of Nelson,[4] which showed that the girdling of pines by the tunnels of the bark beetles was insufficient to account for the rapid death of the tree. He showed by experimental inoculations that the blue-stain fungi would kill pines in a relatively short time without the help of the beetles, death being caused by the stoppage of sap flow through the stained wood. Nelson was able to isolate the blue-stain fungus from the bodies of beetles, and he concluded that it was commonly introduced under the bark by them.

Using material furnished by Craighead, as well as other material collected from various parts of the United States, Rumbold (*17*) found that *Ceratostomella pini* Münch was constantly associated with the attacks of *Dendroctonus frontalis* Zimm. and *D. brevicomis* Lec., and that a new species, *C. ips* Rumbold, was associated with *Ips grandicollis* and *I. calligraphus* Germ.

None of the above-named authors studied in detail the nature of the symbiosis between the beetles and the blue-stain fungi. However, a recent paper by Grosmann (*7*), who was working in Germany, deals in considerable detail with the nature of the symbiosis between bark beetles and fungi. She pointed out that the bark beetles carry yeasts as well as the blue-stain fungi, a fact also demonstrated by

[4] NELSON, R. M. EXPERIMENTS WITH BLUESTAIN FUNGI IN SOUTHERN PINES. Thesis, Ph.D., Univ. Minn. 1930. (In press.)

Person (*16*). Grosmann concluded that the insects are in no way dependent upon either the blue-stain fungi or the yeasts. They were considered as commensals.

RESULTS OF THE EXPERIMENTS

EXPERIMENTAL EVIDENCE THAT BLUE-STAIN FUNGI ARE INTRODUCED INTO THE LOGS BY BARK BEETLES

In the study of the relation of an insect to the spread and development of a disease, it is the authors' opinion that, in order to prove conclusively that an insect is an agent of dissemination and inoculation, the disease should be produced experimentally by visitation of the insect under controlled conditions with adequate checks. Although frequent or constant association of the insect with the disease may leave little doubt as to the role played by the insect, the proof is not complete until the relationship has been experimentally demonstrated. Insofar as the writers know this has not been done for the bark beetles and blue stain. One of the objects of these experiments was to determine to what extent bark beetles are dissemination and inoculation agents of blue stain.

The exposed logs that were not caged were found to be infested by bark beetles the latter part of May, only a few days after they were cut and put into position. The development of these and other beetles and the associated fungi was studied by frequent examination of extra logs exposed for that purpose.

On September 18, 1931, approximately 4 months after the experiment was started, the first set of 16 logs was removed and examined. The bark was removed from each log and the degree of insect infestation and the amount of blue stain and other fungus infection were noted. In doing this a 5-inch section of each end of the 40-inch log was disregarded, all notes being made on the central 30 inches. Since there was some variation in the size of the logs, the surface area of this region was recorded for each log. The degree and nature of insect and fungus infestation of each log are given in table 1. Additional evidence confirming the data given in table 1 was obtained from similar logs opened in the two following years and from logs opened while studying the progressive development of beetles and fungi, but since the evidence of association is so clear cut the detailed notes are given for one series only.

It will be seen from table 1 that blue stain always followed the attack of the 2 species of *Ips* and was absent from the logs that were protected from the insects by wire cages. Also, in those logs that became infested with only a few bark beetles that managed to get into the cages, the stain was limited to the immediate vicinity of the *Ips* tunnels, while the remainder of the log was free from stain. One log from each of the six different treatments was photographed, and these are shown in figure 2. Of particular interest is the log representing series D, in which is shown one nuptial chamber of *I. grandicollis* with one short side channel. Observe that blue stain has developed around this tunnel but is absent elsewhere. In figure 3 are shown cuts into logs from series E and F showing the development of blue stain in logs infested with *Ips* and the absence of stain in logs free of insect infestation.

237

TABLE 1.—*Degree and nature of insect infestation and fungus infection of the logs 4 months after the beginning of the experiment*

Log no.	Treatment and other data	Insect infestation	Fungus infection	Remarks
1	Not caged; no end treatment; surface area 735 square inches; tree no. 5.	Ips pini, 11 broods; I. grandicollis, 7 broods; Monochamus sp., 11 tunnels; Ithagium sp., 3 larvae; buprestid larvae, 2; a few small unidentified tunnels.	Blue stain abundant, but overgrown by dense mycelial mats of Peniophora gigantea; Ceratostomella perithecia source; yeast and a few unidentified fungi present; some green mold (Trichoderma koningi) in older tunnels; bark very loose.	Peniophora apparently entered through exposed ends, and by rapid invasion of sapwood inhibited the normal development of blue stain.
2	Not caged; no end treatment; surface area 787.5 square inches; tree no. 7.	I. pini, 7 broods; I. grandicollis, 12 broods; Monochamus sp., 8 tunnels; buprestid larvae, 2.	Essentially the same as no. 1.	Essentially the same as no. 1.
3	Not caged; no end treatment; surface area 712.5 square inches; tree no. 5.	I. pini, 18 broods; I. grandicollis, 8 broods; Monochamus sp., 12 tunnels; buprestid larvae, 3; Ithagium sp., 2 larvae.	do	Do.
4	Not caged; no end treatment; surface area 682.5 square inches; tree no. 3.	I. pini, 18 broods; I. grandicollis, 7 broods; Monochamus sp., 17 tunnels; buprestid larvae, 5; Ithagium sp., 3 larvae.	do	Do.
7	Not caged; ends and limb scars sealed with pitch and burlap; surface area 817.5 square inches; tree no. 2.	I. pini, 43 broods; I. grandicollis, 17 broods; Monochamus sp., 15 tunnels; Ithagium sp., 3 larvae; buprestid larvae, 30.	Blue stain and yeast abundant and closely associated with Ips tunnels; other fungus infection insignificant or absent; bark loose.	Moisture content of the log much greater than that of logs with ends not sealed.
8	Not caged; ends and limb scars sealed with pitch and burlap; surface area 697.5 square inches; tree no. 6.	I. pini, 51 broods; I. grandicollis, 4 broods; Monochamus sp., 17 tunnels; buprestid larvae, 11.	do	Do.
9	Caged; ends and limb scars sealed with pitch and burlap, surface area 712.5 square inches; tree no. 6.	None	No blue stain present; 2 small spots of inner bark stained with a fungus forming small black sclerotia but no spores; apparently entering through minute cracks in the bark; bark not loose.	Do.
10	Caged; ends and limb scars sealed with pitch and burlap; surface area 705 square inches; tree no. 2.	do	No blue stain or other fungus infection; 100 percent clean; bark not loose.	Do.
11	Caged; no end treatment; surface area 735 square inches; tree no. 2.	I. grandicollis, 3 broods	Blue stain present only about tunnels of I. grandicollis. Some infection with a white basidiomycete (P. gigantea) entering through exposed ends; bark not loose.	One end of the cage was closed with muslin, a method which proved not to be always proof against smaller beetles; slower development of Peniophora as compared to logs 1–4 probably due to absence of Ips.
12	Caged; no end treatment; surface area 742.5 square inches; tree no. 7.	I. grandicollis, 3 broods, which developed only to egg-channel stage; Pissodes sp., 17 pupal chambers.	Blue stain and yeast associated with Ips egg channels but absent elsewhere; small amount of infection by Peniophora near exposed ends; bark not loose.	Do.

238

13	Not caged; ends and limb scars sprayed at intervals with ethyl mercury chloride; surface area 840 square inches; tree no. 5.	I. pini, 31 broods; I. grandicollis, 10 broods; Monochamus sp., 10 tunnels; buprestid larvae, 11; Rhagium sp., 4 larvae.	Blue stain and yeast abundant; spreading and fruiting to within 1 inch of ends, where it was checked by spray applied to end of log; some Trichoderma and other secondary fungi present; stain associated with Monochamus and buprestid tunnels only when these made contact with Ips tunnels; bark loose.	Spray applied at intervals to end of logs very effective against fungus infection, at the same time allowing the log to dry as rapidly as logs with no end treatment.
14	Not caged; ends and limb scars sprayed at intervals with ethyl mercury chloride; surface area 795 square inches; tree no. 7.	I. pini, 29 broods; I. grandicollis, 11 broods; Monochamus sp., 11 larvae; buprestid larvae, 5; Rhagium sp., 1 larva.	do	Do.
15	Caged; ends and limb scars sprayed at intervals with ethyl mercury chloride; surface area 862.5 square inches; tree no. 7.	None	One small spot of stain associated with crack in bark; fungus not identified, but not Ceratostomella; bark not loose.	Do.
16	Caged; ends and limb scars sprayed at intervals with ethyl mercury chloride; surface area 825 square inches; tree no. 5.	I. grandicollis, 4 broods, all on upper side of log.	Blue stain and yeast associated with Ips tunnels but absent elsewhere on log; bark not loose.	These beetles apparently entered through the end of cage covered with muslin.

As will be discussed in more detail later, cultures were made of the fungi found in these and certain other logs. It is sufficient to say here that blue-staining fungi were always found developing and spreading from the bark-beetle tunnels and that the evidence justifies the conclusion that they were introduced into the logs by the beetles and that they were rarely or never introduced in any other way. In addition to the blue-staining fungi, a characteristic yeast was found constantly associated with the beetle attacks. Several different kinds of bacteria, also, were isolated from freshly made tunnels, but these were not consistently present. In the older tunnels several

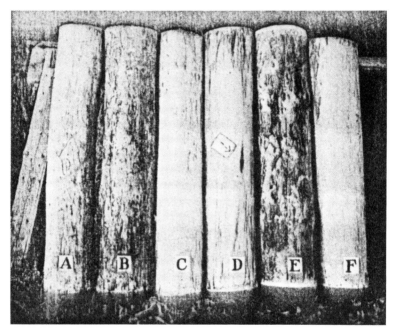

FIGURE 2. One log from each of the six series; the arrow on the log from series D points to an area of blue stain surrounding an incomplete tunnel made by a single *Ips* beetle that managed to get through the cage.

other fungi were often present, the most common of which was a species of *Trichoderma*. It is very probable that these were also introduced by beetles or other insects, but they develop more slowly than the blue stain and are secondary in nature, apparently not being able to penetrate extensively into the woody tissue. The most common fungus entering through the exposed nontreated ends of the logs was *Peniophora gigantea* (Fr.) Massee. This fungus was not present in any of the logs with sealed or treated ends, but developed abundantly under the loosened bark of the logs with exposed ends and caused a rapid decay of the sapwood. Fruiting bodies were often found on the underside of the infected logs. Sporophores of this and other fungi sometimes grew out through holes made in the bark by insects, but there was no evidence that they were consistently introduced by bark beetles.

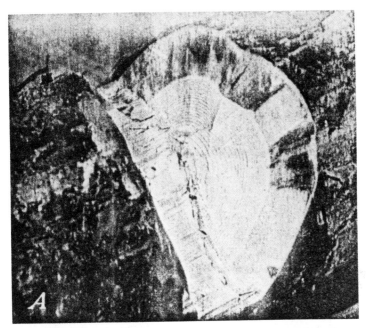

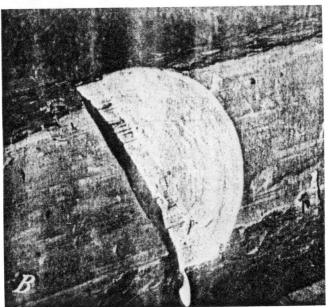

FIGURE 3.—Two logs cut to show presence or absence of stain in the sapwood: *A*, A log from series E, not caged; *B*, a log from series F, caged.

As a further check on the association of blue-stain infection and bark-beetle infestation, a log of each series was sawed in cross section as shown in figure 4. With the aid of a planimeter the area of blue-

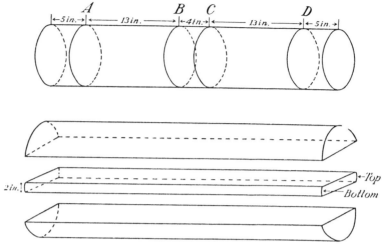

FIGURE 4.—Diagram to show how logs were cut for the measurement of the amount of stained sapwood.

stained wood, showing in the cross sections *A*, *B*, *C*, and *D*, was measured and calculated in terms of percentage of total area of sapwood in cross section. A plank 2 inches thick was sawed from each of the other logs as shown in figure 4. In the same manner the area

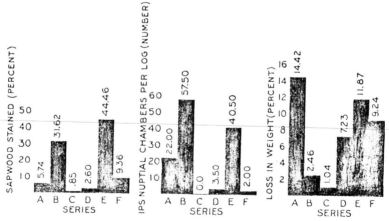

FIGURE 5.—Amount of blue stain in the logs of the different series, and the relation of insect infestation and moisture content of the wood to the prevalence of blue stain.

of stained wood, as revealed in longitudinal section, was calculated. The results of these measurements and also the degree of beetle infestation are shown graphically in figure 5. It will be seen that the amount of stain is closely correlated with the amount of bark-beetle infestation, except in the check logs 1, 2, 3, and 4. The extremely small amount of stain found in these logs that were heavily attacked by bark beetles was difficult to understand until it was noted that the wood-rotting fungus *Peniophora gigantea* had penetrated practically all of the sapwood and, by its very rapid development, had inhibited the normal development of blue stain. This explanation of the absence of blue stain in these logs was verified the following season by observing the development of the fungi in similar logs at frequent intervals throughout the season.

Since it has been shown that the development of blue stain is influenced by the moisture content of the wood (*4*, *13*) and since the loss of water from the logs was influenced by the different treatments, the logs were weighed at frequent intervals until they were opened. Figure 5 shows graphically the percentage of loss in weight by the logs during the first summer of the experiment. This loss, for practical purposes, may be considered to be due almost entirely to loss of water. As a further check on the moisture content of the logs, six increment borings were made from a log of each series just before the bark was removed for examination. The approximate percentage of moisture in each sample (oven-dry basis) was as follows: A, 69; B, 110; C, 102; D, 70; E, 55; and F, 58. Although the nature of this determination is subject to considerable error, the relative values agree closely with the data obtained from the loss of weight. Since blue stain develops well at any moisture content between 55 and 110 percent, it is improbable that moisture content was a limiting factor in blue-stain development in these experiments. It is obvious from the data given in figure 5 that there is no correlation between the amount of blue stain and the moisture content of the logs of the different series.

Because of the several kinds of insects that entered the uncaged logs and the resulting overlapping of their tunnels, it was often difficult to interpret with assurance the significance of the fungi found associated with the tunnels. In the case of the bark beetles this difficulty was in part overcome by the fact that a few beetles entered the cages of logs 11, 12, and 16, which resulted in these logs being infested with a few isolated broods. In order further to overcome this difficulty additional logs were caged, with ends sealed or sprayed, and into each cage a few beetles of a single species were introduced. In all of these logs blue stain developed abundantly about all of the *Ips* tunnels and was absent on other parts of the log, verifying the conclusion that the blue-stain fungi are commonly introduced into the logs only by the bark beetles.

ASSOCIATION OF BARK BEETLES AND FUNGI

Parallel with the experiments reported above, the more intimate relationships between bark beetles and fungi were studied. Logs infested with bark beetles were opened at frequent intervals and the progress of fungus infection determined by microscopic and cultural studies. At the same time, insects in all stages of development were killed, fixed, and embedded in paraffin and were later studied by histological methods. In this manner, a fairly complete picture of the association between the bark beetles and the fungi was obtained. For the sake of brevity the results of both studies are presented together and the association is described in chronological sequence following the life cycle of the insects.

As stated in the foregoing, two species of bark beetles, *Ips pini* and *I. grandicollis* attacked the logs soon after they were cut and put in

place. Because of the similarity of development and fungus association of the two species, they will be discussed together, any observed
differences being pointed out as the occasion demands.

The life history of these bark beetles is, briefly, as follows: Pupae
and some of the young adults hibernate under the bark of logs or trees
attacked during the previous summer. Young adult beetles often
emerge from infested trees in the late fall months and enter the litter
and duff under the trees and spend the winter there. They come out
early the following spring and attack fresh trees or logs. The males
find suitable logs or trees, and then each bores a hole through the
bark (fig. 6, A, a) and excavates a broad, flat chamber in the inner
bark and cambium region. This chamber is known as the "nuptial
chamber" (fig. 6, A, b). Several females soon join the male in this
chamber and each female constructs a long tunnel known as an "egg
tunnel", extending out from it (fig. 6, A, c). The pattern in which
these egg tunnels radiate from the nuptial chamber is characteristic
of the species. As the female extends her egg tunnel she makes small
niches or pockets along each side of it (fig. 6, A, d). An egg is placed
in each of these niches and covered with boring dust or frass. The
eggs hatch in a few days and the young larvae begin burrowing tunnels
(fig. 6, A, e) in the inner bark at approximately right angles to the egg
tunnels. These larval tunnels increase in size as the larvae grow.
The larvae become full grown and ready to pupate in about 3 weeks.
Each larva then excavates a small oval chamber at the end of its
tunnel. This is the pupal chamber (fig. 6, B). The larva then
transforms to the pupal stage and later to the adult, the length of this
transformation period varying with the season of the year. The
young adults do not immediately emerge from the log but burrow
about under the loosened bark, feeding extensively. After this period
of feeding, they bore exit holes through the bark and fly away in search
of a new tree or log. There are 2 generations a year in Minnesota,
1 emerging in midsummer, the other in fall and early spring.

The life histories and habits of *Ips pini* and *I. grandicollis* are rather
similar. One of the chief differences is in the arrangement of their
tunnel patterns. In the case of *I. pini* there are usually 3 to 6 egg
tunnels, each made by a different female, radiating in a star-shape
pattern from the nuptial chamber. *I. grandicollis* forms usually
only 2 or 3 egg tunnels from each nuptial chamber, and these tunnels
extend in a longitudinal direction very nearly parallel with the grain
of the wood. This difference in tunnel pattern is important because
the extent of the circumference of a log involved by a brood of *I. pini*
is naturally considerably greater than that invaded by *I. grandicollis*.
Since the blue-stain fungi grow most slowly in a tangential direction,
the more spreading tunnels of *I. pini* usually result in a greater cross-
sectional area of blue-stain infection and consequently a more rapid
death of infested trees.

In May and early June 1931 many beetles were caught as they
alighted upon the logs cut from a freshly felled Norway pine. Some
of these were killed and fixed for histological study. Cultures were
made from some, and others were dissected and examined under the
microscope. Microscopic examination of these beetles frequently
disclosed fungus spores adhering to the legs, wings, and other external
parts. Several different kinds of spores were found, but the most
abundant and most characteristic were at once recognized as ascospores

of the *Ceratostomella* found in the logs infested by the two species of *Ips*. This fungus has since been described and named by Rumbold (17) as *Ceratostomella ips*. Cultures made from the beetles, both internally and externally, yielded this fungus along with certain

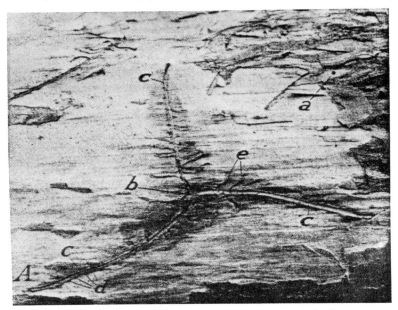

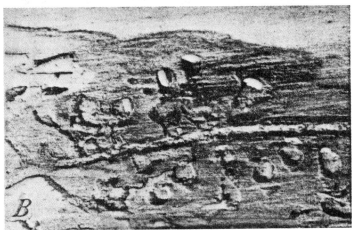

FIGURE 6.—*A*, Portion of a Norway pine log with bark removed to show tunnels of *Ips pini*: *a*, An entrance hole; *b*, nuptial chamber; *c*, 1 of 3 egg channels; *d*, egg niches; *e* larval tunnels; *B*, pupal chambers and pupae of *I. grandicollis*.

characteristic yeasts. Bacteria and other fungi were frequently obtained, but *C. ips* and the yeasts were universally present. The most frequently occurring fungus other than these two was *Trichoderma koningi* Oudem. found, also, in nearly all of the old bark-beetle tunnels. The universal occurrence of these fungi in and on the bodies

245

of the beetles caught as they were alighting on the freshly cut logs supports the evidence that the fungi are introduced into the logs by the insects.

Among the fungi isolated from the beetles and from the stained wood adjacent to the beetles were several cultures closely resembling *Ceratostomella ips*, but bearing only conidia. The conidia were often formed on typically *Graphium*-like coremia, but on malt agar the sporophores were more commonly shortened to form tuberculate clusters. These were cultured on various media and under various conditions, but they could not be induced to form perithecia. These cultures could be identified only as species of *Graphium*. On account of the similarity of these cultures to *C. ips*, it was thought that they might be the haploid form of this fungus. (Buisman (*3*) has recently shown that when several strains of *G. ulmi* are mixed in culture, perithecia of *Ceratostomella* are formed.) But when several of these cultures were mixed, no perithecia were formed.

As a further check on the identity of these imperfect forms a single perithecium of *Ceratostomella ips* was placed in a drop of sterile distilled water until the ascospores oozed out of the ostiole. With the aid of a Chambers micromanipulator 15 individual ascospores were picked up and cultured. Nine of these single ascospore cultures produced perithecia in abundance and also formed a few conidia. Six of the cultures formed conidia and were similar in all respects to the *Graphium* cultures isolated previously. When each of these six cultures was grown in combination with each of the remaining imperfect cultures only conidia were formed. Moreover, when an imperfect culture was grown on agar side by side with a perfect form each retained its characteristic type of fructification. If the imperfect forms were haploid and the perfect forms diploid, there was no evidence of diploidization of the haploid form. It would appear from this evidence that the *Graphium* cultures isolated from stained wood and from the beetles were specifically identical with *C. ips* but lacked the ability to form perithecia.

Histological study of the beetles also revealed the universal presence of spores of the blue-stain fungi, both externally and internally. The beetles were killed and fixed in Dietrich's solution in a partial vacuum. They were embedded in paraffin, and sections 12 to 15 microns thick were cut and stained with the Gram-Weigert stain. This procedure revealed the ascospores of *Ceratostomella ips* adhering in clumps to various parts of the exoskeleton and also scattered throughout the intestinal tract (fig. 7). In many specimens fragments of perithecia were found, showing that the beetles feed upon these fruiting bodies. Staining reactions gave no indication that the spores were digested or otherwise injured by passage through the body of the insect. To test this point further a number of beetles were caught in sterile glass vials and held until pellets of feces were obtained. Some of these were plated on 1-percent malt-extract agar, and cultures of *C. ips* were obtained from a high percentage of them. Examination of the pellets under the microscope also disclosed the characteristic ascospores of this fungus. When the pellets were crushed and placed in hanging drops of sterile water, the spores germinated and grew normally, thus proving conclusively that they were not injured by passage through the intestinal tract of the beetles.

Cultures made from the bark and sapwood adjacent to freshly made nuptial chambers yielded *Ceratostomella ips* and yeast in nearly every

246

case, showing that the spores germinate soon after they are introduced. In all such chambers pellets of feces are found adhering to the walls of the chamber. The moist bark evidently furnishes sufficient moisture for germination of the spores and subsequent growth of the fungi. Although no proof can be presented, it is quite probable that spores adhering to the exoskeleton of the beetles are brushed off on the moist wood, where they would germinate and start infection.

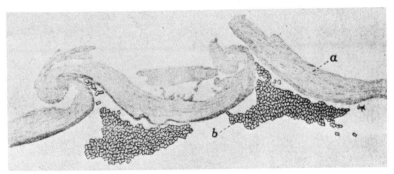

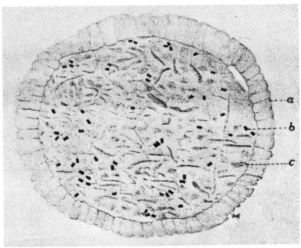

FIGURE 7.—Detailed drawings showing the spores in and on the body of mature beetles: *A*. Masses of ascospores adhering to the abdomen of a beetle, exoskeleton (*a*), masses of ascospores (*b*); approximately × 400; *B*, cross section of the midintestine, showing (*a*) wall of intestine, (*b*) ascospores of *Ceratostomella ips*, (*c*) partly digested wood fragments; approximately × 400.

Another interesting means of distributing the inoculum within the tunnel was discovered while beetles caught on the surface of the logs were being dissected. It was observed that from one to a dozen or more small mites were attached to the ventral part of the thorax or in the concave wing declivities of nearly all the beetles examined. These obviously had attached themselves to the beetles before they emerged from the old infested logs. Careful examination showed mites running about in nearly all freshly made tunnels. They were also found in great abundance in old tunnels. Apparently, they leave the beetles when they enter the log and feed on the fungi and decomposing bark tissue. When the beetles of the new brood are ready to emerge, some of the mites attach themselves to the beetles and are thus carried to new trees or logs. Microscopic examination of the mites taken from the beetles, as well as cultures made from them, showed that spores of the blue-staining fungus were often disseminated by them.

Of the various fungi introduced into the log by the bark beetles, the yeasts apparently develop most rapidly at first. When the outer bark is removed from a freshly made tunnel, such as the one shown in fig-

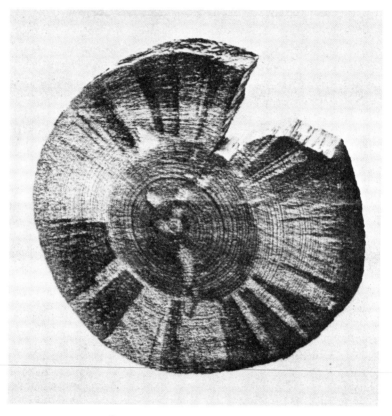

FIGURE 8.—Section cut from a log of Norway pine to show the development of blue stain in the sapwood

ure 6, A, it is seen that the inner bark is stained brown for some distance around the tunnel. Isolations from the advancing border of this stained bark frequently yield pure cultures of yeast, while the blue-staining fungi can be found only in the bark and wood closer to the tunnel. As time goes on, the blue-stain fungi spread rapidly in the sapwood and inner bark. The rate of spread is most rapid in a radial plane, up and down the log as well as toward the center. In advanced stages stained areas appear as wedges in the sapwood when seen in cross section (fig. 8). The blue stain, however, does not affect the heartwood and its radial development ceases sharply when the heartwood is reached.

As stated above, the eggs of the bark beetles are deposited singly in small niches in the sides of the egg channel. Each egg is covered with a soft plug of sawdust. Cultures made from this sawdust plug show that it is always contaminated with yeast and other fungi. When the eggs are aseptically removed and placed on agar, it is evident they also are frequently surface-contaminated with yeast, *Ceratostomella*, and other fungi. The eggs are very delicate and easily injured, but a limited number of cultures made from surface-sterilized eggs show that they are internally sterile. As the young larvae develop and bore out a tunnel in the inner bark, the tissue surrounding the tunnel is stained brown. Yeasts can nearly always be found in the stained tissue, but such tissue is often sterile, indicating that the brown stain may be due in part to oxidation. When larvae were killed and embedded in paraffin, stained sections often revealed yeast cells in their intestinal tracts. In many cases, however, no yeast was found in the bodies of the larvae.

Shortly after the larvae pupate the blue-stain fungi begin to sporulate. The nature and amount of sporulation is more or less dependent upon the immediate environment. By this time the bark usually is becoming loose and there is a space of varying width between it and the wood. If the log is exposed to direct sunlight, its upper surface may dry out and there may be little surface growth or fructification of the fungi.

Ceratostomella ips forms two kinds of spores. Conidia are formed usually in the typical *Graphium* manner and coremia are often found in the old egg channels, the larval tunnels, or in the pupal chambers (fig. 9, *A*). The spores are often formed in the pupal chambers while they are still occupied by the pupae, so that the newly formed beetles are surrounded by a mass of sticky conidia. *C. ips*, however, in nature produces perithecia more commonly than conidia. The perithecia are formed frequently on the sides of the old egg channels, with their long black beaks pointing toward the center of the channels (figs. 9, *B*, and 10). They may be formed also in any crack in the inner bark or even completely embedded in the soft, partially decayed tissue of the inner bark. When moisture conditions are right, the ascospores ooze from the beaks of the perithecia in white sticky masses (figs. 9, *B*, and 10).

When transformation is complete the newly formed beetles begin feeding. They wander through the old egg channels (fig. 9, *B*) and also make new feeding tunnels in the inner bark. In doing this they take many spores into their digestive tract and many more stick to the external parts of the body, so that, when the beetles emerge from the log, they are thoroughly infested with fungus spores.

Although *Ceratostomella ips* was the blue-staining fungus most frequently associated with the bark beetles, another apparently undescribed fungus frequently was found that caused a stain indistinguishable from that caused by *C. ips*. When this fungus was present it usually predominated, and in many tunnels examined *C. ips* apparently was entirely absent. The fungus was first observed fruiting in the pupal chambers of *Ips pini* and was later found associated with several broods of *I. grandicollis*. Only the conidial fructification has been observed, and this is formed most frequently in the pupal chambers and in the adjacent larval tunnels. Sporulation begins shortly after pupation and, by the time the mature beetle is formed, the walls of the pupal chamber are lined with a white waxy mass of conidia (fig. 11). Observations have shown that these conidia often form part of the first food consumed by the newly

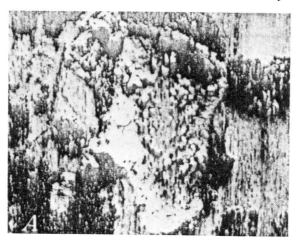

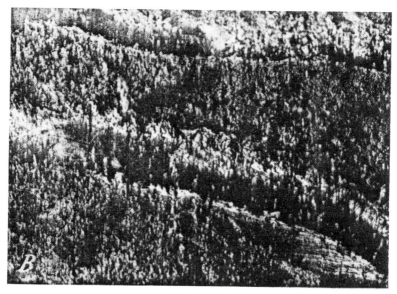

FIGURE 9. *A*, *Graphium*-like coremia formed by *Ceratostomella ips* in a pupal chamber of *Ips pini*, approximately × 10. *B*, Bark beetle (*I. grandicollis*) in an old egg channel; note the perithecia of *C. ips* lining the tunnel, with their beaks bearing glistening masses of spores all pointing toward the center of the channel. Such beetles become contaminated with the spores both internally and externally.

formed beetle. The rather large hyaline globose to pyriform conidia (fig. 12, *A*) are formed on the ends of short, erect palisaded sporophores, forming a compact cushion (fig. 12, *B*). In its general aspects this fungus resembles the so-called "ambrosia" fungi described by Hubbard (*10*), Neger (*14*), Schneider-Orelli (*18*), and others and associated with the ambrosia beetles. Cultures of the fungus were obtained by picking up single conidia and also by making

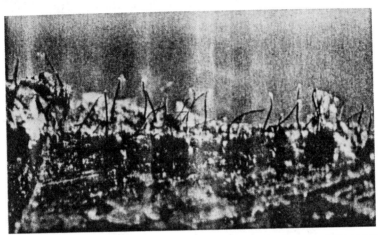

FIGURE 10. —Perithecia of *Ceratostomella ips* in a beetle tunnel; note the glistening mass of sticky ascospores on the tips of the perithecia.

tissue cultures from blue-stained wood adjacent to the beetle tunnels. At least two different strains of the fungus were isolated that differed somewhat in spore size but were identical in other respects. The

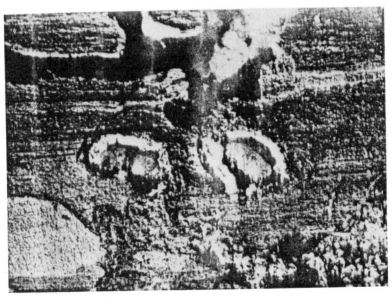

FIGURE 11. —Two pupal chambers of *Ips pini* showing immature beetles surrounded by masses of spores of *Tuberculariella ips*.

spores of one strain were somewhat smaller and more globose than those of the other. There was considerable variation in size and shape of spores in any given culture. Some were distinctly globose,

251

while others were long and pyriform. Spores formed on agar cultures also were distinctly more globose than those formed in nature. The spores ranged from 7.9μ to 22.5μ in width and from 13.3μ to

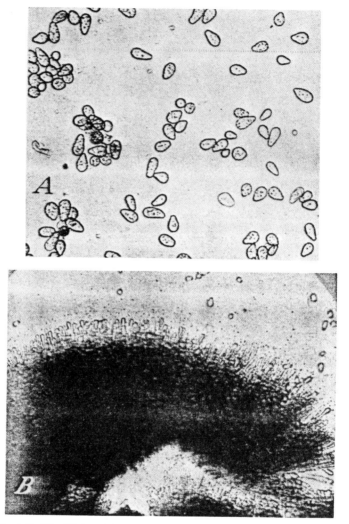

FIGURE 12.—A, Conidia of *Tuberculariella ips;* approximately × 130. B, Sporodochium of *T. ips* showing the palisade arrangement and terminal position of spores; approximately × 50.

23.8μ in length. The sporodochia were white and waxy, but there was no distinct mucus holding the spores together. The fungus appears to be a species of the genus *Tuberculariella* Von Höhnel (9). Because of its close association with the two species of *Ips*, the name *Tuberculariella ips* is proposed. A brief technical description is given below.

Tuberculariella ips, n.sp.

Conidia hyaline, globose to pyriform, usually apiculate at the narrow end, ranging from 7.9μ to 22.5μ in width and from 13.3μ to 23.8μ in length, borne singly and successively at the ends of unbranched septate conidiophores; sporodochia white and waxy but not mucilaginous. Young colonies on agar colorless, later changing to black; scant gray aerial mycelium; young hyphae hyaline, old hyphae brown; mycelium 2.7μ to 6.7μ in diameter. In agar cultures conidia borne terminally on simple branches of the mycelium; sporodochia sometimes formed in old cultures.

On sapwood of *Pinus* spp. infested with *Ips pini* Say or *I. grandicollis* Eichh. at Itasca Park, Arago, Minn. Causes distinct blue stain of sapwood, and fruits abundantly in pupal chambers and larval tunnels of the insects.

LATIN DIAGNOSIS

Sporodochia alba cerea haud glutinosa; conidia hyalina, globosa vel pyriformia, plerumque apiculata ad extremitatem angustiorem, 7.9μ—22.5μ lata, 13.3μ—23.8μ longa, ad apices conidiophororum simplicium septatorum singulatim iterum atque iterum lata.

Coloniae in "agar" cultae primum hyalinae deinde nigres centes, mycelio aerio tenui griseo hyphis primum hyalinis deinde brunneis; mycelio 2.7μ—6.7μ crasso, conidiis ad apices ramorum simplicium mycelii latis; sporodochiis interdum in culturis antiquis factis.

As stated above, the newly formed beetles frequently find themselves completely surrounded by masses of the conidia of this fungus. Numerous observations have shown that the beetles often feed upon these spores, frequently completely cleaning out the pupal chambers before leaving them. Dissections and histological studies also have shown large numbers of these spores in the intestinal tracts of the beetles (fig. 13). Although some of the spores appear to be destroyed by the passage, many of them evidently are not injured. A thick gelatinous cell wall usually is present on such spores stained in the intestinal tract, and the spores show no signs of injury. Microscopic examination of freshly emerged beetles shows spores adhering to the external parts of the beetles, but, unlike the ascospores of *Ceratostomella ips*, they are readily washed off when the beetles are passed through the solutions in preparation for embedding in paraffin.

By artificial inoculation it was proved that this fungus would cause typical blue stain indistinguishable from that caused by *Ceratostomella ips*. The fungus was grown also on many different kinds of media under different conditions, including irradiation with ultraviolet light, in an unsuccessful effort to induce the production of sexual spore forms. It appears, then, that the fungus is another true blue-staining fungus actively spread by these two species of bark beetles. The same fungus has been found also in association with *Ips pini* in white-pine windfalls. The factor or factors influencing the prevalence of the two blue-staining fungi and determining which one will predominate are not known.

As previously mentioned, cultural experiments showed that yeasts are universally associated with the bark beetles. They are the first to multiply extensively in the bark adjacent to freshly made tunnels. Yeasts also have been isolated from the sapwood, but here they are soon outgrown by the blue-staining fungi. The yeasts are present in great quantity in the inner bark in later stages of the beetles' development and are taken into the bodies of the mature beetles during their feeding period just prior to emergence from the log. The histological studies show yeast cells in varying amounts always

253

present in the food contents of the intestinal tracts of freshly emerged beetles.

On several occasions small masses of oblong hyaline conidia were found in the old tunnels of *Ips pini*. Cultures made from single spores formed brown mycelial cultures on malt agar but did not produce blue stain on wood. Examination of the mycelium showed the presence of clamp connections, and older cultures formed what

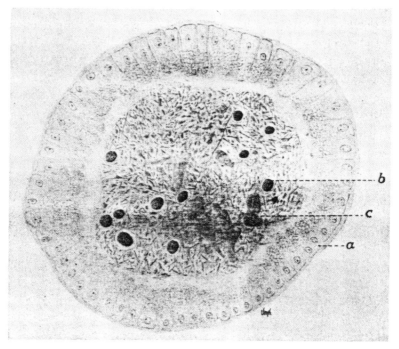

FIGURE 13.—Highly magnified section of the intestinal tract of a mature beetle (*Ips pini*) showing the presence of viable spores of *Tuberculariella ips: a*, Intestinal wall; *b*, conidium of *T. ips; c*, partly digested wood fragments. Approximately × 75.

appeared to be abortive poroid fruiting bodies. The identity of the fungus and its significance are not known.

In isolating fungi numerous bacterial colonies were found in the plates. These were so variable and inconsistent in their occurrence that they were considered of little significance.

In addition to the bark beetles and the mites previously mentioned, a number of insects of various types frequently were found inhabiting old tunnels. They were mainly predators or parasites of the bark beetles. Since these insects enter the logs only after the bark beetles and associated fungi have become thoroughly established, it is thought that they are of secondary importance only.

DISCUSSION

The facts presented above show quite clearly that blue-staining fungi are definitely associated with *Ips pini* and *I. grandicollis* and that they are disseminated and introduced into trees or felled logs by these beetles. The nature of the fructification of the blue-staining fungi makes it appear highly improbable that wind is of any significance in disseminating them. The results of the controlled experiments with caged and uncaged logs, some with sealed ends and some with ends exposed, bear out this conclusion. Although the blue-staining fungi are the most obvious ones associated with the beetles, cultural studies show that other fungi are present with more or less regularity, even when other insects are absent. When one looks at the inner bark of a log at the time beetles are emerging and sees the many different kinds of fungi growing and sporulating, it is obvious that several different fungi must be disseminated with some degree of regularity. It is possible that some of these organisms are of greater significance than would be indicated by general observations. On the other hand, evidence, both cultural and histological, tends to show that the blue-staining fungi and the associated yeast fungi are predominant, both in the amount of inoculum carried by the bark beetles and in the rapidity of their development in the log.

As would be expected, other fungi develop as the disintegration of the inner bark advances and as the bark is loosened from the wood. These, without doubt, play a part in the ultimate destruction of the log and cannot be ignored completely. The most common of these "secondary" fungi is the green moldlike fungus identified as *Trichoderma Koningi*. It fruits abundantly in the old tunnels before and after the beetles have emerged. The spores are borne loose and dry in a manner favoring wind distribution, but since it has been isolated from the bodies of freshly emerged beetles, probably it also is frequently disseminated by them.

The constant association of fungi with these bark beetles naturally raises the question of the symbiotic relationships between them. As previously mentioned, Grosmann (7) has already considered this question in her study, which dealt primarily with *Ips. typographus* L. and to a lesser extent with several other species of bark beetles. The blue-staining fungus associated with *I. typographus* was described by Grosmann and named *Leptographium penicillatum*. In addition, 2 or 3 characteristic yeasts were always present. Grosmann reached the conclusion that no true symbiosis existed between the beetles and their associated fungi. She concluded from her experiments that the beetles were not dependent upon the blue-stain fungi and that if any benefits were derived from the association they were all in favor of the fungus. She also concluded that the yeasts were in no way necessary for the development of the beetles and were to be considered as commensals.

Although the writers have not made extensive experiments dealing with the nutrition relations of the bark beetles and the associated fungi, observations and histological studies make it seem very unlikely that the beetles utilize the fungi extensively as food. In the examination of several hundred prepared slides of insects in all stages of development there was no indication that the fungi were digested. Yeast cells were often found in the intestinal tract of the larvae, but they showed no signs of disintegration and appeared to pass through uninjured. They were frequently entirely absent, and when present did not appear to be multiplying rapidly. No fungi of any sort were found inside the body of the pupae. In adult beetles both yeast cells and spores of the blue-staining fungi were generally present, but they, likewise, appeared to be uninjured. Since neither of these fungi destroy wood to any appreciable extent and apparently do not multiply in the body of the insects, it is highly improbable that they digest the wood particles taken in by the insects. The feeding experiments of Grosmann (7) would tend to show that the action of the fungi on the tissues of the bark do not make it more suitable as food for the beetles. Since her experiments did not include the entire life cycle of the insects and were not carried out under fungus-free conditions, this conclusion cannot be accepted as beyond question.

One other factor, apparently overlooked by Grosmann, is the effect of the fungi on the immediate environment of the developing brood of beetles. Until it is possible to bring about the development of a brood of beetles in bark entirely free of fungi, it cannot be safely concluded that the fungi do not in some way influence favorably the development of the beetles. In the writers' experiments in which logs were protected from insects by cages and from fungus infection by sealing or spraying the ends, the bark did not separate from the wood as did that of infested logs. When the tissue of such bark as a medium for beetle development is compared with that overgrown by fungi and separating from the wood, it is readily seen that the two environments are strikingly different. Moreover, most conifers secrete resin into freshly made wounds, and in living trees such resin secretions are often able to overcome the attack of individual insects or broods. Many bark beetles are known to attack living trees most successfully when the trees are weakened by drought or other factors. It is very probable that reduced resin flow or moisture content of the inner bark may be the determining factor in such cases. Nelson [5] has shown that the blue-stain fungi, in the absence of beetles, interrupt the flow of sap in infected trees, causing a rapid decrease in moisture content and usually resulting in death within a few months. Obviously this reduces the flow of resin. Thus beetles aided by the blue-stain fungi are able to attack certain trees which without such aid they could not successfully attack. Such benefits derived from the fungi by the beetles would certainly come within the broader concept of symbiosis, as generally used. That the fungi derive benefit from the association through dissemination by the beetles and by introduction into the tissues of the inner bark is obvious from the facts mentioned above. Their special adaptation to dissemination in this way would indicate a symbiotic relationship of long standing.

Person (16) has demonstrated recently that the inner bark of western yellow pine when fermented by the yeast associated with *Dendroctonus brevicomis* Lec., is more attractive to this beetle than the nonfermented bark. This fact is offered as an explanation of the selection of certain trees for attack by the beetle. Person believes that, in trees weakened by drought or other abnormal conditions, a limited amount of respiratory fermentation results in the production of volatile aldehydes or esters that attract a few beetles in the immediate vicinity of the trees. These introduce the yeast, which increases the rate of fermentation and results in an increased amount of the attractive substance sufficient to attract beetles from a greater

---

[5] Nelson, R. M. See footnote 4.

256

distance. If this explanation is correct, the yeasts also must be considered as truly symbiotic with the beetles.

Buchner (2) and others have described several wood-inhabiting beetles that possess special anatomical modifications of the female definitely adapted to insure the perpetuation of symbiotic fungi by contamination of the egg either before or after oviposition. When this study was started it was suspected that some such structure would be found in the bark beetles. Careful study of many sections of the insects in all stages of development has, however, revealed no such structures. This accords with the observations of Grosmann (7) on *Ips typographus*. Transmission of the fungi from one generation to another apparently is accomplished entirely as indicated previously, namely, by means of spores and yeast cells either adhering to the external parts of the insect or passing through the intestinal tract and being expelled in the feces in newly made tunnels. Male and female beetles appear equally effective in introducing the fungi. Both yeasts and blue-stain fungi have been isolated from freshly made nuptial chambers containing only the male insect. The fungi have been isolated also from the bodies of both male and female beetles. In several instances in caged logs large patches of blue stain developed from nuptial chambers into which no females entered.

SUMMARY

A study of two species of bark beetle (*Ips pini* Say and *I. grandicollis* Eichh.) and the fungi associated with them has been made as the first part of a general investigation of the interrelations of insects and fungi in the deterioration of felled logs of Norway pine.

Experimental evidence is presented showing that these bark beetles introduce blue-staining fungi into the logs and that the fungi are rarely, if ever, introduced in any other way.

Two different blue-staining fungi were found associated with these bark beetles. The most prevalent of the two is *Ceratostomella ips* Rumbold, the fungus isolated by Rumbold from the galleries of *Ips calligraphus* and *I. grandicollis*. The second apparently has not previously been reported. It is briefly described in this paper as *Tuberculariella ips*, n.sp.

Certain cultures of *Graphium* isolated from stained wood and from the beetles proved to be identical with *Ceratostomella ips*, although they could not be made to produce perithecia. Of 15 cultures derived from single ascospores of *C. ips*, 6 formed only conidia and were identical with the *Graphium* cultures previously isolated. The remaining 9 cultures formed both conidia and perithecia. Perithecia were not produced when the 6 *Graphium* cultures were mated in all combinations.

In addition to the blue-staining fungi, characteristic yeasts were constantly associated with the beetles.

The fungi are introduced by either male or female beetles, and they begin to grow in the inner bark and sapwood soon after introduction. The yeast fungi grow more rapidly at first in the inner bark, but the blue-stain fungi spread more extensively in the sapwood.

Mites are frequently introduced into the logs by the beetles. The mites attach themselves to the underside of the thorax and in the concave wing declivities, where they are not easily brushed off.

257

When the beetles enter a log some of the mites leave the beetles and move about in the tunnels as they are constructed. Yeast cells and spores of the blue-staining fungi were found adhering to the bodies of the mites. The mites probably aid in distributing the spores about the beetle tunnels.

The blue-staining fungi sporulate profusely during the pupation of the bark beetles. *Ceratostomella ips* forms perithecia more commonly than conidia, but typical *Graphium* coremia are often found in the old egg channels or in the pupal chambers. The perithecia of *C. ips* are usually formed on the walls of the old egg channels with their beaks pointing toward the center of the channels. When moisture conditions are favorable, the spores ooze from the tips in sticky masses. The newly formed beetle leaves its pupal chamber and feeds extensively under the bark before emerging. In doing this it brushes against the sticky spores which adhere to the body of the beetle. Examination of the contents of the intestinal tract of beetles shows that ascospores and even parts of the perithecia are eaten. Large quantities of spores and yeast cells are found in the intestinal tracts of the beetles. These bear no signs of injury, and germination experiments show that they are still viable after passage through the body of the beetles.

The second blue-stain fungus forms masses of sticky conidia in the pupal chambers and in the old egg channels during the pupation period. These spores also adhere to the bodies of the beetles and are passed through the intestinal tract uninjured.

Yeast cells frequently are found in the intestinal tract of the larvae, where they also are apparently not injured. No fungi were found inside the body of the pupae.

Histological study of the mature beetles revealed no anatomical modification to insure transmission of the fungi to the young.

The eggs of the beetles were internally sterile, although yeast and fungus mycelium were abundant in the sawdust plugs covering the eggs in the niches.

Although no nutritional symbiosis could be demonstrated between the beetles and their associated fungi, the relationship is considered as one of true symbiosis in the broader sense. The fungi obviously derive benefit in being disseminated by the beetles and in being introduced into the inner bark of the logs or susceptible trees. The blue-staining fungi, by inhibiting the flow of sap, in all probability make living trees more favorable for beetle development, and by aiding in the decomposition of the inner bark cause it to separate from the wood, creating a more favorable environment for the development of the insect broods. Until a brood of beetles can be reared in a fungus-free log, it cannot safely be concluded that the fungi are not necessary for the normal development of the beetles.

LITERATURE CITED

(1) BOYCE, J. S.
    1923. THE DETERIORATION OF FELLED WESTERN YELLOW PINE ON INSECT-CONTROL PROJECTS. U.S. Dept. Agr. Bull. 1140, 8 pp., illus.
(2) BUCHNER, P.
    1930. TIER UND PFLANZE IN SYMBIOSE. Aufl. 2, völlig umgearb. und erweiterte von Tier und Pflanze in Intrazellularer Symbiose. 900 pp., illus. Berlin.

(3) BUISMAN, C.
   1932. CERATOSTOMELLA ULMI, DE GESCHLACHTELIJKE VORM VAN GRA-
      PHIUM ULMI SCHWARZ. Tijdschr. Plantenziekten 38: 1–5, illus.
(4) COLLEY, R. H., and RUMBOLD, C. T.
   1930. RELATION BETWEEN MOISTURE CONTENT OF THE WOOD AND BLUE
      STAIN IN LOBLOLLY PINE. Jour. Agr. Research 41: 389–399,
      illus.
(5) CRAIGHEAD, F. C.
   1928. INTERRELATION OF TREE-KILLING BARK BEETLES (DENDROCTONUS)
      AND BLUE STAIN. Jour. Forestry 26: 886–887.
(6) GRAHAM, S. A.
   1925. THE FELLED TREE TRUNK AS AN ECOLOGICAL UNIT. Ecology 6:
      397–411, illus.
(7) GROSMAN, H.
   1930. BEITRÄGE ZUR KENNTNIS DER LEBENSGEMEINSCHAFT ZWISCHEN
      BORKENKÄFERN UND PILZEN. Ztschr. Parasitenk. 3: [56]–102,
      illus.
(8) HARTIG, R.
   1878. DIE ZERSETZUNGSERSCHEINUNGEN DES HOLZES DER NADELHOLZ-
      BÄUME UND DER EICHE IN FÖRSTLICHER, BOTANISCHER UND
      CHEMISCHER RICHTUNG. 151 pp., illus. Berlin.
(9) HÖHNEL, F. VON
   1915. BEITRÄGE ZUR MYKOLOGIE. IX. ÜBER DIE GATTUNG MYXOSPORIUM
      LINK. Ztschr. Gärungsphysiol. 5: [191] 215.
(10) HUBBARD, H. G.
   1897. THE AMBROSIA BEETLES OF THE UNITED STATES. U.S.Dept.Agr.,
      Div. Ent. Bull. (n.s.) 7: 9–30, illus.
(11) MacCALLUM, B. D.
   1922. SOME WOOD-STAINING FUNGI. Brit. Mycol. Soc. Trans. 7: 231–236,
      illus.
(12) MÜNCH, E.
   1907–8. DIE BLAUFÄULE DES NADELHOLZES. Naturw. Ztschr. Forst u.
      Landw. 5: 531–573, illus., 1907; 6: 32–47, 297–323, illus., 1908.
(13) ————
   1909. UNTERSUCHUNGEN ÜBER IMMUNITÄT UND KRANKHEITSEMPFÄNG-
      LICHKEIT DER HOLZPFLANZEN. Naturw. Ztschr. Forst u. Landw.
      7: 54–75, 87–114, [129]–160, illus.
(14) NEGER, F. W.
   1911. ZUR ÜBERTRÄGUNG DES AMBROSIAPILZES VON XYLEBORUS DISPAR.
      Naturw. Ztschr. Forst u. Landw. 9: 223–225, illus.
(15) NELSON, R. M., and BEAL, J. A.
   1929. EXPERIMENTS WITH BLUESTAIN FUNGI IN SOUTHERN PINES. Phyto-
      pathology 19: 1101–1106.
(16) PERSON, H. L.
   1931. THEORY IN EXPLANATION OF THE SELECTION OF CERTAIN TREES BY
      THE WESTERN PINE BEETLE. Jour. Forestry 29: 696–699.
(17) RUMBOLD, C. T.
   1931. TWO BLUE-STAINING FUNGI ASSOCIATED WITH BARK-BEETLE INFES-
      TATION OF PINES. Jour. Agr. Research 43: 847–873, illus.
(18) SCHNEIDER-ORELLI, O.
   1911. DIE ÜBERTRÄGUNG UND KEIMUMG DES AMBROSIAPILZES VON XYLE-
      BORUS (ANISANDRUS) DISPAR f. Naturw. Ztschr. Forst u. Landw.
      9: 186–192, illus.
(19) VON SCHRENK, H.
   1903. THE "BLUING" AND THE "RED ROT" OF THE WESTERN YELLOW
      PINE, WITH SPECIAL REFERENCE TO THE BLACK HILLS FOREST
      RESERVE. U.S.Dept.Agr., Bur. Plant Indus. Bull. 36, 40 pp.,
      illus.
(20) WILSON, M.
   1922. THE BLUING OF CONIFEROUS TIMBER. Roy. Arbor. Soc. Trans. 36:
      82–92.

TRANSMISSION OF THE DUTCH ELM DISEASE PATHOGEN BY SCOLYTUS MULTISTRIATUS AND THE DEVELOPMENT OF INFECTION

K. G. Parker, Philip A. Readio, Leon J. Tyler, and Donald L. Collins[1]

It has been demonstrated that elm bark beetles (family Scolytidae) transmit the pathogen, *Ceratostomella ulmi* (Schwarz) Buisman, to healthy elm trees (4, 5). Fransen and Buisman included the lesser European elm bark beetle, *Scolytus multistriatus* Marsham, in their experiments and C. W. Collins *et al.* (2), working in the United States, also obtained transmission to healthy trees by this species. Inoculations made during the early part of the growth period resulted in a higher percentage of infections than those made in middle or late summer (5). Fransen (4) considered that he was able to trace infection to certain feeding scars made by scolytid beetles. May (7) found that *C. ulmi* could be isolated from scars from which short brownish streaks extended into the twig and from scars "in which no apparent infection had occurred."

Coremia of *Ceratostomella ulmi* have been observed in maternal tunnels and pupal cells of both *Scolytus scolytus* F. and *Scolytus multistriatus* (6, 8). Fruiting structures (mostly coremia) have frequently been observed in the maternal galleries and pupal cells of *S. multistriatus* in diseased trees in and around New York City. Also, they have been observed in dead wood from trees not killed by the Dutch elm disease, and in healthy logs exposed to beetle attack in the field. A discussion of this and a review of the literature are given by Donald L. Collins *et al.* (3). The beetles become infested with the fungus, mostly on their outer surfaces, from the coremia in the pupal cells. Also, the fungus has been isolated from their intestinal tracts (1).

MATERIALS AND METHODS

Cultures of Beetles

1. To make isolations of the pathogen from the surfaces and from the intestinal tracts of beetles they were collected singly in sterile test tubes. The individual adult beetle was then: (a) immersed in a sterile drop of water in a Petri dish for 30 minutes, (b) immersed in a 1 to 1,000 mercuric bichloride solution for 2 minutes, and (c) rinsed in sterile water. The intestinal tract was then removed and macerated in a drop of sterile water in a Petri dish. Acidified potato-dextrose agar was poured into the plates

[1] Thanks are due the Boyce Thompson Institute for Plant Research for making available facilities for doing much of the work reported here. Dr. W. H. Rankin, in charge of Dutch Elm Disease Control for the New York State Department of Agriculture and Markets, and members of his staff, assisted in locating and collecting material. Dr. D. S. Welch made suggestions regarding the work and critically read the manuscript. Others who assisted in the work are L. L. Pechuman, Seth Pope, and Henry Dietrich.

containing the surface washings and the intestinal tracts. It may be pointed out that the method of dissection obviated any chance of contamination of the intestinal tracts from the few spores that might have escaped the mercuric bichloride treatment.

2. To determine the fungus load carried by beetles used in certain of the transmission experiments the beetle-infested logs were first placed in small screen cages. Soon after emergence had begun beetles were collected daily under aseptic conditions, each in a separate sterile test tube. Each beetle was macerated in a drop of sterile water in a Petri dish, one dilution made, and acidified potato-dextrose agar poured into the plates.

Cultures of Plant Tissues

The method as described was used both for field-collected and experimental material. The experimental trees were completely dissected in searching for infected tissue. If any brown discoloration was found in the wood some of the discolored tissue was excised and planted on potato-dextrose agar in Petri dishes. If discolored tissue was not found each feeding scar made by the beetles was cultured separately. If only a small amount of discolored tissue was present, both it and the scar were cultured, but in separate plates. Where the discolored tissue involved more than one scar, the scars were not cultured. The recovery of *Ceratostomella ulmi* from discolored (brown) wood was considered as proof of infection. Where the fungus was recovered from the scars only, it was considered that infection had not taken place, but that transmission of the fungus by the beetles had occurred. On this basis a distinction between "infection" and "transmission only" is made in the tables.

Methods of Inoculation

1. *By Naturally Infested Beetles.* Wood, producing beetles infested with *Ceratostomella ulmi*, was enclosed with healthy trees in out-of-door cages 2½ feet wide by 5 feet long by 6 feet tall. The side walls were of wire screen and the roof was of glass. Eight trees were placed in each cage. After allowing periods of 3 to 10 days for the beetles to emerge, the logs were removed.

2. *By Artificially Infested Beetles, in the Study of Development of Infection.* The beetles were collected and immediately surface-disinfested as follows: They were (a) dipped in water, (b) in 50 per cent ethyl alcohol, (c) immersed in 1 to 1,000 mercuric bichloride solution for 2 minutes, and (d) rinsed 3 times in sterile distilled water. After this treatment the beetles were placed on filter paper in sterile Petri dishes to dry. After drying they were placed in large sterile test tubes with elm twig cultures of *Ceratostomella ulmi* bearing numerous coremia and conidiophores. After being allowed to crawl over the cultures the beetles were taken out and placed on healthy trees. To do this a cage made of celluloid closed at each end with muslin was fastened over the top of the tree and 5 beetles were

placed in the cage. The trees in experiments 1 and 3 were inoculated out-of-doors and those in experiment 2 were inoculated in the greenhouse. The latter were moved out-of-doors in November following their inoculation in August. Otherwise, all trees were held in screen or cheesecloth cages out-of-doors during the summer months until they were examined. During the winter they were all stored out-of-doors.

Experimental Trees

With one exception the trees used in all experiments were 2-year-old budded nursery stock, 6 to 8 feet tall. They were potted in the fall for use the following spring. In experiment 1 of the study of development of infection, 40 of the trees inoculated were 3 years old and had been potted in the spring of the year previous to their use. All trees were in fair to good vigor at the time they were inoculated and, in general, continued extension of shoot length until about July 1.

RESULTS OF CULTURES

Isolations from Beetle Intestinal Tracts

In order to determine whether *Ceratostomella ulmi* occurred in the intestinal tracts of *Scolytus multistriatus*, cultures were made from beetles as they emerged from wood taken from diseased trees. Of 669 such cultures, 509, or 76.1 per cent, produced the fungus from surface washings and 96, or 14.3 per cent, from the intestinal tracts. The number of colonies in plates made from the intestinal tracts was much smaller than in those from surface washings.

Isolations from Beetle-feeding Scars Collected in the Field

In September, 1935, branches bearing feeding scars of scolytid beetles were collected from apparently healthy elm trees in an area of severe disease incidence. These branches were brought to the laboratory and cultures made of the scars. The fungus was isolated from a short discolored streak near one scar. In addition to this it was obtained from 10 of 1,102 scars cultured where no invasion was found beyond the scar tissue. The 10 scars yielding *Ceratostomella ulmi* came from 6 of the 14 trees represented.

On March 24, 1936, similar collections were made from the same location. Of 612 scars cultured *Ceratostomella ulmi* was obtained from 15.

In 1937 and in succeeding years cultures were made of similar material collected at several other locations. *Ceratostomella ulmi* was obtained from scars from most collection stations located near points where trees infected with the Dutch elm disease had been found.

RESULTS OF INOCULATION EXPERIMENTS

Transmission by Naturally Infested Beetles

In these experiments, logs used as beetle sources had previously yielded beetles 50 to 65 per cent of which carried spores of the fungus.

One tree in experiment 1 was discarded because of extensive discoloration in the wood not caused by *Ceratostomella ulmi*.

TABLE 1.—*Transmission by naturally infested beetles*

Experiment	Dates trees inoculated	Dates trees examined	Trees				Feeding scars		
			Number examined	Number with transmission only	Number infected	Number cultured	With *C. ulmi*		
							Number	Per cent	
1	8 on July 1 and 8 on July 4, 1937	Sept. 17–18, 1937	15	5	5	414	25	6.0	
2	8 on May 28 and 16 on June 8, 1938	Aug. 29–31, 1938	24	9	5	291	23	7.9	
	Uninoculated	Aug. 31, 1938	10	0	0	....	......	......	

At the time the trees in experiment 1 were examined, the fungus had invaded the wood throughout one tree. Most of the leaves had dropped and there was considerable dead wood in this tree. On 3 others 10 to 25 per cent of the leaves were wilted or had dropped. There were several dead twigs and branches. The discolored tissue varied in extent from 10 to 25 inches along the various branches. In some instances the infected twigs had died, the fungus being obtained from the dead tissue.

At the time the trees in experiment 2 were examined, 4 of the infected trees showed leaf symptoms such as defoliation, drying, and green wilt. On 1 of these trees most of the branches were dead and there were several dead twigs on the other 3 trees. In 2 trees most of the wood was discolored; in others there was less discoloration. In 1 tree the only discolored tissue was in 1 new shoot, with about 12 inches of the tip involved.

Development of Infection

In 1936 and 1937 experiments were designed for the purpose of determining whether, if the trees be left standing, infections may eventually take place in trees bearing scars in which the fungus persists for 1 or more seasons.

Experiment 1. Twenty trees were inoculated on each of the dates June 30, July 1, 2, and 3, 1936, with beetles that had been on the cultures for 2 hours. After the beetles had been on the trees 7 days, they were removed and cultured singly.

Recovery of the fungus from the beetles after their removal from the trees was very good, a few hundred colonies being obtained from each beetle.

Experiment 2. Sixty trees were inoculated, 20 on each of the dates August 26, 27, and 28, 1936. The method was similar to that used in experiment 1.

TABLE 2.—*Development of infection following transmission by beetles*

Experiment	Dates trees inoculated	Dates trees examined	Trees			Feeding scars			
			Number examined	Number with transmission only	Number infected	Number present	Number cultured	With *C. ulmi*	
								Number	Per cent
1	June 30, July 1, 2, and 3, 1936	July 14–17, 1936	19	14	0	115	114	31	27.2
		Oct. 13 and 14, 1936	20	10	6[a]	112	106	37	34.9
		Sept. 6, 1937	19	12	4	124	110	49	44.5
		June 23, 1938	18	13	1	109	94	41	43.6
	Uninoculated	June 23, 1938	10	0	0	0	......	......	......
2	Aug. 26, 27, and 28, 1936	Oct. 2–4, 1936	20	13	0	172	167	28	16.8
		Sept. 6, 1937	20	16	0	178	157	49	31.2
		June 27 and 28, 1938	20	15	0	166	149	30	20.1
	Uninoculated	June 28, 1938	10	0	0	0	......	......	......
3	June 15 and 16, 1937	July 20, 1937	18	12	5	73	71	34	47.9
		Sept. 14, 1937	18	9	7	66	63	35	55.6
		July 7, 1938	18	12	5	69	65	36	55.4
		Oct. 19, 1939	28	16	4[b]	104	78	42	53.8
		July 23–25, 1940	28	16	3[c]	104	84	37	44.0
	Uninoculated	July 25, 1940	20	0	0	0	......	......	......

[a] Includes a tree that wilted and was examined July 31, 1936.

[b] Does not include 1 tree with a dead branch, which probably had been infected but from which *Ceratostomella ulmi* was not obtained when cultures were made in October, 1939.

[c] Does not include 1 tree that wilted and apparently was invaded throughout by the fungus in 1937 but from which *Ceratostomella ulmi* was not obtained in cultures made from living discolored wood in July, 1940.

264

Recovery of the fungus from the beetles after removal from the trees was slightly less successful than in experiment 1.

Experiment 3. One hundred twenty trees were inoculated, 60 on June 15 and 60 on June 16, 1937. The beetles were left on the cultures overnight (about 22 hours) and were removed from the trees after 6 days.

Recovery of the fungus from the beetles after removal from the trees was almost as good as in experiment 1.

At various dates, as indicated in table 2, trees from the different experiments were cut and examined. Each lot examined was selected so as to represent the whole as to number of feeding scars.

In experiment 1 only 1 tree wilted. In experiment 2 no wilt occurred. In experiment 3, 1 tree was wilted by July 6, 1937. By August 7, after 18 trees had been cut for examination, wilt had occurred on 5 other trees, varying in extent from $\frac{1}{5}$ to $\frac{3}{4}$ of the leaves on each tree.

DISCUSSION

In the experiments here reported *Ceratostomella ulmi* became established in many beetle feeding scars without the occurrence of true infection. It is shown in table 2 that infection did not occur in the trees inoculated in August, 1936, although the fungus could be isolated from feeding scars on these trees nearly 2 years after inoculation. Cultures made a few weeks, or at various intervals up to 2 or 3 years after the trees had been inoculated, indicated little or no difference in the percentage of scars containing the fungus in viable condition. On the other hand, there appeared to be no initiation of infection after a few weeks following the inoculations. That is, if *C. ulmi* was introduced into a feeding scar by the beetles and invasion of the adjacent tissue did not take place within a few weeks, infection never resulted from that inoculation. The fungus remained viable in the scar tissue on some trees more than 3 years without invading the trees.

In several infected trees in these experiments all discolored tissue was dead at the time of examination. If the cultures were made from such trees within the growing season of the year in which they had been inoculated *Ceratostomella ulmi* was isolated from the dead part but not from the live parts below. In a few instances it was not obtained from the proximal part of the dead portion, although it was viable in the distal part.

There was some indication that the number of trees showing infection by cultural examination 2 or 3 years after inoculation was smaller than when the examination was made earlier. In no case did the fungus invade tissue produced in years subsequent to the year of inoculation.

The results of these experiments and the ease with which the Dutch elm disease pathogen can be isolated from feeding scars collected from trees in the field indicate that a great many inoculations made by the feeding activities of the beetles do not result in true infection.

SUMMARY

Cerastomella ulmi was obtained from the outer surfaces of *Scolytus multistriatus* adults in higher percentage than from their intestinal tracts. Likewise, the numbers of colonies in the cultures were much greater.

Transmission of the fungus to potted healthy elm trees by the beetles in their feeding activities was readily obtained. The fungus was reisolated from feeding wounds on uninfected trees as long as 3 years following inoculation.

Infection was obtained on trees inoculated during the late spring and early summer. Inoculations made later in the season induced infection less frequently or not at all.

There was evidence that the fungus sometimes died in infected trees. Sometimes the infected twig died without the entire tree becoming invaded.

LITERATURE CITED

1. BETREM, J. G. De iepenziekte en de iepenspintkevers. Tijdsch. over plantenziekten 35: 273–288. 1929.
2. COLLINS, C. W., W. D. BUCHANAN, R. R. WHITTEN, and C. H. HOFFMAN. Bark beetles and other possible insect vectors of the Dutch elm disease *Ceratostomella ulmi* (Schwarz) Buisman. Jour. Econ. Ent. 29: 169–176. 1936.
3. COLLINS, DONALD L., K. G. PARKER, and HENRY DIETRICH. Uninfected elm wood as a source of the bark beetle (*Scolytus multistriatus* Marsham) carrying the Dutch elm disease pathogen. N. Y. (Cornell) Agr. Exp. Stat. Bull. 740. 1940.
4. FRANSEN, J. J. Enkele gegevens omtrent de verspreiding van de door *Graphium ulmi* Schwarz veroorzaakte iepenziekte door de iepenspintkevers, Eccoptogaster (Scolytus) *scolytus* F. en *Eccoptogaster* (Scolytus) *multistriatus* Marsh. in verband met de bestrijding dezer ziekte. Tijdsch. over plantenziekten 37: 49–62. 1931.
5. FRANSEN, J. J., and CHRISTINE BUISMAN. Infectieproeven op verschillende iepensoorten met behulp van iepenspintkevers. Tijdsch. over plantenziekten 41: 221–239. 1935.
6. GROSSMAN, HÉLÈNE. Beiträge zur Kenntnis der Lebensgemeinschaft zwischen Borkenkäfern und Pilzen. Zeitschr. für Parasitenk. 3: 56–102. 1930.
7. MAY, CURTIS. Outbreaks of the Dutch elm disease in the United States. U. S. Dept. Agr. Circ. 322: 1–19. 1934.
8. WOLLENWEBER, H. W., and C. STAPP. Untersuchungen über die als Ulmensterben bekannte Baumkrankheit. Arb. Biol. Reichsanst. für Land- und Forstwirtsch. 16: 283–324. 1928.

Insect Transmission of Ceratocystis Species
Associated with Aspen Cankers

T. E. Hinds

Ceratocystis canker of aspen (*Populus tremuloides* Michx.) caused by the fungus *Ceratocystis fimbriata* Ell. & Halst., was first confirmed in Minnesota by Wood & French (13) in 1962, although the cankers, whose cause was unknown at the time, had been reported earlier from the western United States (2, 4, 9, 11).

Insect transmission of *Ceratocystis* species is common; two specific studies have demonstrated ability of insects to transmit *C. fimbriata*. Crone & Bachelder (6) obtained infection on London plane tree in 6 of 11 trials by placing beetles on cultures of the fungus prior to using them as inoculating agents. Insects collected from diseased plane trees, however, only transmitted *C. fimbriata* directly in two of seven trials. Moller & DeVay (12) provided circumstantial evidence for transmission of *C. fimbriata* by insects to almond. They isolated the fungus from field-collected insects, and transferred insects reared on cultures of the fungus to healthy trees. They demonstrated direct transmission and subsequent infection with two of the many insect species tested. The exclusion of insects and mites by a screen covering fresh bark wounds prevented infection and canker development on the trunks of control trees.

The fact that *C. fimbriata* is insect-transmitted in other hosts suggested that insects may be involved in the transmission of *C. fimbriata* in aspen, particularly as insects are commonly present on or about Ceratocystis cankers on aspen, and infection normally occurs at trunk wounds (7). This paper reports on studies conducted to investigate this possibility.

MATERIALS AND METHODS.—To attract insects, aspen trees in two areas of the Roosevelt National Forest, Larimer County, Colo., were wounded biweekly throughout the summers of 1967 and 1968. An area of bark about 10 X 10 cm was cut loose from the trunk with a hatchet on each of two trees. Insects attracted to each wound were collected with an aspirator biweekly and put in separate vials.

PHYTOPATHOLOGY, 1972, Vol. 62, pp. 221-225.

Those to be used for disease transmission studies were collected individually in sterile gelatin capsules. Specimens of each apparent species of insect were preserved in alcohol, and most were identified by the Insect Identification and Parasite Introduction Research Branch, Entomology Research Division, USDA, Beltsville, Md. The staphylinids were identified by Ian Moore, El Cajon, Calif.

RESULTS.—*Association of insects with trunk wounds.*—Time of insect emergence in the spring was unknown; trunk wounds made the first week in June did not attract insects until 3 weeks later. Wounds made in July, August, and the first week in September, however, attracted adult insects within a few days. The wounds became infected with different species of *Ceratocystis* soon after insect visitation, and a succession of perithecial formations was apparent. Mature perithecia of *C. alba* DeVay, Davidson, & Moller formed in 4-5 days; *C. moniliformis* (Hedgc.) C. Moreau, in 5-7 days; *C. fimbriata* and *C. populina* Hinds & Davidson, in 7-10 days; *C. tremulo-aurea* Davidson & Hinds, in 10-14 days; and *C. crassivaginata* Griffin, within 21 days. Perithecia of the various species were frequently intermixed on wounds, but those of *C. alba* soon disintegrated after maturing. Sapwood invaded with *C. moniliformis* appeared pink for the first few days, then turned the characteristic blue-black discoloration similar to that caused by other species of blue-stain fungi. Infected wounds had the unique ester odors typical of *C. fimbriata* and *C. moniliformis* in culture.

Wounds attracted insects (Table 1) throughout the summer. Nitidulids usually appeared first, followed in a few days by staphylinids and flies. Of the nitidulids, three species of *Epuraea* and *Colopterus truncatus* were most abundant and most frequently collected. Morphological differences between the three *Epuraea* species are minor, and they are combined here for discussion. Insects mated and oviposited under the loose bark, and larvae of the nitidulids, staphylinids, and flies were common. Adult nitidulids died after oviposition. Nitidulid eggs hatched in ca. 1 week, and larvae matured in about 3 weeks, and dropped to the ground to pupate. At least two generations were produced during the summer, and larvae of the last generation overwintered as pupae in the soil at the base of the trees. *Glischrochilus moratus* and *G. vittatus*, while not so numerous, were present throughout the summer, and were more common in September and October. *Chymomyza aldrichi* adults, larvae, and pupae were common on wounds throughout the summer, whereas adult Gelechiidae, Oecophoridae, and Tachinidae occupied wounds only

268

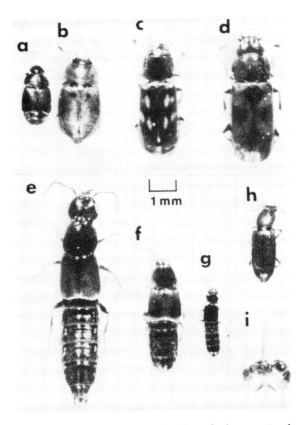

Fig. 1. Insects commonly found on fresh aspen trunk wounds in Colorado. Nitidulids: **a)** *Colopterus truncatus;* **b)** *Epuraea erichsoni;* **c)** *Glischrochilus vittatus;* and **d)** *Glischrochilus moratus;* staphylinids: **e)** *Quedius raevigatus;* **f)** *Quedius* sp.; and **g)** *Nudobius corticalis;* the root-eating beetle: **h)** *Rhizophagus brunneus;* and Pomace fly: **i)** *Chymomyza aldrichi.* Scale same for all insects.

during cold weather. *Trypodendron retusum* and *Idiocerus lachrymalis* were collected on healthy bark adjacent to wounds. Numerous other insects visited the wounds, particularly during cold periods, but were not common enough to collect for culturing and identification.

Insect-Ceratocystis associations.—For isolation of fungi, individual insects were placed in petri dishes containing a 2% Fleischmann's diamalt and 2% Difco-Bacto agar medium within 2 hr after collection. The insects were allowed free movement in the plates for 24 hr to several days, after which they were pushed down into the agar.

The carrot technique recommended by Moller &

TABLE 1. Frequency of *Ceratocystis* spp. associated with insects collected from fresh aspen trunk wounds in Colorado

Insect family and species	No. insects cultured	Ceratocystis spp. recovered				
		C. fimbriata	C. populina	C. moniliformis	C. crassivaginata	C. pilifera[b]
		%	%	%	%	%
Nitidulidae (sap-feeding beetles)						
Epuraea spp.[a]	51	16	90	13	2	
Colopterus truncatus Randall	50	44	41	11	2	3
Glischrochilus moratus Brown	10	40	100		10	20
Glischrochilus vittatus Say	35	49	94	9	14	17
Rhizophagidae (root-eating beetles)						
Rhizophagus brunneus Horn	41	32	83	29	15	17
Staphylinidae (rove beetles)						
Nudobius corticalis Casey	50	38	88	18	12	4
Quedius raevigatus Gyllenhal	31	26	100	26		
Quedius sp.	28	11	71	7		2
Drosophilidae (Pomace flies)						
Chymomyza aldrichi Sturtevant	27	22	70	22		15
Tachinidae (Tachina flies)						
Nowickia sp. [probably *N. latifrons* (Tothill)]	10		30			

270

Aphididae (aphids, plant lice) *Pterocomma pseudopopulea* Palmer	3	66		33	33
Gelechiidae (Gelechid moths) *Anacampis niveopulvella* Chamberlin	8	50	12		
Oecophoridae (moths) *Ethmia coloradella* Chamberlin	2		50		50
Scolytidae (bark beetles) *Trypodendron retusum* LeConte	5	40	80		
Cicadellidae (leafhoppers) *Idiocerus lachrymalis* Fitch	27	37	52	19	
Anthocoridae (minute pirate bugs) *Anthocoris musculus* Say	3	33	100		33

a Three species of *Epuraea*: *E. avara* Randall; *E. erichsoni* Reitter; and *E. terminalis* Mann.
b 1968 collections only.

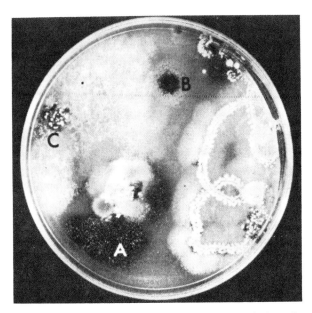

Fig. 2. Petri dish culture with numerous colonies of *Ceratocystis,* bacteria, yeasts, and other fungi 1 week after the introduction of an insect; **a)** *C. fimbriata;* **b)** *C. populina;* and **c)** *C. moniliformis.*

DeVay (12) was used for the initial screening of insects for *C. fimbriata.* The method was effective, but too selective. Placing live insects directly in plates containing diamalt agar medium allowed growth and identification of the various species of *Ceratocystis* involved.

The nitidulids frequently laid eggs which hatched in the plates. Larvae and adults would consume perithecia, aerial mycelium, and yeast growing in the plates, but larvae seldom pupated; they died and became overgrown with fungi. Nematodes introduced by the insects were also common in some plates.

The insects (Fig. 1) often carried one or more species of *Ceratocystis;* it was not unusual to obtain at least three from a single insect. In addition to *C. fimbriata, C. crassivaginata, C. moniliformis, C. pilifera* (Fries) C. Moreau, and *C. populina* were frequently isolated. The common insects collected and the frequency of the various species of *Ceratocystis,* as obtained from plate cultures, associated with them are listed in Table 1.

It was not possible to identify all fungi which grew in the plates. It was not unusual to have 50 or more colonies of *Ceratocystis* in a plate (Fig. 2). Also, fast-growing species, such as *C. moniliformis,* would

272

cover a plate within 10 days and obscure colonies of other species. *Ceratocystis crassivaginata*, which usually requires about 3 weeks for production of perithecia, was usually obtained only by subculturing. *Ceratocystis pilifera* was first detected in plates near the end of the 1st year of screening; consequently, identifications of this species in Table 1 pertain only to the 1968 collections. Although this fungus has a wide range of hosts including *P. tremuloides*, this is apparently the first report of its association with an insect. *Ceratocystis alba* grows slowly, and seldom produces perithecia on diamalt agar; consequently it was not detected in the plates.

Ceratocystis populina was first to produce perithecia in culture and the easiest to identify, which may account for its being the most frequently isolated species from all insects. *Ceratocystis tremulo-aurea* was isolated once from *Rhizophagus brunneus*, whereas *C. minor* (Hedgc.) Hunt was isolated once each from *Anthocoris musculus* and *Glischrochilus vittatus*. Of the 381 insects plated, 36 (9%) were so completely overgrown with other fungi that the presence of *Ceratocystis* could not be verified.

Inoculation via insect vectors.—Ceratocystis infection of fresh trunk wounds in the field, and the frequency of *Ceratocystis* spp. associated with insects attracted to these wounds, suggested that some insects were vectors of the fungi. To demonstrate insect transmission, 3-year-old aspen sprouts growing in the greenhouse were inoculated in July 1968 by placing two live, field-collected insects of the same species in a small aseptic bark wound (slit to the cambium). The slit was then covered with an adhesive tape bandage. The covering and insects were removed after 10 days. Controls consisted of bark slits and covering only.

Cankers were produced at all bark slits into which insects were inserted. None developed in the controls. Necrotic bark tissue surrounding the inoculation wound and *Ceratocystis* perithecia were evident when the insects and bandages were removed. Many insects were still alive at the end of 10 days. Canker formation and stem girdling, depending upon stem size, were evident 7 weeks later, and continued until the end of the growing season. By then, all insect-inoculated stems, with the exception of two inoculated with *Colopterus truncatus*, were girdled. The stems were cut for microscopic examination of perithecia at the inoculation site, and for isolation of fungi from canker tissue. Table 2 lists the insects used, number of inoculations made, and fungi associated with the cankers.

TABLE 2. Transmission of *Ceratocystis* spp. by field-collected insects to aspen in the greenhouse

Insect	No. inoculations	No. times *Ceratocystis* isolated from canker tissue		No. times *Ceratocystis* perithecia observed at inoculation site				
		C. fimbriata	C. populina	C. fimbriata	C. populina	C. alba	C. crassivaginata	C. moniliformis
Epuraea spp.	18	7	4	14	16	18	3	3
Colopterus truncatus	10	1	1	1	6	6	0	0
Nudobius corticalis	11	3	2	7	10	10	0	1
Quedius sp.	5	0	0	3	6	4	0	1
Q. raevigatus	4	1	2	1	2	2	0	0
Rhizophagus brunneus	9	5	3	4	8	8	1	2
Control	10	0	0	0	0	0	0	0

TABLE 3. *Ceratocystis* spp. isolated from insects emerging in the spring

Insect	No. insects	No. times *Ceratocystis* spp. isolated			
		C. fimbriata	C. populina	C. pilifera	C. alba
Epuraea spp.	20	6	15	4	1
Colopterus truncatus	1	1	1	0	1
Nudobius corticalis	32	9	4	0	7
Quedius raevigatus	10	0	0	0	0
Rhizophagus brunneus	2	0	0	0	0

Presence of fungi in insect.—A modification of Batra's technique (3) of "fractional sterilization" of insects was used to determine whether *Ceratocystis* species were present within the nitidulid *Glischrochilus vittatus*. This modification consisted of placing the insects alternately in moist and dry sterile chambers for three 24-hr periods each, prior to their placement on diamalt culture media.

Of nine surface-sterilized nitidulids, *C. fimbriata* was isolated from five, *C. populina* from nine, *C. pilifera* from three, *C. moniliformis* from one, and *C. crassivaginata* from one.

Persistence of fungi in insect.—Because *Ceratocystis* spp. were able to survive within *Glischrochilus vittatus*, the following study was made to determine their ability to overwinter in pupae.

Newly emerging insects were collected in the spring by placing muslin cloth and plastic cages (140 X 140 cm) on the ground in May 1969 around infected trees at two areas. Cage edges were embedded 15-30 cm into the ground and secured around the tree base with plastic tape. A zipper in the cloth and a covered jar lid ring in the plastic provided access to the cage's interior. Insects began to emerge the 1st week in June, and were trapped within the cages on a freshly cut piece of aspen. Insects were individually collected twice weekly during the month, and placed on culture media in petri dishes within 2 hr. Culture media used were diamalt agar and diamalt agar with the addition of 0.5% Difco yeast extract.

The various insects collected from eight ground cages and the species of *Ceratocystis* they carried as determined from cultures are given in Table 3. Identity of *Ceratocystis* fungi was often obscured by fast-growing soil fungi.

Acquisition of fungi from soil.—To determine whether *C. fimbriata* was present in the soil, samples were collected in mid-August from the soil at the base of two infected trees in each of two areas. Each sample was thoroughly mixed, and a small portion placed between carrot discs. Soil also was placed on fresh sterile aspen blocks (3 X 3 cm) on moist filter paper in petri dishes. All inoculations were incubated at 100% humidity at room temperature, and checked weekly for 3 weeks.

None of the 150 soil samples incubated between carrot discs yielded *Ceratocystis*. At the end of 3 weeks, only six *C. populina* colonies appeared on four of the 138 aspen blocks tested. No other species of *Ceratocystis* were detected.

DISCUSSION.—The habits of the various insects found on fresh aspen trunk wounds are variable and incompletely known. Nitidulids are generally considered saprophagus and mycetophagus. Adults and larvae of the *Epuraea* and *Colopterus* species observed in this study fed on mycelium and perithecia, as did the larvae of *Chymomyza aldrichi*. Larvae and adults of certain *Glischrochilus* and *Rhizophagus* species are predaceous on xylophagus insects (1). Predation was not observed. These insects were active in the fungus mats formed on the sapwood. Tachinidae are parasitic on many lepidopterous insects, which may account for their presence in wounds. The staphylinids are known predators, and were observed preying on the nitidulids collected in this study. Numerous aphids, nematodes, and mites were found in fresh wounds, but their role is unknown in the etiology of canker formation.

Several species of *Ceratocystis* soon form perithecia on fresh wounds, and the insects which frequent these wounds become contaminated with spores of these fungi. The fact that at least five species of *Ceratocystis* were transmitted by insects used in greenhouse studies confirm their potential as transmitting agents. The relative importance of each insect species is still uncertain, however. It has been shown that *C. fimbriata* causes cankers (7, 13, 14), but observations on 3-year-old field inoculations with *C. populina* and *C. crassivaginata* indicate that they too may cause cankers.

Others have determined the acquisition and persistence of *C. fimbriata* in or on vectors (6, 12). Hussain (8), who worked with aspen canker insects in Colorado, used Bretz's technique (5) to surface-sterilize 12 larvae of *Epuraea*, 22 adult *Epuraea*, and 15 adult *Colopterus truncatus* before placing them on culture media. *Ceratocystis fimbriata* was isolated from eight larvae, seven adult *Epuraea*, and six adult *Colopterus truncatus*. *Ceratocystis populina* was isolated from 12 larvae, 16 adult *Epuraea*, and two adult *Colopterus truncatus*. Hussain concluded that the adult nitidulids carried the two fungi internally. Hussain also cultured eight *Epuraea* and two *Colopterus truncatus* adults which had just emerged from pupae in the soil. *Ceratocystis fimbriata* was isolated from all of the newly emerged insects. His evidence that the fungus could pass through one generation suggested that it could overwinter in pupae. Hussain (8) might have recovered additional species of *Ceratocystis* had his insect isolates been subcultured. During the latter part of this study, *C. alba* commonly formed perithecia, and its identification was confirmed when the diamalt yeast extract medium was used. Had this medium also been used throughout the study, *C. alba* would probably have been recovered in the initial surveys (Table 1).

Soil fungi carried by the insects collected from the ground cages quickly covered some of the culture plates. Over half the plates were so overrun that species of *Ceratocystis* could not be isolated. Soil fungi were also common in the other plates, but the *Ceratocystis* spp. were identified before plates were completely overrun.

Moller & DeVay (12) investigated the possibility that *C. fimbriata* might be present in orchard soil. Using a carrot disc technique, they recovered the fungus from soil only occasionally, and then only under specific conditions. They concluded that "the soil apparently serves as a limited inoculum source, if at all". P. D. Manion (*personal communication*) occasionally isolated the organism from soil in greenhouse pots using sterile aspen blocks as a culture medium (10). No definite conclusions concerning soil as a source of inoculum can be drawn from this limited study in Colorado. The fact that *Ceratocystis* has been isolated from soil indicates the fungus may be able to survive there.

Nitidulid beetles, which are sap- and fungus-feeding insects, are ideally adapted for transmission of *Ceratocystis* spp. Although nitidulids were not commonly found on Ceratocystis cankers in early spring when *C. fimbriata* produces perithecia and ascospores, they readily infected fresh trunk wounds. Active cankers may thus be of secondary importance as an inoculum source, and the insects themselves the reservoirs of primary fungus inoculum.

LITERATURE CITED

1. ARNETT, R. H., JR. 1963. The beetles of the United States. Catholic Univ. Amer. Press. Wash., D.C. 1112 p.
2. BAKER, F. S. 1925. Aspen in the central Rocky Mountain region. U.S. Dep. Agr. Bull. 1291. 46 p.
3. BATRA, L. R. 1963. Ecology of ambrosia fungi and their dissemination by beetles. Kans. Acad. Sci. Trans. 66:213-236.
4. BOYCE, J. S. 1961. Forest pathology [3rd ed.]. McGraw-Hill Book Co. New York. 572 p.
5. BRETZ, N. L. 1966. Improved laboratory methods for rearing the boll weevil. J. Econ. Entomol. 59:374-376.
6. CRONE, L. J., & S. BACHELDER. 1961. Insect transmission of canker stain fungus Ceratocystis fimbriata f. platani. Phytopathology 51:576 (Abstr.).
7. HINDS, T. E. 1972. Ceratocystis canker of aspen. Phytopathology 62:213-220.
8. HUSSAIN, N. G. 1968. The role of nitidulids in the transmission of Ceratocystis canker of quaking aspen. M.S. Thesis. Colo. State Univ. 138 p.

9. LONG, W. H. 1918. An undescribed canker of poplars and willows caused by Cytospora chrysosperma. J. Agr. Res. 13:331-343.
10. MANION, P. D., & D. W. FRENCH. 1967. Nectria galligena and Ceratocystis fimbriata cankers of aspen in Minnesota. Forest Sci. 13:23-28.
11. MEINECKE, E. P. 1929. Quaking aspen. A study in applied forest pathology. U.S. Dep. Agr. Tech. Bull. 155. 33 p.
12. MOLLER, W. J., & J. E. DEVAY. 1968. Insect transmission of Ceratocystis fimbriata in deciduous fruit orchards. Phytopathology 58:1499-1508.
13. WOOD, F. A., & D. W. FRENCH. 1963. Ceratocystis fimbriata, the cause of a stem canker of quaking aspen. Forest Sci. 9:232-235.
14. ZALASKY, H. 1965. Process of Ceratocystis fimbriata infection in aspen. Can. J. Bot. 43:1157-1162.

INTRODUCTION TO SECTION V:
VIRUS RELATIONSHIPS

Viruses are more dependent upon insect vectors than any other pathogen. Vector-virus relationships are many and varied. These are summarized very well in a review paper by Maramorosch (1963). Chewing insects play a relatively minor role in virus transmission and we have chosen the paper by Walters (1952) which describes the transmission of three viruses by grasshoppers to focus attention on the role of chewing insects in virus transmission. Insects with piercing-sucking mouthparts are most important as virus vectors and they receive major attention in this collection. Close biological relationships ranging from transovariol passage from generation to generation, multiplication in the vector and even apparent attacks on the vector by the viruses they carry exist among insects and the viruses. These aspects of virus transmission are treated in the papers of Sylvester (1969), Jensen (1959), and Maramorosch (1952).

The recent association of mycoplasma-like organisms with diseases long believed to be induced by viruses has opened a new dimension in the study of insect-pathogen relationships. Many of the close biological relationships once thought to exist between insects and viruses may actually be an insect-mycoplasma-like organism relationships rather than insect-virus relationships. We have chosen the paper by Maramorosch, Shikata and Grandos (1968) to summarize the possible insect-mycoplasma relationships.

The scope of insect transmission has been expanded in this collection of papers to include the important role of mites as virus vectors and we have chosen the papers by Slykhuis (1955) to summarize this topic.

ARTHROPOD TRANSMISSION OF PLANT VIRUSES[1,2]

By Karl Maramorosch

Arthropod-borne plant viruses are among the most important, most complex, and most extensively distributed plant disease agents in the world. The economically important diseases they cause, as well as the intriguing mechanisms by which they survive and propagate, have attracted numerous workers to this constantly expanding field.

The vectors of any one plant virus are almost always restricted to one of the major taxa, such as the aphids, the leafhoppers, the whiteflies, the thrips, the mealybugs, the beetles, the treehoppers, the mites, or the nematodes (29). Although a number of records to the contrary can be found in older literature, they are not well established and ought to be reinvestigated in the light of the bulk of evidence that supports the above rule. Like any broad generalization, this rule may have a small number of exceptions. Black (29) pointed out that a second broad generalization has wide validity: a plant virus is almost always transmitted by only one of the principal types of transmission, that is, either by the circulative, the stylet-borne, or the propagative type. One of the possible exceptions to this rule will be discussed in the case of the aphid-borne transmission of potato leaf roll virus. Some beetle-borne viruses may also be transmitted in more than one way, but, nevertheless, the rule has wide validity.

Because of space limitations, the present review makes no attempt to cover the field in a comprehensive manner. The reader will be referred to numerous excellent recent reviews of plant virus transmission. It will be our aim to focus attention on certain aspects that, in the opinion of this reviewer, are either salient or controversial, or that have not been covered adequately elsewhere. While outstanding discoveries of fundamental nature could fairly easily be assembled from the literature, as could also the controversial and stimulating problems, coverage of some lesser-known work presented a more difficult task at first. However, the unselfish cooperation of numerous colleagues in many countries made our undertaking much easier than it appeared in the beginning. In most instances, the subject could be brought up-to-date through personal communications, articles in galley proof, or through the kind permission of authors to quote from their manuscripts in press. I would like to thank all those who helped in the

[1] The survey of the literature pertaining to this review was concluded in June, 1962. The author has omitted numerous conributions which, but for restriction of space, should rightfully be included.

[2] Recent work by the author and his associates, discussed in this review, has been sponsored in part by United States Public Health Service Grants No. E-1537 and E-4290, and by a National Science Foundation Grant No. G-17663.

ANNUAL REVIEW OF ENTOMOLOGY, 1963, Vol. 8, pp. 369-414.

preparation and gathering of the materials and who sent important information. They are not responsible, however, for my errors or conclusions. Special thanks are offered to Professor Teikichi Fukushi of the Hokkaido University, and Dr. Tosi Take Iida of the National Institute of Agricultural Sciences, Tokyo, who provided translations, abstracts of, and comments on recent work published in Japanese. Without this extensive collaboration the material presented in this review could not have been assembled.

APHIDS

The largest number of vectors of plant viruses are among the aphids. Transmission by aphids has been reviewed by various authors in recent years. The reader is referred to the most important reviews on this subject by: Bawden (7), Bradley (37), Broadbent (47), Broadbent & Martini (49), Carter (52), Heinze (86), Kennedy (98), Kennedy et al. (99, 100), Posnette (159), Rochow (170), Smith (198, 199), Sylvester (214, 215, 216), and Watson (233).

Aphids transmit plant viruses in several ways. Controversial conclusions, based on intuition and induction, have stimulated a re-examination of the findings and conclusions concerning the transmission processes. The contributions made in recent years by Sylvester in California have played a most important role in clarifying the issues and in the battle to regain orderly concepts. Sylvester's systematic work with aphids which transmit virus during single probes gave the foundation for the method that played an important role in subsequent aphid vector experiments in many laboratories. Although many attempts have been made to bring order into the somewhat confused picture, the mechanisms of aphid transmission, the reasons for vector specificity, and the multiplication of certain viruses in aphids are still only partly understood.

Types of aphid transmission of plant viruses are characterized by two extremes: one, commonly termed nonpersistent or mechanical, in which aphids can acquire and transmit virus within a matter of seconds or minutes, but soon lose the ability unless they have access to another virus source; the other, usually called persistent or nonmechanical, where aphids often require hours for acquisition and transmission, but where they can continue to transmit virus for many days after removal from the virus source.

The growing number of intermediates, that is, of viruses that are neither persistent nor nonpersistent in the precise meaning of the term, induced Kennedy et al. (100) to abandon such empirical criteria as virus retention in aphids, and, instead, to consider actual routes of virus transport in the vector. Only two such routes, or mechanisms, have been recognized so far. Watson (233) designated them as external and internal: "external" means that the viruses are carried at the tips of stylets and infectivity is lost when the insect molts; "internal" is used for viruses that are ingested and can be recovered from the hemolymph, from which they reach the salivary glands. This second kind is not characterized by loss of virus during molting. Kennedy *et al.* have changed the terms of Watson to the more appropriate terms "stylet-borne" and "circulative." The latter has been adopted from Black's criterion of certain leafhopper-borne viruses (29). The term "circulative," as applied here to aphid-borne viruses, comprises viruses described by Day & Irzykiewicz as "vector-latent" (60). The circulative viruses are acquired by aphids through their mouth parts, accumulated internally, with or without multiplication in the vector, then passed through the insect tissues and introduced into plants again via the mouth parts of the insect. In the case of potato leaf roll virus, evidence suggests that it is a propagative virus, that is, that it has a biological cycle and that it multiplies in its vector. The terms "propagative" (multiplying in their insect vectors) and "circulative" are not mutually exclusive (29). Stylet-borne viruses are carried inside the labial groove, where there is a close interaction between insect saliva, virus, and plant juice. The stylet-borne viruses include most of those described in the literature under the term "semipersistent" and "nonpersistent," while circulative viruses include the "persistent" viruses. Whether all semipersistent viruses should be grouped together and whether all of them are stylet-borne, is still questionable. The term "semipersistent" was originally introduced by Sylvester to describe the vector-virus relationship between beet yellows virus and its vector *Myzus persicae*. Recent evidence, presented by Sylvester & Bradley (216a) and by Bradley & Sylvester (41a), indicated that beet yellows virus may not be stylet-borne and that it therefore belongs to the circulative viruses. However, no evidence has as yet been presented to indicate that this virus is being retained through a molt. It is not known whether the virus could be carried from insect to insect in a serial passage.

The cauliflower mosaic virus, considered at one time to be nonpersistent, semipersistent, or even as both nonpersistent and persistent (91a), can now be classified definitely as stylet-borne. Recent experimental evidence in support of this conclusion comes from the work of Orlob & Bradley (152a), Day & Venables (60a), and Cook (55a). The uneven distribution and low concentration of the virus in infected plants, together with the striking behavioral differences between the two vectors, *M. persicae* and *Brevicoryne brassicae* (Linnaeus), accounted for earlier difficulties in classifying the virus as stylet-borne.

The new system of classification and the terms used by Kennedy *et al.* (100) have so many advantages over those generally used that they will most likely become widely accepted in the future.

Another important point made by Kennedy *et al.* (100) concerns the taxonomic determination of vectors. This problem is of paramount importance in all groups of arthropod vectors. While great care is taken by experimenters to exclude all but one species from a laboratory test of transmission, it would seem imperative to take similar care in respect to the identity of that species. The authors suggest the preservation in a museum collection of some of the specimens used in transmission tests. The accession number or reference should also be quoted in the publication.

This proposal was made by F. F. Smith as early as 1937, when he pointed out that the identity of many insect vectors was uncertain and suggested that some plan be developed for preserving the proved insect vectors of viruses (195). It would at the same time be worthwhile to preserve the viruses, whenever possible. For instance, Allard's *Macrosiphum solanifolii* (Ashm.) (= *M. euphorbiae* Thomas) specimens are preserved in the Smithsonian Institution in Washington, but it is no longer possible to establish whether the virus, transmitted by these insects, was in reality the common tobacco mosaic virus (TMV), as reported in 1914 (2). Subsequent tests, and an extensive search for a vector of TMV, have failed to yield results.

Stylet-borne transmission.—Many attempts have been made in the last decade to explain the intricacies of virus transmission by aphids, and to account for the specificity in the "mechanical" transmission process. In 1952, Bradley postulated that aphids transmit nonpersistent viruses by an essentially mechanical process and that virus contamination of the stylets occurred during saliva-free penetrations (35). No explanation was attempted at that time for he specificiy of aphid vectors. In 1954, Day & Irzykiewicz proposed a "mechanical-inactivator-behavior" hypothesis, that linked specificity with stylet contamination by virus particles and selective inactivation of virus on the stylets by labile components of the saliva with possible differences in the behavior of vectors (60). Sylvester, in 1954, (213a) reviewed the subject of nonpersistent aphid transmission, and also proposed essentially the same hypothesis as Day & Irzykiewicz, but did not include the behavioral component. He assumed specificity to be a function of "compatibility" between the virus, saliva which introduced it, and the host plant region inoculated. In the same year, a third hypothesis was presented by van der Want in The Netherlands (231). It was assumed that vectors acquire virus during brief punctures of epidermal cells only when little or no saliva is produced. With the increase of saliva production and the formation of the salivary sheath during deeper penetrations of the leaf, no virus can be acquired. As the transmission of a stylet-borne ("nonpersistent") virus requires only a few seconds, it is most unlikely that the virus passes through the digestive tract in that short period. Therefore, van der Want postulated that the stylet-borne virus becomes attached in one way or another to the outer surface of the stylets from which it may be removed only by washing or elution. He suggested that the fine structure of the outer surface of the stylets may differ between aphid species, which would account for the differences in vector efficiency.

Bradley & Ganong (40, 41) showed that a number of stylet-borne viruses are carried on the tip of the stylets, in the distal part, that does not exceed 15 μ in length. The experiments leading to the conclusion that only the distal portion of the stylets carries virus particles have been so convincing

284

that the explanation of Bradley became widely accepted. Bradley himself tried unsuccessfully to disprove the conclusions, when he found that the tips of stylets are not the inert structures they were earlier assumed to be (38). He found that certain treatments of the stylet tips, for instance with an electrostatic charge, could inhibit feeding and at the same time allow reproduction of the vectors to continue as if the aphids were feeding (39). It should be pointed out that nonfeeding aphids rarely reproduce. It appears that the stylets have nerves within them and perhaps chemoreceptors similar to those found on the labellum of the blow fly.

In 1958, van Hoof examined the fine structure of aphid stylets with the electron microscope and found considerable differences between different aphid species (92). The structure of the tips of maxillary and mandibulary stylets was of particular interest for virus transmission. It was found that hooks of different shape, depending on the species of aphid, were present on one side of the maxillary stylets. The mandibulary stylets were found to have very fine ridges, often extending over the margin of the stylets. The proximal parts of the mandibulary stylets were relatively smooth. Thus, confirming the hypothesis of van der Want, the tips of the stylets, with their ridges and furrows, seem to provide the vehicle for the virus particles. This idea got further support from Bradley's experiments (36) in which it could be demonstrated that penetration through a membrane over a plant surface reduced the efficiency of both acquisition and inoculation probes but that subsequent membrane-free inoculation probes were not affected. The longer the acquisition penetration, the more likely was the salivary material to coagulate and lock the sheath within the plant. If this occurred, the only virus-contaminated areas are the surfaces of the stylets that break through the sheath and are withdrawn through the gel-like sheath material. Long penetration would tend to eliminate salivary plug transport, and contaminated stylets would be drawn through a close-fitting tube that would tend to remove the adhering virus particles. The hypothesis of the plug transport has originally been proposed by Sylvester (216).

The penetration of the stylets into the leaf tissues is associated with the secretion of the salivary sheath. Sylvester (215) pointed out that the exact function of this sheath has not been established experimentally. Adams & McAllan (1) reported that the saliva contains several enzymes but it is not known whether the middle lamella of plant cells is being dissolved by it, or whether the saliva aids the penetration and feeding of aphids in any other way. It is not even known with certainty whether or not all penetrations made by aphids are preceded, accompanied, or followed by salivary secretion.

Recently Bradley has stressed the important part played by the behavior of vectors (37). Evidently aphids carry stylet-borne viruses on or within the tips of their mouth parts, and transfer them to other plants mainly during the early stage of probing, when only the first layer of the epidermis has been penetrated. The percentage of transmission can be greatly increased by keeping the aphids off plants for a while just before placing them on the source. Watson (232) discovered this remarkable effect and attributed it to "preliminary fasting" that caused physiological changes within aphids. Feeding was believed to reverse these changes. While Watson's reasoning about the mechanism of virus transmission had a profound effect on further research and furthered our understanding of aphid vectors, it was taken for granted for two decades in spite of lack of evidence for physiological changes. Watson used the term "fasting" to depict all that happens to aphids when they are forcibly removed from plants and then confined in a glass dish where they must wander about on a strange surface that they cannot penetrate. This not only causes aphids to fast, but, as pointed out by Bradley (37), it also upsets, frightens, disturbs, and affects them in other ways and so it is likely to affect their transmission of viruses. Also Watson's term "feeding" referred to much more than the ingestion of food and the resulting effects, though most aphid workers who followed her methods restricted their experiments to the feeding proper. In 1949, Sylvester demonstrated for the first time that an aphid normally transmits virus just as well after a brief probe on the source as after longer periods on it (213). The precise methods pioneered by Sylvester made it possible to obtain optimum transmission of some viruses with aphids that have spent as little as 5 min off plants before being placed on the source.

Bradley (37) noticed that for a few minutes after aphids are disturbed from feeding it is difficult to tell whether they really probe or merely rest on the leaf surface. Many actually appear to probe, but do not. There is a gap between the tip of the labium and the leaf. Rough handling, a sharp noise, a strong beam of light or an object moving near the aphids will disturb them and prevent their probing. Even with aphids that have been off plants for some time, probing behavior affects transmission of certain viruses. Probes of less than a minute are better than longer ones. With great care in handling, Bradley succeeded in getting recently collected aphids to make brief probes and in such instances the insects transmitted virus nearly as often as those that had been off plants for some time. These results, obtained with potato virus Y and *Myzus persicae* (Sulzer) showed that there was no effect of fasting on virus transmission as long as all aphids behave in the same way and probe the test plant within the first 2 min. This experiment focused the attention of virus workers on the probing behavior of aphids, or, as someone jokingly remarked, on the importance of aphid psychology in virus transmission. Behavior does not cease to be a factor once probing begins, although any differences, as in the mode of stylet penetration or salivation, are then hidden.

Another almost dogmatic belief, recently disproved by Bradley (37), is the assumption that aphids that have been off plants for some time and are then allowed to stay on the source of virus more than a few minutes, afterwards transmit less and less virus as the result of their "feeding." Bradley found that the epidermis between veins is usually several times richer as a source of virus than is the area over the secondary veins. Just how much this is responsible for the fewer transmissions obtained as the time on the source increases has yet to be shown. Sylvester (personal communication) pointed out that the decrease in virus transmission that follows feeding may be a function of the site chosen as well as the function of other factors; it remains to be shown which of these is the actual cause in a causal chain.

The movement of virus from cell to cell after it has been introduced by a vector and the form in which it is being introduced are not yet clearly understood. It is difficult to decide how much of the development of early infection can be interpreted in terms of cell-virus interaction and how much in terms of virus spread (63, 113). It was suggested by van Hoof (92) that perhaps the aphid-transmissible, stylet-borne viruses were carried in the form of viral nucleic acid, rather than of protein-coated virus particles. Sylvester (216) expressed the view that removal of the protein coat with subsequent preservation of infectivity would be quite feasible in the internal environment of the vectors of circulatory viruses. Evidence in support of these assumptions is lacking thus far.

Circulatory and propagative transmission.—The circulatory aphid-borne viruses are much less common than the stylet-borne viruses. Less than a dozen have been described and only a few have been studied carefully. The most interesting experiments in this group were carried out with the potato leaf roll virus, a circulatory-propagative virus.

Until recently, the only plant viruses shown to multiply within their respective insect vectors were several leafhopper-borne viruses. In 1955, Heinze demonstrated that aphids can withstand severe wounding afflicted during needle inoculations of plant extracts (85). Day, in 1955 (59), presented experiments which, although inconclusive, focused the attention of entomologists and plant pathologists on the possibility that circulatory aphid-borne viruses and, in particular, potato leaf roll virus, may perhaps multiply in *Myzus persicae*.

In 1958, Stegwee & Ponsen (202) presented data from which they concluded that potato leaf roll virus does multiply in its aphid vector. The authors did not use extracts from crushed whole aphids, because they found this material unsuitable. Instead, they used aphid hemolymph. First it was found that when the insects were injected with hemolymph obtained from virus-containing aphids, approximately 50 per cent of the injected insects became infective after an average minimum incubation period of 20 hr. When the hemolymph was diluted with saline solution, the incubation period was as much as seven to ten days. Insects rendered infective by needle inoculation remained infective and did not lose their ability to transmit. Afterwards, a serial passage was attempted. Virus-free aphids, maintained on Chinese cabbage immune to leaf roll, were injected with hemolymph of virus-containing aphids and maintained for the following seven days on Chinese cabbage. After this period, a small amount of their hemolymph was in turn injected into another group of virus-free aphids and this procedure was repeated 15 times at seven-day intervals. In every passage the presence of virus could be demonstrated by testing a few injected aphids on susceptible plants. In the serial passage experiments the calculated dilution of the original inoculum, if no multiplication had occurred, would have reached 10^{-21}, while the dilution end-point of leaf roll virus in hemolymph was found to be 10^{-4}. Therefore, the authors concluded that the virus had multiplied in the injected *Myzus persicae*.

In 1960, Stegwee (200) reported that *Myzus persicae* can acquire potato leaf roll virus during a 10-min acquisition feeding period on *Physalis floridana,* but very few insects became infective after such short feeding. When the acquisition period was increased, the number of infective aphids also increased. Although virus could be detected in aphids 8 hr after they were placed on diseased *Physalis* plants, another 8 to 16 hr were required before aphids were able to transmit. According to Stegwee, less then half of this time is needed for the virus to reach the blood, and the remaining period is required to build up the necessary concentration of virus in the salivary glands. It seems logical to assume that the building up of concentration in the salivary glands is the result of virus multiplication in the vector. It was found that temperature had a profound effect on the incubation and transmission of the virus. When insects were maintained at 35°C, no infectivity developed. The optimal temperature was found to be 20°C and the maximum 30°C. Unless tests are carried out under controlled conditions, comparisons between different experiments are of little significance.

Ponsen (personal communication) was unable to find histological differences between virus-carrying and virus-free aphids. On the other hand, Schmidt (180, 180a) working with the same virus-vector system, and, in addition, with other viruses, like beet yellow-net and pea-enation virus, found pronounced differences in the shape and size of nuclei in the alimentary tract. The nuclei were much smaller and abnormal in shape in viruliferous aphids. Gradations in nuclei of aphids carrying yellow-net virus were reminiscent of those found by Littau & Maramorosch (111, 112) in aster leafhoppers *Macrosteles fascifrons* (Stål) infected with aster yellows virus; however, it seemed that the changes were more pronounced in females, while in aster leafhoppers the changes were primarily found in males. Rutschky & Campbell (173) examined *Macrosiphum granarium* (Kirby) with and without barley yellow dwarf virus. The number of irregularly contoured nuclei varied considerably more in the infected group than in the noninfected, but the means were comparable, so that gross morphological differences in the fat bodies of infective and noninfective aphids were not suitable for diagnostic purposes in determining the presence or absence of the virus in any individual aphid.

Ehrhardt (62) noted metabolic changes in *Myzus persicae* after the aphids acquired leaf roll virus. Eight hours after virus acquisition, a 30 per cent decrease in oxygen consumption was observed in viruliferous insects. The lowest respiration rate was reached after 30 hr, the rate remaining at this low level for the following two and one-half days. It seems likely that there is a relationship between virus multiplication in the aphid vector and the respiratory rate of the insects.

The success of Stegwee & Ponsen (202) in carrying out their serial passage experiment seemed to have been the result of using insect hemolymph rather than extracts of insects. Harrison (84) injected potato leaf roll virus in extracts from crushed *Myzus persicae* into virus-free aphids and reported that the ability of aphids to transmit was gradually lost because of the exhaustion of the supply of virus in the insect. Virus was recovered by the injection technique from aphids after 24 to 48 hr of acquisition feeding, when the insects presumably were not yet infective; no virus could be recovered from crushed insects after they began to transmit the virus. This was considered as evidence for a decrease in virus content of the aphids and against the possibility of virus multiplication in the vector. The observation of Harrison that a rapid decrease occurred in the transmitting ability is at variance with the findings of Stegwee (201) and also with the earlier findings of MacCarthy (114).

The improvements in the aphid injection technique made by Rochow in recent years (170) should permit easy repetition of the serial passage experiment with different dilutions of aphid hemolymph. The method of transferring blood from one aphid to another is likely to circumvent the hazard of inactivation and to permit the demonstration of leaf roll virus in the blood long after the acquisition feeding. It is hoped that such experiments will soon be made and that the controversial findings will thus be clarified.

Another seemingly controversial issue is concerned with the presence or absence of an incubation period in the transmission of potato leaf roll virus by *Myzus persicae*. Kirkpatrick & Ross (102), Klostermeyer (103), and de Meester-Manger Cats (137) found that the transmission can be carried out within minutes after the aphids acquired virus from diseased plants. On the other hand, MacCarthy (114), Day (59), and Heinze (87) do not support these results. Day suggested that the differences in efficiency among strains of aphids could explain the discrepancy. In preliminary tests with North American and European aphids, Heinze was unable to detect such a difference (unpublished results). However, as pointed out by MacCarthy (114), there appears to be no reason why, through the acquisition of a very large amount of virus from a good source of inoculum (for instance, *Physalis floridana,* used by Kirkpatrick & Ross), and in optimal conditions for acquisition and transmission, the interval between acquisition and transmission could not have been eliminated in a few cases. The circulatory-propagative virus could be transmitted for brief periods by vectors in a stylet-borne manner. This would occur at the beginning of a series of test feedings and would soon cease, being later followed by transmission of the propagative virus. This possibility has not yet been supported by experimental evidence in the case of potato leaf roll virus. However, with aster yellows virus, which has been shown beyond doubt to be a propagative virus, transmission without incubation has been obtained by Maramorosch through the injection of massive doses of virus (118). Injected insects transmitted on the day of injection and later stopped transmitting. Because of premature death of insects which received large volumes of inoculum, it was not possible to establish whether they would have regained infectivity upon completion of incubation. The immediate transmission of aster yellows virus and of leaf roll virus might have been caused by the massive doses acquired by the vectors, but there has been no indication of a stylet-borne phase in the immediate transmission of leaf roll virus; such a phase was definitely excluded in aster yellows virus because it had been acquired through injection.

Variation within aphid species.—Three kinds of variation within an aphid species have been recognized. The first kind concerns variations in virus transmission among different clones or strains of one species. The second deals with variations among various developmental stages. The third type distinguishes variations among different forms of one species.

In 1947, Bawden & Kassanis (8) suggested that only occasional individuals of *Myzus persicae* might be vectors of potato virus C in contrast to most individuals of this species which are unable to transmit the virus.

Until 1955, variability among aphids had received very little attention, and most reports on variation within one aphid species have appeared in the last seven years. Stubbs' experiments (205) demonstrated the variation between different cultures of *Myzus persicae* in their ability to transmit a circulatory yellows virus from spinach. Stubbs found that his cultures retained their ability or inability to transmit virus in successive experiments, and he emphasized the importance of this finding. Williams & Ross (238) reported variability among clones of *M. persicae* in the transmission of potato leaf roll virus, also a circulatory virus. Björling & Ossiannilsson (17) found that two circulatory viruses were transmitted with varying degrees of efficiency by 100 strains of three aphid species, *M. persicae*, *Aphis fabae* Scopoli, and *Myzus ascalonicus* Doncaster. In the case of *M. persicae*, the Swedish workers were able to group 85 strains in a series ranging from 10 to 80 per cent transmission of beet yellows virus.

Rochow (167) described variation among clones of *Toxoptera graminum* (Rondani) in the transmission of the circulatory barley yellow dwarf virus. Collections from Wisconsin and Illinois were found to transmit the virus fairly efficiently, while a Florida collection was virtually inactive. The inactive clone of *T. graminum* in this case had a slightly different beak tip from that of the active clones.

Simons (187) showed that variation among clones is not restricted to the transmission of circulatory viruses but may occur also among stylet-borne viruses. He also found that a clone of *Aphis gossypii* Glover efficient in transmitting one virus will not necessarily be efficient in transmitting another virus.

Differences among developmental stages of *Macrosiphum geranicola*

(Hille Ris Lambers) in the transmission of the circulatory virus of filaree red leaf were noted by Anderson (4). Young nymphs seemed to acquire the virus more readily than did adults. The minimum latent period was shorter in nymphs than in adults. The same applies to pea-enation mosaic (186a).

Recently, variation in virus transmission by different forms of one species has also been reported. Paine & Legg (156) obtained transmission of hop mosaic virus by the spring winged form of *Phorodon humuli* (Schrank), but not by the wingless summer form. Orlob & Arny (152) found that only oviparae and fundatrigeniae of *Rhopalosiphum fitchii* (Sanderson) were capable of transmitting the circulatory barley yellow dwarf virus, while four other forms of the same aphid species failed to transmit the virus. Orlob (151) found that oviparous females of *Macrosiphum euphorbiae* (Thomas) and *Brevicoryne brassicae* (Linnaeus) transmitted both potato virus Y and cabbage virus B, as did apterous viviparous females. However, a difference among forms of *Aphis nasturtii* Kaltenbach was detected in the transmission of potato virus Y. Migratory forms, such as gynoparae, males, and fundatrigeniae transmitted efficiently, while no transmission was obtained by oviparae and fundatrices.

Variation among aphid species involves the problem of why one species is a vector of a particular virus while another species is not. This question of specificity has not yet been solved, but some recent experiments may help to explain certain aspects of specific virus transmission by aphids. Badami (5) found that a strain of the stylet-borne cucumber mosaic virus was readily transmitted by *Myzus persicae* at first, but that it lost this property (vector transmissibility) during transfers in a greenhouse. The isolate remained transmissible by *Myzus ascalonicus* and *Aphis gossypii*, but not by *M. persicae*. The latter remained an efficient vector of other isolates of the same virus. This indicated that the basis for this type of vector specificity involved a change in the virus and not in the vector. Similar loss of adaptation or affinity to insect vectors has been discovered in leafhopper-borne viruses (25).

Rochow (169, 170) made one of the most important contributions to our knowledge of variation in the transmission of barley yellow dwarf virus. This virus belongs to the circulatory type (155). Variations between the transmitting ability of two vector species, *Rhopalosiphum padi* (Linnaeus) and *Macrosiphum granarium* (Kirby) were first noted by Toko & Bruehl (218, 219), and later by Rochow (165), Slykhuis *et al.* (194), Smith (197), and Watson & Mulligan (234). Rochow showed that one strain of the virus was transmitted efficiently by *M. granarium* but was not transmitted regularly by *R. padi* or *Rhopalosiphum maidis* (Fitch). A second strain was transmitted efficiently by *R. padi* but not transmitted regularly by *M. granarium* or *R. maidis*. The third strain was transmitted fairly efficiently by *R. maidis* but not transmitted regularly by *M. granarium* or *R. padi* (166).

Two specialized techniques were used by Rochow in a brilliant series of experiments that made possible many kinds of tests not available for other aphid-virus combinations. The first technique was the transmission of barley yellow dwarf virus to aphids through semipermeable animal membranes (168). This technique has been used for many years with some leafhopper-borne viruses (9) and with arthropod-borne animal viruses, and has now been used for the first time as a simple qualitative test for an aphid-borne virus in liquid preparations. The second technique was the needle injection method, which has become a standard procedure for leafhopper-borne viruses (122) since its introduction by Storey in 1933 (204). This technique has also been widely used for yellow fever transmissions to mosquitoes (Whitman, personal communication). The barley yellow dwarf virus was transmitted by this injection method to aphids from extracts of viruliferous aphids and from the sap of infected plants (138). Although injected aphids often transmitted virus within one day, an inoculation test feeding period of five days was found most suitable.

An indication of the specificity of the two strains of barley yellow dwarf virus was given by results of a continuing transmission series that began in 1957 and has been carried to date through 32 serial transmissions. One strain was transmitted to 144 of 146 plants by *Macrosiphum granarium,* but to none of 97 plants by *R. padi.* In contrast, in parallel tests with the second strain, *Rhopalosiphum padi* transmitted virus to 132 of 137 plants, but *M. granarium* transmitted this virus strain only to 1 of 95 plants (170). These data suggest an absolute specificity for transmission of one strain by *M. granarium* and a nearly absolute specificity for transmission of the other strain by *R. padi.* The same specificity was also found when aphids were fed virus extracts through membranes, and when the insects acquired the two strains of virus by injection instead of by feeding. This relationship was independent of the source of inoculum—it held for virus from infected plants as well as from viruliferous aphids. Since Rochow's colony of *R. padi* continued to transmit some virus isolates very efficiently, the explanation of the observed specificity could not be based on poor transmitting ability. Tests of collections of aphids from different parts of the United States provided additional evidence that the specificity was not based on intrinsic peculiarities of the colonies but that the major basis for the variation rested with the virus and not with the aphids.

Rochow found that the virus in "nonvectors" reached the hemolymph, so that the gut wall does not seem to be a barrier in this system as it is in some leafhopper systems (190, 204). All results seem to indicate that the virus is extremely variable and that existing strains of the virus differ in the efficiency with which each aphid species can transmit them. The strains can be divided into two groups. Viruses of one are transmitted efficiently by *Rhopalosiphum padi.* Some strains of this group are not transmitted by *Macrosiphum granarium,* while other strains are readily acquired, but only occasionally transmitted by *M. granarium* (171). Still other strains may be transmitted as efficiently by *M. granarium* as by *R. padi.* The second group of strains is transmitted efficiently by *M. granarium,* but very rarely, if at all, by *R. padi.*

Transmission and nutritional factors.—The way in which food plants are maintained determines not only the amount of transmission but also the reproducibility of results and a large amount of experimental variation. Swenson (212) pointed out that investigation of the basis of difference in efficiency of transmission of a virus by two aphid species seems premature until one can account for a variation of 10 to 90 per cent efficiency within one species. One complete gap in plant virus studies is the effect of various environmental and nutritional factors on susceptibility of plants to virus inoculation by insects. Information has been obtained for susceptibility to mechanical inoculation, but it is not known whether these results are parallel to susceptibility to the same viruses introduced by vectors. This lack of information is the more striking because most plant viruses are transmitted in nature by insects. We have, therefore, a great variety of crop plants exposed to numerous viruses but no knowledge of the relation of crop environment and nutrition to virus spread.

Kennedy stated that aphids appear ideally fitted for spreading viruses in the field and that one might, therefore, expect far more spread than actually occurs. (98).

Transmission and food uptake.—Björling *et al.* (16) were the first to use radioactive tracers in the field studies of insect vectors of plant viruses. Aphids labeled with P^{32} were released in the field and the movement and dispersal observed. Interesting experiments have been carried out recently with virus transmission and radioactive tracers in Japan. Nishizawa *et al.* (146) fed *Myzus persicae* for 24 hr on *Raphanus sativus,* infected with mosaic and labeled with P^{32} and S^{35}. Afterward, the aphids were transferred for 20 min to one lot of healthy seedlings, and for 24 hr to a second lot. Although P^{32} was transferred to all plants on which the aphids fed, virus transmission occurred only in some instances. Even when aphids were starved for 6 hr after they had fed on diseased plants, they still transmitted P^{32} to all seedlings. Sulfur-35 was found in the rostrum, pharynx, salivary gland, and alimentary tract of the insects. Nishizawa *et al.* (145) found that aphids fed on P^{32}-labeled diseased radish plants for 5 or 10 min, would infect up to six successive seedlings in 10-min transfers, while they continued to transmit P^{32} up to the tenth seedling. Obviously, the amount of P^{32} acquired in 10-min feeding was considerable and the autoradiographic test sensitive enough to detect minute amounts. On the other hand, when acquisition feeding on labeled diseased plants was reduced to 1 min or 30 sec, no appreciable difference could be found between virus transmission and P^{32} transmission.

Shirahama found, in 1950, in Japan that cucumber mosaic virus is transmitted to radish seedlings by alatae of *Myzus persicae* and *Rhopalosiphum pseudobrassicae* (Davis) mostly between the hours of 8:00 to 10:00 a.m. and 3:00 to 5:00 p.m., and that the aphids rarely visit radishes at noon, early in the morning, or at night (185). It would be interesting to find whether transmission and feeding under controlled greenhouse conditions are correlated, or independent of each other. In a leafhopper vector of aster yellows virus (131) the two processes seem to be independent.

Nishi (144) found an inhibitor to tobacco mosaic virus in radish plants that were infested by *M. persicae* and *R. pseudobrassicae*. The number of local lesions produced on *Nicotiana glutinosa* was reduced 50 per cent by the inhibitor emitted by the aphids into the radish plants. Nishi found that this inhibitor could withstand 95°C for 10 minutes. Day & Iszykiewicz reported an inhibitor of tobacco mosaic virus in the saliva of *Lygus oblineatus* (Say) (60). Although inhibitors of plant viruses were demonstrated in insect juices, their action could only be demonstrated through mechanical inoculation tests. Inhibitors failed to act whenever applied to insect stylets. Orlob (personal communication) found that this inhibition is specific for TMV, and that the saliva does not inhibit transmission of cauliflower mosaic virus when applied to the stylets of viruliferous cabbage aphids.

Citrus wound-tumor virus.—The first tumor-producing plant disease caused by an aphid-borne virus was recently described by Wallace & Drake (229). The causative virus is transmitted to citrus by *Myzus persicae* and by *Aphis gossypii*. The latter was described as a vector by Weathers & Laird (236). The virus also causes vein-enation on infected plants (67, 115, 228). On semi-hard or woody stems, galls develop either spontaneously near the thorns or at places of mechanical injuries. Wounding induces woody galls on stems and roots. When roots of diseased plants were wounded by means of pin punctures, galls developed at most of the wound sites. There are many similarities between the citrus wound-tumor virus and the leafhopper-borne wound-tumor virus discovered by Black (20, 21, 97).

LEAFHOPPERS AND PLANTHOPPERS

Leafhoppers (Cicadellidae) comprise the second largest group of vectors of plant viruses, exceeded only by aphids in the number of transmitting species and transmitted viruses. In Japan, leafhoppers were linked definitely with the spread of plant disease agents as early as 1902, when the entomologists Onuku and Murata discovered that *Nephotettix apicalis* var. *cincticeps* (Uhler) was responsible for the transmission of rice stunt (29). The transmission of sugar beet curly top virus was studied in the United States for nearly as many years as rice stunt was studied in Japan. It is somewhat surprising that no leafhoppers were known as vectors of plant viruses from Western Europe until 1953, although they were known earlier in Russia. In 1953, two leafhopper vectors were described from The Netherlands. The first was *Macropsis fuscula* (Zetterstedt), the vector of Rubus stunt virus (61); the second was *Euscelis plebejus* (Fallen), found to transmit an obscure clover virus (119). Since then, a number of leafhopper vectors have become known from Western Europe, and several species have been studied in Central and Eastern Europe.

The subject of leafhopper-borne viruses has been thoroughly reviewed in recent years. The reader is referred to the most comprehensive discussions of the subject by Black (29, 30). Some other reviews that cover the subject are by Black (23, 24, 27), Köhler & Klinkowski (104), Maramorosch (121, 122, 128, 129), Smith & Brierley (196), and Völk (227).

Circulatory transmission.—Leafhopper-borne viruses are either circulatory or propagative. As already pointed out, the terms are not mutually exclusive. Although sugar beet curly top virus is retained through molts and can be transmitted for many days after a single short acquisition feeding, a good deal of evidence has been obtained to indicate that this virus is circulatory without being propagative. It is today much more difficult to provide evidence for absence of multiplication than for the existence of multiplication, but critical data support the view that the virus does not undergo multiplication in *Circulifer tenellus* (Baker). Bennett & Wallace (9) demonstrated a progressive decrease of the virus content, following a short acquisition feeding. The decrease was measured by feeding extracts of leafhoppers to nonviruliferous leafhoppers and testing the latter on beet seedlings. This decrease, which seems to be the most significant finding in support of lack of multiplication, has also been found by Harrison (84) for potato leaf roll virus in *Myzus persicae*, and yet, in the latter case, the work of Stegwee & Ponsen (202) provided strong evidence for propagative transmission. This clearly shows how difficult it is to demonstrate lack of multiplication. Freitag (70) and Bennett & Wallace (9) found a consistent decrease in transmission of curly top virus by individual leafhoppers, independent of the natural decrease due to age. Old and poorly transmitting leafhoppers could regain infectivity by renewed feeding on a diseased plant. These findings are quite different from those obtained with propagative leafhopper-borne viruses such as wound-tumor or aster yellows virus. In preliminary experiments, Maramorosch (unpublished data) has been unable to transmit the beet curly top virus serially in the vector. Moreover, Bennett & Wallace (9) found a proportional relationship between the length of acquisition feeding and the transmitting ability of individual leafhoppers, which, again, is in striking contrast to results obtained with aster yellows virus (107), in which the length of virus acquisition had only a slight effect on transmission. Kunkel (107) pointed out that, in one respect, the beet leafhopper and the aster leafhopper behave similarly toward the viruses they transmit. Even after relatively long infective feeding periods, some individuals of both species fail to become viruliferous. This is readily explained in the case of the aster leafhopper by assuming that some individuals are much less susceptible to infection by aster yellows virus than are others. If beet leafhoppers having a short infective feeding period take up a small charge of virus and those having a long infective period take up a large charge, it is difficult to understand why some individual leafhoppers that would become viruliferous if allowed a very long infective feeding period acquire no virus at all during an interval as long as six days on a diseased plant.

Propagative transmission.—The propagative leafhopper-borne viruses are transmitted specifically by one or a number of leafhopper vectors. Most of them cannot be successfully inoculated directly into plants and most are very unstable outside the living plant or insect cell. There is no evidence that the virus in the insect vectors is in a different form from that in the infected plants, but, in some instances, it has been demonstrated that the virus occurs in higher concentration in insects. Nevertheless, insect extracts as well as plant extracts have failed in most cases to inoculate very susceptible plants. Until very recently, the only methods to assay the viruses depended upon obtaining insect-transmitted infections in plants. No detection by serology, electron microscopy, or by cytopathological or other effects on vectors were available for any viruses in this category.

There are many propagative leafhopper-borne viruses which infect their leafhopper vectors and multiply in them just as they infect plants and multiply in their respective plant hosts. In most cases, the infection of the leafhopper is not apparent. There are two techniques which provide unquestionable evidence for multiplication of viruses in vectors. The first is the serial passage technique in which the virus is carried from insect to insect by injection until the dilution attained exceeds with certainty the maximum dilution of the starting material that can be successfully inoculated. This technique was used successfully by Maramorosch (117) with aster yellows virus and its vector, *Macrosteles fascifrons* and by Black & Brakke (31) with wound-tumor virus in *Agallia constricta* Van Duzee. As mentioned earlier, it was also used with an aphid-borne virus by Stegwee & Ponsen (202). The second technique to prove multiplication is by transovarial passage of virus from generation to generation of vectors until the dilution attained exceeds with certainty the maximum possible without multiplication in the insect. Black (22) estimated that a dilution of 10^{-12} should be exceeded in such a passage to provide evidence for virus multiplication. This technique was first used by Fukushi (72, 73) in his classical experiments on multiplication of rice stunt virus in *Nephotettix apicalis* var. *cincticeps*. The clover club leaf virus, discovered by Black (19) in *Agalliopsis novella* (Say), was transmitted transovarially for more than five years through 21 generations, providing proof that this virus also multiplied in its insect vector (22). Clover club leaf virus (123) and rice stunt virus (74, 101) can also be transmitted to their respective vectors by injections, but this technique has not been used for serial passages. Shinkai (182) transmitted rice stripe virus transovarially to 40 generations of *Delphacodes striatella* (Fallen), a planthopper belonging to the Delphacidae. Yamada & Yamamoto (240, 241) carried this virus through 24 passages in the same vector. In the case of rice stripe virus, as in rice stunt and clover club leaf virus, it was found that leafhoppers varied genetically in their ability to transmit virus. The greatest proportion of infective progeny occurred among descendants of the active, or susceptible, insects, while the least proportion of infective progeny was found among the progeny from inactive, or non-susceptible, insects. Crosses between the two resulted in an intermediate proportion of transmitting insects. Nymphs from females that had just acquired virus before ovipositing required an incubation period before transmitting, while those from infective females could transmit immediately after hatching. The virus did not pass through the sperm and almost all progeny of infective females received the virus. Shinkai (183) recently carried rice stunt virus transovarially through *Deltocephalus (Inazuma) dorsalis* Motschulski, as well as through *Nephotettix cincticeps*. In the course of the serial passage through *D. dorsalis*, the number of infective leafhoppers in the progeny decreased from generation to generation, and some leafhoppers seemed to be killed prematurely by the virus infection.

Almost every year in the last decade new reports appeared of transovarially transmitted viruses in leafhoppers, which make it probable that this phenomenon is quite common. In the case of wound-tumor virus and potato yellow dwarf virus, transovarial passage is limited to less than 5 per cent (25) unless special selection and breeding for transovarial transmission is carried out (140). Grylls (82) found that rugose leaf curl virus passes to a high percentage of the progeny of infective *Austroagallia torrida* (Evans). Prusa *et al.* (162) found in Czechoslovakia that oat sterile-dwarf virus does not pass through the egg of *Delphacodes pellucida* (Fabricius), whereas the wheat striate virus carried by the same vector was shown to pass transovarially. Shinkai, in Japan, demonstrated recently (184) that the virus causing stripe disease of rice passed to a high percentage of the progeny of infected *Delphacodes striatella* (Fallen) females, while the black-streaked dwarf virus, transmitted by the same plant hopper, does not pass to the progeny. *Delphacodes pellucida*, described as a vector of maize rough dwarf virus from Israel (83) has not been tested adequately to establish whether or not the virus passes transovarially to the progeny. Recently, Lindsten (110) described the transmission of oat striate and of oat dwarf tillering virus by *Delphacodes pellucida*. Both viruses overwinter in their insect vector. The oat striate virus is probably identical with the European wheat striate mosaic virus. The dwarf tillering virus, transmitted transovarially from infective females to their offspring, is similar to, or identical with, the virus that causes sterility and dwarfing of oats in Czechoslovakia (162).

Two species of planthoppers have been described as vectors of the virus causing hoja blanca disease of rice. Alarming losses are caused by the disease in several Latin American countries. Galvez *et al.* (79, 80) studied the virus-vector relationships in Colombia. They found that *Sogata orizicola* Muir and *S. cubana* Crawford were able to acquire the virus in a single day of acquisition feeding, and could transmit it after an incubation period of from seven to nine days. There were indications that the virus passed transovarially to the progeny of infective females. It was found that less than 10 per cent of randomly collected *S. orizicola* was able to transmit the virus, and that among the progeny of infective females the percentage of active transmitters was much higher. This is suggestive of genetically controlled active and inactive races (203) and the genetic variation in the efficiency to transmit the virus (18). Planthopper vectors retained infectivity throughout their life.

Morphology of leafhopper-borne viruses.—No direct evidence exists at present for an eclipse period during the cycle of propagative viruses in insects. The possibility that an eclipse period really exists has been discussed by Maramorosch (120) and by Black (29). The existing evidence on the reproduction of other viruses would suggest that an eclipse period is part of the virus cycle of reproduction in the plant and in the insect. The presence of soluble viral antigen of wound-tumor virus in both insect and plant supports this probability. Wound-tumor virus was the first propagative virus characterized morphologically. Brakke *et al.* (43) showed that virus particles obtained from insects and those obtained from plants were similar in size and structure.

Thus far, none of the viruses transmitted transovarially to the progeny of infective females have been transmitted through the sperm of infective males. This may be explained by the assumption that these viruses are primarily concentrated in the cytoplasm and not in the nucleus. Direct evidence for the presence of rice dwarf virus in the cytoplasm of insect cells was recently obtained by Fukushi *et al.* (78) and Fukushi (unpublished data), who, for the first time, was able to photograph virus particles in ultrathin sections of an insect vector. Fukushi's electron micrograph (Fig. 1) reproduced here with his permission, clearly demonstrates the presence of large clusters of the rice dwarf virus in crystal-like arrangements in the cytoplasm, while no virus particles are present in the nucleus, nor in the mitochondria. The visualization of a plant virus within cells of its vector is one of the most outstanding contributions of recent years. It was expected as a logical outcome of the evidence that has accumulated over the years for the multiplication of this and several other viruses in their leafhopper vectors, but it remained for Fukushi, who provided the first direct evidence for such multiplication, to obtain the first electron micrographs. Fukushi *et al.* (78) also were able to obtain electron micrographs of the virus in plant cells.

Another plant virus was recently characterized morphologically by Herold *et al.* (89). In a personal communication, Bergold informed this reviewer that the virus had since been identified as corn mosaic, transmitted by *Peregrinus maidis* (Ashmead). Virus particles found in thin sections of corn leaves, were uniform in shape and size, 242 mμ in length and 48 mμ in diameter, with a membrane and a dense rod-shaped central core. The particles were concentrated in the cytoplasm of plant cells.

During 1962, Black, Hills, and Markham (personal communication, paper in press) obtained very detailed electron micrographs of purified wound-tumor virus. The photograph (Fig. 2), furnished by Black *et al.*, shows individual particles of about 60 mμ in diameter. The virus definitely contains RNA, and no DNA has been detected. This finding is of great importance, because until now it was not known what kind of nucleic acid any of the dual host—"plant-insect" viruses isolated from insect vectors contained. The sedimentation rate of the virus was found to be 510 Svedberg units. Recently, further studies were made on the morphology of the wound-

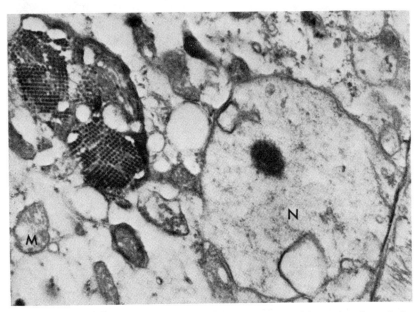

Fig. 1. Clusters of rice dwarf virus particles in an ultrathin section through the abdomen of an infective *Nephotettix apicalis* var. *cincticeps*. N represents the host cell nucleus, and M the mitochondria. × 33,000. Unpublished. Courtesy Prof. T. Fukushi, Hokkaido University, Japan.

tumor virus. Bils & Hall (12) reported that the virus is about 60 mμ in diameter and has the shape of an icosahedron. The surface of the virus consists of 92 subunits about 7.5 mμ in diameter. The virus core stained heavily with uranyl acetate, agreeing with Black's finding that it consists of RNA. The core comprises about 20 per cent of the volume of the virus particle. Dr. Albert B. Sabin (personal communication) called the attention of this reviewer to the striking similarity in the number of subunits of wound-tumor virus and animal viruses of ECHO type 10, now known as reoviruses. Future work will undoubtedly be directed towards a study of possible relationships between these reoviruses and wound-tumor virus.

Earlier work in Japan by Yoshii & Kiso (243) indicated that rice dwarf virus was also an RNA virus, because RNA isolated from dwarf diseased rice plants was infectious when injected into the abdomen of leafhoppers. The authors reported that even ingested RNA rendered leafhoppers infective. The RNA preparation was inactivated by RNase. The authors did not test the RNA content of purified preparations, nor did they study RNA from insect vectors.

Strains of aster yellows virus.—Thirty years ago only two strains of

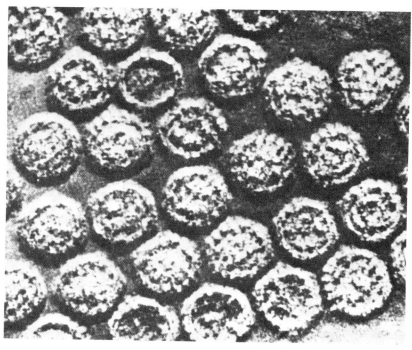

FIG. 2. Fine structure of wound-tumor virus. The individual virus particles are 60 mμ in diameter and contain RNA. Unpublished. Courtesy Drs. L. M. Black, G. J. Hills and R. Markham, The Agricultural Research Council, Cambridge, England.

aster yellows virus were recognized in the United States, and the existence of the virus and its vectors in other parts of the world was not known. Today, at least five strains of aster yellows virus have been isolated and studied in California (Freitag, personal communication), and two distinct strains are known to occur in the eastern United States. Aster yellows virus is known to be transmitted most efficiently by *Macrosteles fascifrons* throughout North America. A number of less efficient vectors have been reported from California. In recent years, additional vectors have also been reported in the eastern parts of the United States and Canada. In Japan, Fukushi reported the presence of aster yellows in 1930 (71) and, more recently, he and Nemoto demonstrated that the leafhopper *Ophiola flavopicta* (Ishihara) acts as a vector in nature (75, 76). Japanese aster yellows virus was transmitted by this leafhopper from tomato to *Nicotiana rustica* and other plants by Oshima & Goto (153) and from carrot to potato, petunia, and China aster by Fukushi & Shikata (77).

In Germany, the disease was described in 1936 by Richter (164) and the vector, *Macrosteles laevis* Ribaut, was reported by Heinze & Kunze (88). *Aphrodes bicinctus* (Schrank) was also suspected as an additional vector. In Poland, in 1958, Kochmann and Książek (personal communication) transmitted aster yellows virus from onions by means of *M. laevis*. It has also been reported in onions from Czechoslovakia (33). In Russia, aster yellows virus has been known for many years as the cause of Koksaghyz yellows, and its transmission by a *Macrosteles* sp. has been studied (174, 175, 211).

Unfortunately, no serological test is available to determine the identity and relationships of strains of aster yellows virus. It was assumed for many years that transmission by *Macrosteles fascifrons* is limited to aster yellows virus, and that positive transmission by this leafhopper identifies the causative agent of a yellow infection as aster yellows virus. Recent investigations showed that *M. fascifrons* acts as a vector of at least one, if not several, other viruses, in addition to transmitting strains of aster yellows virus. The signs of disease and the host range of different strains, as well as of other yellows-type and big-bud type viruses are not adequate as distinguishing criteria. Until a serological test becomes available, the identification of strains must depend on cross-immunity tests in plants and in *M. fascifrons*.

In 1929, Severin found that aster yellows in California was readily transmitted to *Zinnia elegans* Jacq. and to celery, which were then thought to be immune from aster yellows from the East (181). Actually, neither *Zinnia* nor celery is immune to the eastern strain (108), but the field resistance is so considerable that before 1950 practically no yellows was reported by celery growers in the eastern states. The two plant species can be infected experimentally with the eastern strain, but only with great difficulty, by confining large numbers of the infective aster leafhoppers on very young seedlings. No infections could be obtained in older *Zinnia* plants, irrespective of the number of insects used. In the last decade western strains of aster yellows virus, or strains that would infect field-grown celery, were isolated in New York, New Jersey, Maryland, and Pennsylvania. In 1952, Magie *et al.* identified western aster yellows in bulbs of gladiolus shipped from Oregon to the East (116). The origin of other isolates from field-grown celery and plantain may never be established but the likelihood is considerable that they also came originally from the West.

In 1955, Kunkel found that the eastern and a western strain of aster yellows could be distinguished by symptom expression in *Nicotiana rustica* plants (108). Differences in the type of growth were strikingly shown by secondary shoots of infected plants. Similar differences were found in *Zinnia* plants. The distinguishing of the aster yellows strains by their symptoms in *N. rustica* enabled Kunkel to demonstrate for the first time that the presence of one virus in a leafhopper may interfere with the transmission of another. When one virus strain became well established in groups of insects or in individual insects, which usually took place 14 days after virus acquisition, the insects were unable to acquire and transmit the second strain (109). This cross-protection by virus strains provides an additional method for testing relationships between yellows viruses. In cases where the same insect vector transmits the viruses to different plants and the cross-immunity cannot be tested in plant hosts, Kunkel's discovery may provide a means of testing for cross-protection. Such a possibility was suggested by Black (29) for testing the possible relationship between California aster yellows and cherry buckskin virus strains, transmitted by *Colladonus geminatus* (Van Duzee) (93). While in aster yellows tests with two virus strains Kunkel found complete cross-protection, Freitag (personal communication), working with five different strains, all of the western type, found a complicated relationship, which could not be explained easily. Whereas some strains seemed to protect against transmission, others did not. These results are not surprising in view of the findings of Maramorosch (124) with two strains of corn stunt virus acquired consecutively by *Dalbulus maidis* (DeLong & Wolcott). When the Rio Grande strain was acquired first, it prevented the transmission of the Mesa Central strain. However, in *D. maidis* protection in the reverse direction is incomplete. It was concluded that the Rio Grande strain was either more virulent or multiplied faster and thus protected the insects from acquiring and transmitting the second strain.

In 1956, Maramorosch (125) found that *Macrosteles laevis,* a vector of aster yellows virus in Europe, would not transmit strains of aster yellows virus of either the eastern United States or of western (Oregon) origin, although the two strains were efficiently transmitted by *M. fascifrons.* Although the two species of leafhoppers are closely related and almost indistinguishable, attempts at hybridization failed.

A virus, transmitted by *M. fascifrons* but distinct from aster yellows, was recently investigated in Canada by Chiykowski (54). In addition to *M. fascifrons,* the virus was also transmitted in Canada to several plant species by *Aphrodes bicinctus* (Schrank) and by *Scaphytopius acutus* (Say). It causes phyllody in clover, similar to the phyllody described from Europe by Frazier & Posnette (68, 69), Bovey (34), Evenhuis (64), Valenta (222), and Musil (139). The vectors of phyllody in Europe include *Euscelis plebejus* (Fallen), *Macrosteles viridigriseus* Edwards, *Aphrodes bicinctus* (Schrank), *Aphrodes albifrons* (Linnaeus), *Macrosteles cristatus* (Ribaut), and *Macrosteles laevis* Ribaut. In Italy, where no vector has yet been found, the clover phyllody disease has been observed by Grancini (personal communication). Chiykowski (54) and Musil (139) pointed out that the incubation period of clover phyllody is much longer than that of aster yellows, when the viruses are studied in the same host plants. Although no conclusive statements are possible about the relationship of the two viruses, their distinctiveness has been established beyond doubt. Chiykowski (54) found that the incubation period in *M. fascifrons* was almost twice as long for clover phyllody virus as for aster yellows virus. He suspected that the phyllody virus had been introduced into Canada from Europe in recent years, which would explain its geographical limitation despite lack of natural barriers to its spread. Limited movement of the leafhopper vectors may be responsible for the slow spread of phyllody.

The rapid spread and increased occurrence of celery yellows in the eastern part of the United States might be explained on the basis of recent findings by Maramorosch (132). Contrary to preliminary findings (129), a shorter incubation period in plants and in insect vectors was found for the celery-infecting strain. The difference was not great, with a minimum incubation period in insects at 25°C of eight days, compared to nine days for the eastern strain. However, the span between the first and the last plant infected with the celery strain in controlled conditions was only two days, compared to eight days for the eastern strain. This shorter span between the first and last day of the disease onset may play an important role in the spread of celery yellows, as cross-immunity prevents reinfection with the slower-multiplying strain.

Loss of transmissibility.—A few years ago, Black (26) discovered that certain leafhopper-borne viruses, maintained for many years in plants through grafting, had lost their affinity to the arthropod vectors, and no longer could be transmitted by their original insect carriers. It seems likely that vectorless strains of viruses have evolved artificially in the laboratory through a process of mutation or gradual selection. However, the possibility of the loss of a stage in the development of the virus cannot be excluded entirely, although at present there is no evidence supporting the existence of such virus forms or of different developmental stages in the life cycle of viruses multiplying in insects and plants.

Virus acquisition and transmission.—In a study of virus acquisition and transmission, Maramorosch (131) found that *Macrosteles fascifrons* seldom acquires virus from older, symptomless leaves of diseased plants. Only 3 per cent of insects became viruliferous in a single day of acquisition feeding on older leaves, while 80 per cent acquired virus from the diseased inflorescence, and 90 per cent from the leafless stem.

Virus transmission was not evenly distributed throughout the day, but occurred in distinct peaks, at 8.00 a.m., 11:00 a.m., 3:00 p.m., 5:00 p.m., and 8:00 p.m. Almost twice as many plants became infected during the afternoon hours, as during the morning hours. The increased transmission coincided with increased uptake of food, as measured by the uptake of C^{14}-labeled glucose, but no definite peaks were found in food uptake. The observed transmission peaks may indicate the existence of an independent mechanism governing virus transmission.

Nagaraj & Black (140) have found that the abilities of *Agallia con-stricta* to transmit wound-tumor virus were unrelated to the abilities to transmit potato yellow dwarf virus. Their experiments indicated that the hereditary mechanisms which determine the abilities of a single leafhopper species to transmit two unrelated plant viruses were inherited independently. Actually, the authors found that the ability to transfer wound-tumor virus from insect to insect transovarially, and that of transferring potato yellow dwarf by insects to plants, depended on either two alleles or two or more genes. It seems that individuals within a vector species, in much the same way as plants, have different specific genetic susceptibilities to virus infection. This conclusion is in accord with findings made by Storey (203) 30 years ago.

Virus interrelationships.—Attempts to define the relationships of yellows type viruses are severely hampered by the lack of a world-wide virus collection. A comparison between some of the European and Canadian viruses was made by Valenta (220, 221, 223, 224). Ryshkow (176) pointed out that the stolbur group of viruses, transmitted primarily by *Hyalestes obsoletus* Signoret, and, in addition, by at least four other leafhoppers, should be separated from the group to which the typical aster yellows virus belongs. The same view was often expressed by the late L. O. Kunkel (personal communication), who called the attention of this reviewer to the big-bud symptoms in tomato plants, caused by stolbur virus and the Australian big-bud virus but not by strains of aster yellows. The finding that several *Macrosteles* species, including *M. fascifrons,* can act as vectors of both types of viruses may necessitate a revision of earlier conclusions concerning the identification of aster yellows virus and of its reported vectors in various regions, including the eastern part of North America.

Serology.—The pioneering work of Black (28) and of Brakke *et al.* (42, 43) on the purification and serology of leafhopper-borne viruses permitted the characterization of several viruses by electron microscopy, while the use of viral antigens made their accurate detection possible. Whitcomb & Black (237) have measured the rate of increase of wound-tumor soluble antigen in the vector, *Agallia constricta* Van Duzee, infected by the injection technique. The titer of soluble antigen increased rapidly between the fourth day, when it could be first detected, and the tenth day, when it reached a plateau at which it remained for many weeks. This rapid increase was caused by the rapid multiplication of the virus in the insect. On the other hand, the infectivity and efficiency of transmission seem to increase gradually, reaching their maximum at about five weeks after the injection of the virus into the vector. Although the level of soluble antigen remains high, the infectivity of the insects decreases in later weeks. Using the precipitin ring test, a method was developed to detect the presence or absence of wound-tumor virus in a single leafhopper. Although all insects injected with large doses of wound-tumor virus showed an increase in soluble antigen, some failed to transmit the virus. Thus, the serological method proved to be much more sensitive in detecting viruliferous insects than was the testing of leafhoppers on susceptible plants.

It is not known in which tissues or organs of the vector the virus multiplies. Fluorescent antibody studies by Nagaraj et al. (141) were perfected so that now a method exists by which the wound-tumor virus can be detected in cross-sections of vectors. However, this technique has not yet revealed the site of viral multiplication. It has been speculated that the fat body which, in the case of some virus infections of vectors, may show cytopathogenic changes, is the place where propagative viruses multiply, but this could not be proven. The mycetome has also been suspected because of symbionts in which the multiplication of viruses could theoretically take place. This possibility was discussed by Black (23), but no indications of changes in the mycetome have been reported until very recently. Nasu (142) observed changes in the mycetome of viruliferous males of the black-streaked green rice leafhopper, Nephotettix sp. As compared with uninfected individuals, viruliferous males carrying rice stunt virus had shrunken mycetomes, in which the internal layers appeared to have hardened. Numbers of infected males up to 67 per cent manifested these changes, and the same individuals showed also changes in their fat body tissues, similar to those described by Littau & Maramorosch (112) in aster yellows vectors. In the green rice leafhopper, Nephotettix cincticeps, also a vector of rice stunt virus, mycetome shrinkage occurred in 75 per cent of infected males.

Deleterious effects of viruses on vectors.—In 1940, Sukhov in Russia found that the planthopper, Delphacodes (Liburnia) striatella (Fallen), a vector of the pseudo-rosette virus "zakuklivanie," had X-bodies in fat body tissues, the salivary glands, and the gut (207, 209). Professor Sukhov kindly supplied two photographs of these crystalline virus inclusions (Fig. 3a, 3b). They were obtained from viruliferous insects maintained for prolonged periods on diseased oats plants. When the intestinal tract of a living plant hopper was removed and placed in a drop of water, the inclusions remained inside the gut, except for occasional particles that escaped through the damaged wall into the surrounding water. The same kind of virus inclusions was found in diseased oat plants (208). No deleterious effects of X-bodies on the vectors has been reported.

In 1956, Littau & Maramorosch (111) described changes in the fat body tissues of Macrosteles fascifrons that were infected with aster yellows virus. The same authors found later (112) that these changes can be detected in males, but not in females, and that they become pronounced only after a few weeks, and not during the beginning of the transmission period. The changes were found in some, but not all, infective males. Nuclei of

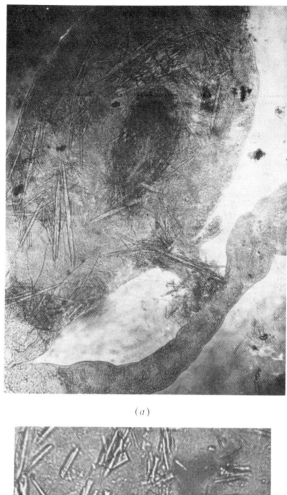

(*a*)

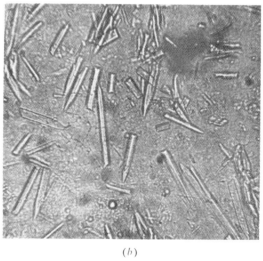

(*b*)

FIG. 3. *a*. Midgut of *Delphacodes striatella* Fallen with X-bodies of the oat rosette ("zakuklivanie") virus. *b*. Virus crystals that escaped through a damaged portion of the gut wall into the surrounding water. Courtesy Prof. K. S. Sukhov, Institute of Genetics, Academy of Sciences, U.S.S.R., Moscow.

the fat body were stellate instead of round, and the cytoplasm appeared sparse. The 1956 report was an indication that a "plant-insect" virus may cause direct harm to its insect host and vector and it focused the attention of workers in different laboratories to this problem. Similar cytological changes in leafhopper and planthopper tissues were found recently by Nasu (142), at the National Institute of Agricultural Sciences, Tokyo, and by Takahashi & Sekiya (217) of the Nagano Agricultural Experiment Station in Japan. The details of these studies will be discussed elsewhere (96, 134). Directly harmful and often killing effects on vectors by plant viruses were described by Jensen (94, 95), Watson & Sinha (235), and more recently by Shinkai (183) with *Deltocephalus dorsalis* Motschulski. Jedlinski (personal communication) working at the University of Illinois in Urbana, Illinois with *Graminella nigrifrons* (Forbes) also found a direct effect on the longevity of insects carrying an oat-infecting virus.

These findings indicate that arthropod vectors are sometimes directly harmed by the viruses that multiply in their bodies. They strengthen the hypothesis of Maramorosch (122) and others, that these viruses may have originated as viruses of insects, originally harmful to their insect hosts; later on some of them have lost their insect pathogenicity and have gradually become adapted to plant hosts.

Consistent changes in oxygen consumption and in the respiratory quotient between viruliferous and virus-free *Nephotettix cincticeps* infected with the rice stunt were found by Yoshii (242). The author concluded that the infection of the vector by the rice stunt virus resulted in an increase of enzyme activities and in an accelerated metabolism. However, viruliferous insects were obtained by maintaining the leafhoppers for at least one month on diseased plants. Therefore, the observed changes in metabolism could have also been caused by the changes in the diet.

Beneficial effects of viruses on insects.—In the course of an investigation of the fate of viruses acquired by nonvector insects, Maramorosch (126) found a surprising relationship between the corn leafhopper, *Dalbulus maidis* and the aster yellows virus. *D. maidis* is a vector of corn stunt virus, but it is unable to transmit aster yellows virus. The insects ordinarily survive and breed well only on corn (*Zea mays* L.) and on a wild grass, teosinte (*Euchlaena mexicana*). When corn leafhoppers were confined to an aster plant with aster yellows, they were not rendered infective; they could survive on diseased as well as on healthy aster plants, whereas normal corn leafhoppers usually die on healthy aster plants within four days. By injecting the hemolymph of infected corn leafhoppers into aster leafhoppers, it was further found that corn leafhoppers acquired and retained the aster yellows virus for prolonged periods. Moreover, they were able to survive not only on healthy asters, but even on carrot, rye, and several other plants that are as unsuitable to normal corn leafhoppers as healthy asters. The ability to live on plants that were formerly unsuitable could be destroyed by subjecting the insects to 36°C for eight days. The same treatment destroys aster yellows virus in aster leafhoppers (106), and it seems likely that the change in the feeding and survival is directly dependent on the presence and action of the aster yellows virus in corn leafhoppers. The mechanism of this unique phenomenon has been studied further by Orenski & Maramorosch (148) and by Orenski et al. (149). The amount of C^{14} and P^{32} taken up from labeled leaves was used as a measure of feeding activity. The uptake of tracers left no doubt that normal corn leafhoppers not only probe on plants that cannot support them, but that they actually take up glucose while feeding on the phloem. The total amount of food taken up from plants other than corn was much lower than that from corn plants. However, the lack of survival was more likely due to indigestion than to starvation, because starved insects, given distilled water, lived a few days longer than insects feeding on strange plants. Corn leafhoppers with aster yellows virus fed slightly better on aster leaves than did normal corn leafhoppers. This difference could only be detected when insects fed on young aster leaves. When the uptake of isotopes from aster leaves was compared in the corn and aster leafhoppers, it was found that corn leafhoppers, with or without the virus, acquired only from 1 to 10 per cent as much isotope from aster leaves as did aster leafhoppers. That seemed to provide further evidence that the survival of viruliferous corn leafhoppers was not caused by an increase in the amount of food taken from aster plants, but by a change in the ability to digest the strange food.

The beneficial effect of a plant virus on an arthropod is a novel finding. Viruses may emerge as being only the pathogenic individuals among a rich collection of transmissible factors, some of which may have been more beneficial to the host organisms than their pathogenic relatives have been harmful. In the course of evolution of viruses, selection of infective nucleoproteins most likely went not only in the direction of pathogenicity but also in the opposite direction, giving rise to beneficial viruses. Work at this new frontier of science has only begun.

Disease symptoms induced by leafhopper feeding.—In 1959, Maramorosch (127) described an ephemeral disease of corn, resembling the Australian Wallaby-Ear disease, and induced by the feeding of *Dalbulus elimatus* (Ball). In Australia, according to Day (personal communication), specimens of *Cicadulina bipunctella* (Matsumura) were collected from different localities and tested for Wallaby-Ear transmission. All were found to induce the characteristic symptoms and no "virus-free" colony could be established. In the Philippines, Maramorosch et al. found that *Cicadulina bipunctella* induced galls on maize and rice plants (135). All insects collected in nature were able to induce galls. According to Ruppel (172), most representatives of the genus *Cicadulina* are either virus vectors or induce plant diseases through their toxins. In Colombia, for instance, *Cicadulina pastucae* Ruppel & DeLong has been associated with the spread of *enanismo* (Gilberto Bravo and Antonio Uwigarro, quoted by Ruppel). The incidence of the disease is greater around borders of cultivated fields, which indicates that the lateral movement of individual leafhoppers is not great, and that they move by short jumps rather than by flights. While *enanismo* is most likely caused by a virus, the same species of leafhopper also induces vein swellings of wheat and barley on the Sabana de Bogota, but does not transmit *enanismo* there. This vein swelling has characteristics of a toxin-induced disease.

THRIPS

The status of thrips-borne viruses has been discussed critically by Sakimura (177, 178). Only one virus is known to be thrips-borne: tomato spotted wilt virus. This virus is world-wide in its distribution. Its relationship to the vector species has been studied since 1927 when Pittman (157) first described its transmission by *Thrips tabaci* Lindeman. The disease and virus have been given various names. In Russia, Razvyazkina (163) described it as "makhorka tip chlorosis virus" (chlorosis of *Nicotiana rustica*), while, in Bulgaria, Kovachevski & Markov (105) called it "tomato bronzing" virus. In addition to *T. tabaci,* three other species have been found to transmit spotted wilt virus: *Frankliniella schultzei* (Trybom) (179), *F. occidentalis* (Pergande) (81), and *F. fusca* (Hinds) (178). The report of *F. insularis* (Franklin), as a vector from Australia, was due to misidentification of *F. schultzei. Thrips tabaci,* common in every region of the world, is believed to be the major vector, while all *Frankliniella* species are regional in distribution. Although *T. tabaci* shows no preference for feeding on tobacco in North America and the Southern Hemisphere, it infects *N. rustica* and tobacco in the Balkans and in Russia. Repeated observations leave no doubt that adult thrips cannot acquire the virus. Acquisition occurs only during the larval stage. When the virus completes its latent period before pupation, larvae may become infective. Razvyazkina (163) reported an inoculation threshold of 5 min, after an acquisition feeding of at least 30 min. Sakimura found an increase in percentage of infection when the feeding periods increased (178). A definite latent period, or incubation period, of the virus in its vector species has been known since the original finding of Bald & Samuel (6). Minima ranging from 3 days (163) in *T. tabaci* to 12 days (178) in *F. fusca* were reported. The shorter periods were found in cases where inoculation was achieved by larvae before pupation, while the longer ones were found in insects that changed into adults. The virus is often retained throughout the life of the vector. Although, in many instances, infectivity is continuous, sometimes it has been found to be erratic, with sporadic transmissions and long periods of no transmissions in between. Obviously, some vectors are poor transmitters, while others are more efficient. No experimental data have been obtained so far on the possible multiplication of the spotted wilt virus in thrips vectors. The inability of the adult insects to acquire the virus has not been clarified either. No conclusive data exist to support or reject the possibility that the virus passes transovarially to a percentage of the offspring. As pointed out recently by Sakimura (178), the virus-vector relationships in thrips-borne viruses have been investigated less vigorously than have those in the aphid- or leafhopper-borne viruses.

All strains of the spotted wilt virus are readily juice transmissible. The virus has a thermal inactivation point *in vitro* at 42°C. and a longevity in extracts of less than 5 hrs at 18°C. It has been identified morphologically by Black (28), and was first believed to be spherical (32). The diameter of the purified particles from plant juices was found to be 85 mµ. Density gradient centrifugation was used for purification of the virus. Its sedimentation rate was established as 590 (Black, personal communication). Best (10, 11), working with strains of spotted wilt virus, reported recombinations obtained in plants infected simultaneously with different strains. However, the markers of the strains used by Best do not permit a definite conclusion as to the production of hybrid strains. No attempts to repeat these experiments or to confirm the findings have been made in vectors inoculated simultaneously with different strains of the virus.

WHITEFLIES

The literature dealing with whitefly transmission of plant viruses has been reviewed by Orlando & Silberschmidt (150) and by Heinze (86). In 1946, Orlando & Silberschmidt solved the mystery of "infectious chlorosis" of *Abutilon thompsonii* that puzzled geneticists and plant pathologists for many decades. The virus disease that could only be transmitted by grafting in Europe and North America was found to spread naturally in Brazil. The whitefly, *Bemisia tabaci* (Gennadius), carried the virus from one *Sida* plant to another but, strangely enough, not from *Abutilon* to *Sida* (186).

Relationships between various tropical viruses and *Bemisia tabaci* have been studied in only a few instances. In India, where whiteflies are probably the most important vectors of plant viruses, *B. tabaci* has been reported as the vector of tobacco leaf curl, tobacco yellow-net virus, and several viruses affecting bean, cucurbits, and other cultivated plants. Varma (226) reported that whiteflies can carry three different viruses simultaneously. In Brazil, Costa & Bennett (57) found that *Euphorbia* mosaic virus was retained by whiteflies for prolonged periods, often for life. In all instances, an incubation period was found in *B. tabaci* that varied from 4 to 5 hr to 24 to 48 hr. Thus, this virus can be classified as circulatory. Great differences were found between individual vectors in their ability to transmit virus. Tests of several hundred individuals revealed that the transmitting ability of females was twice that of males (57). The same was found for the transmission of infectious chlorosis virus (150). In the latter, a feeding period of 30 min was adequate for virus acquisition, and the ability to produce infection seemed to increase with prolonged acquisition feeding time. Studies carried out by Bird (14) in Puerto Rico indicated that *B. tabaci* transmits a chlorosis virus to *Sida* plants, that is either closely related or identical with the chlorosis virus of *Sida* in Brazil. Bird found that whiteflies acquired virus during a 15 min acquisition feeding and that the virus was retained by the vector for long periods. Results of transmission tests with *Sida* and *Jathropa* virus indicated that at least two races of *B. tabaci* were present in Puerto Rico. One of these races was recently reported to transmit two new viruses, not related to either *Sida* chlorosis or *Jathropa* mosaic (15). Flores & Silberschmidt (66) pointed out that whitefly-borne viruses frequently induce diseases with strikingly similar symptoms in host plants, although the viruses may not be closely related. In the absence of serological tests, cross-protection tests have been used with symptomatology. The authors concluded from their results that cross-protection alone did not provide adequate criteria for the determination of whitefly-borne virus strains. In 1957, Silberschmidt *et al.* (186) met with difficulties in transmitting the chlorosis virus from *Abutilon* to *Sida rhombifolia* by means of vectors, although the virus could easily be transmitted by the same vectors from *Sida* to *Sida*. Therefore, the authors postulated that strains of "infectious chlorosis" virus probably originated from a virus population that found favorable conditions for multiplication in some specific hosts in which other strains became suppressed. By this mechanism of strain evolution, *Abutilon* would have selected a strain that produced severe mottling in that species, while retaining only a mild degree of pathogenicity for *Sida*. According to this hypothesis, the virus strain that infects *Leonorus* plants would have an even lesser degree of affinity to the original host plant, *Abutilon*. A further step in this evolution of virus strains would be represented by *Euphorbia* mosaic and by *Jathropa* mosaic. While this hypothesis deals primarily with virus adaptations to plants, the affinities of virus strains to *Bemisia tabaci* should also be considered. The low degree of transmissibility of chlorosis virus from *Abutilon* to *Sida*—only 4 per cent, according to Silberschmidt's results (186)—might indicate a step in the progressive loss of vector transmissibility (26).

MEALYBUGS

The transmission of plant viruses by mealybugs has been studied in great detail in Africa, where, in Ghana and Nigeria, the important swollen shoot disease of cacao was found to be mealybug-borne. Posnette (158) pointed out that the swollen shoot virus probably began to spread from indigenous jungle trees to cacao in plantations many years ago, soon after extensive plantings had become established. The disease had not been known before 1922, and not been definitely recognized before 1936. In 1950 it was estimated that more than 15 million trees succumb every year. Many virus strains have been isolated. The swollen shoot virus is carried by several species of mealybugs, which are tended and dispersed by ants, as well as by wind and by natural migration. Mealybugs require several hours feeding on an infected plant before they become infective, but can then infect a healthy plant in less than one hour. According to Posnette and co-workers

311

(160, 161), the transmitting efficiency of the most important vector, *Pseudococcus njalensis* Laing, increased with prolonged feeding on diseased plants. Maximum efficiency was obtained after an acquisition feeding of 10 hr. When longer acquisition periods were allowed, mealybug infectivity decreased. Usually, infectivity of vectors was lost very soon and not more than two plants could be inoculated consecutively by the same mealybug. However, the apparently stylet-borne virus could be retained up to 36 hr when the insects which acquired virus were prevented from immediate feeding. Swollen shoot is probably the most destructive economically of all plant virus diseases because of the high price of cacao beans and the amount of yearly devastation.

Pineapple wilt in Hawaii has been the subject of controversy for many years, ever since its outbreaks became linked with mealybugs. The fact that the same species of mealybugs existed in many locations where pineapples were grown, while wilt appeared only in some, but not in others, pointed to the possible virus etiology. The disease has been linked by Carter with the feeding of two species, *Dysmicoccus neo-brevipes* Beardsley and *D. brevipes* (Cockerell) (53). At first it was assumed that the wilting of pineapple was caused by a toxin introduced into plants by mealybugs. It was observed that usually only large numbers of feeding insects would cause wilt, while small numbers failed to produce the symptoms. In addition, control measures with insecticides were found to reduce and almost eliminate the spread of the disease, which also seemed to support the hypothesis of an insect toxin, rather than a virus. In 1951, Carter revised his original interpretation when he discovered that mealybugs could induce wilt only after first feeding on a "source" (diseased) plant (50). In 1952, Carter postulated that mealybugs carry a transmissible "latent factor," separate and distinct from the wilt-inducing toxin (51). Carter did not use single insects in his experiments, but, on the basis of his massive inoculations versus inoculations with small numbers of insects, one is led to believe that the efficiency of mealybugs in the transmission of the infectious agent of wilt is rather poor. This reviewer favors the substitution of the term virus source for Carter's term "positive" source, because the experimental data leave little doubt that a virus is involved. The main reasons for this assumption are that (*a*) unless mealybugs feed on diseased plants, they are unable to infect healthy seedlings; and (*b*) mealybug infectivity is lost when the insects feed on healthy plants or when they continue to probe on inoculated leaves. In other words, mealybugs acquire virus by feeding on plants infected with wilt, and soon lose infectivity. This is similar to the relationship between the cacao swollen shoot virus and its mealybug vectors (158). It appears that pineapple plants can be rendered more susceptible to infection by exposing them to feeding of large numbers of virus-free mealybugs. Moreover, pineapple plants can become symptomless carriers of the virus (53). These findings have not only theoretical but also practical implications. They resulted in the control of the disease in Hawaii through the use of insecticides, and through the propagation of wilt-resistant varieties.

In Puerto Rico, Bird (13) found that a single specimen of *Dysmicoccus brevipes* could transmit wilt virus to healthy susceptible pineapple seedlings when the mealybugs were confined to test plants for 24 hr. Disease symptoms appeared after three months. The virus could also be acquired by mealybugs from apparently recovered plants, which no longer showed symptoms of wilt.

TREEHOPPERS

Treehoppers (Membracidae) had not been known to transmit plant viruses until 1958, when the first authenticated account of pseudo-curly top virus transmission by a *Micrutalis* sp. appeared. Simons & Coe (189) found in Florida that the treehopper vector efficiently transmits the virus. Transmission is highly specific. A close relative of the vector, *Micrutalis calva* (Say), seems to be unable to transmit the virus (130). Simons (188) studied the relationship between the virus and its vector. He found that the acquisition and inoculation threshold periods were less than 1 hr. A latent period of 24 to 48 hr was found. Virus retention seemed correlated with length of acquisition feeding, and there was no evidence of virus multiplication in the vector. The circulative virus showed many similarities to the sugar beet curly top virus in its relationship to the vector as well as in host symptomatology. The weed *Solanum gracile* (Link) is a host for the tree-hopper and also for the virus. The discovery of the membracid vector of pseudo-curly top virus is of great interest because the disease may become of economic importance. The finding that plant vectors occur among families and groups that until now have not been known to comprise virus vectors should be kept in mind by those who search for transmitters of disease agents. It is now realized that vectors of viruses are not limited to the "old" groups but may as well occur among unsuspected taxa.

MITES

Mite transmission has been recently reviewed by Slykhuis (192, 193). Currant reversion in England was the first plant disease suspected since 1927 to be caused by mite-borne virus (3, 136). With presently available techniques, further work on currant reversion ought to be carried out, to find out whether the disease symptoms would persist after the plants are freed from mites through chemical treatments. Such treatments can remove mites completely, and in their absence graft experiments ought to be carried out to test the viral nature of the disease. No experiments have been reported on the possible effect of virus-free mites obtained from eggs hatched on healthy plants, nor on the acquisition of virus by such mites.

Eriophyid mites are now known to transmit at least six different plant viruses. The Eriophyidae are a distinct group with no close relation to other mite groups. They feed by sucking plant juices, puncturing the plant cells with their slender stylets. Their stylets are inside a groove of the rostrum that has two pads at its apex, serving as ducts for the saliva. Independent movement of the mites is very limited because of their small size and vulnerability to desiccation. Although some mites can be transported by beetles, the main means of dispersion is wind (191). Eriophyid mites are dependent on specific young host tissues and their feeding causes little if any injury. Mite injury may, though, simulate virus symptoms and more than once have such injuries been ascribed to "air-borne" viruses. Slykhuis found that the mite *Aceria tulipae* Keifer can transmit two viruses simultaneously, wheat streak mosaic virus and wheat spot mosaic virus (193).

Fig mosaic was suspected to be mite-borne in 1933 (55) and the vector, *Aceria ficus* (Cotte), was discovered in 1955 by Flock & Wallace (65). Also in 1955, Wilson *et al.* reported the transmission of peach mosaic virus in California by *Eriophyes insidiosus* Keifer and Wilson (239). There are several other viruses suspected of being mite-borne. Among them is cherry mottle leaf virus in California studied by L. S. Jones (personal communication).

As far as is known, none of the mite-borne viruses passes transovarially to the progeny, but all seem to persist in the mites through the molts. Slykhuis (193) noticed that nymphs acquire wheat streak mosaic virus, while adults do not. This is reminiscent of the thrips acquisition of tomato spotted wilt virus, and indicates a biological relationship.

The small size of mite vectors creates a difficult problem in the study of virus-vector inter-relationships of this group. It can be expected that the number of known viruses and vectors will soon increase with improved techniques and mounting interest in mite-borne viruses.

TOBACCO MOSAIC VIRUS TRANSMISSION

Although tobacco mosaic virus (TMV) has been one of the first viruses studied, its transmission in nature has never been explained adequately. The controversial reports have recently been reviewed by Broadbent (48). It is now generally accepted that the virus is not transmitted by sucking insects, though it may be occasionally transmitted by biting ones. Some earlier workers stated that aphids were vectors and this work warranted retesting. Recently Orlob (personal communication, to be published) failed to verify the following insects as vectors of the virus: *Macrosiphum euphorbiae* (Thomas) and *Myzus persicae* (91); *Pseudococcus citri* Risso (143, 147); *Pentatrichopus fragaefollii* (Cockerell) (56). It has been the general consensus of opinion that the careful work of Miss Hoggan (91) was carried out with either a virus other than TMV, or with an unusual strain of TMV. The virus was necrotic to pepper, while most strains cause only a mottle on this host plant. Teakle & Sylvester (217a) demonstrated that both *M. persicae* and *Myzus circumflexus* (Buckton) were able to inoculate TMV into plant cells if the virus was first placed on the leaf surface. Orlob found that in the transmission of TMV the aphid stylet cannot be considered as a "micro-needle." Attempts to transmit the virus by placing it on the stylet of the aphid failed. Virus could be recovered from the stylets of fasting aphids, but not after they had fed. In contrast, the virus was transmitted when tissues were punctured by means of a micro-needle having the approximate size of an aphid stylet. No infection was obtained when virus was put on the stylets of leafhoppers, plant bugs, and mealybugs. Only the potato flea beetle *Epitrix cucumeris* Harris transmitted the virus when its mouth parts were treated with virus suspension. The flea beetles lost infectivity within a short period (one day), indicating a mechanical type of transmission. The beetles, that move freely among tobacco plants, act as efficient vectors under experimental conditions. Orlob found no cross-protection of two strains of tobacco mosaic virus in the tarnished plant bug, and was able to recover both strains, in spite of the fact that they were retained by the insects and could be demonstrated by infectivity tests and by electron microscopy to be present in the intestines and feces. Day & Irzykiewcz recovered infectious TMV from macerated aphids. Ossiannilsson (154) also found TMV particles in the gut of *Myzus persicae*, and even in a leafhopper fed on diseased plants, and he suggested that aphids may acquire the virus occasionally when probing. No particles could be found in stylets cut off from aphids which had fed for a long time on infected plants. This ingenious method was also used by van Soest & de Meester-Manger Cats (225) who cut off the stylets of *M. persicae* feeding on an infected plant, collected the droplets emerging from the stylets and tested for activity by inoculating tobacco, by a serological method, and by examination under an electron microscope. However, no TMV could be detected.

Walters (230) demonstrated TMV transmission from tobacco to tobacco by the grasshopper *Melanoplus differentialis* (Thomas). Sukhov & Vovk (210) reported transmission by caterpillars of *Plusia gamma* (Linnaeus). In these instances, the virus is probably mechanically transferred by the biting mouth parts. A rather unusual kind of mechanical transmission was discovered recently by Costa *et al.* (58), when the virus was found to be transmitted by the ovipositors of the leafminer flies *Liriomyza langei* Frick.

The transmission of TMV by caterpillars was studied in great detail by Brčák in Czechoslovakia (44, 45, 46). The author found that the feces of *Barathra brassicae* (Linnaeus), which were previously fed on leaves with TMV, contained approximately 50 per cent of the original titer of the virus. However, during the passage through the intestines, the virus was strongly inhibited by enzymes. This inhibition was reversed in the intestines before the feces were excreted by the caterpillars. The author attempted to transmit TMB by means of *Pseudococcus maritimus* (Ehrhon) and *Trialeurodes vaporariorum* Westwood but no transmission could be obtained by means of these insects.

An interesting paper by Sugiura & Hirayama (206) on the transmission of TMV by caterpillars has been overlooked by most reviewers and recent workers on this subject. The authors found that caterpillars of *Barathra brassicae* transmitted TMV to 15 per cent of test plants. Fasting gradually decreased the ability of caterpillars to transmit the virus. After 24 hr of fasting only 4 per cent of the test plants became infected. When caterpillars that carried TMV on their mouth parts were feeding on healthy plants for more than 3 hrs, they no longer were able to infect tobacco plants. As ascertained by local lesion counts, the fluid vomited by the caterpillars which had fed for 48 hrs on diseased plants contained approximately $\frac{1}{3}$ of the TMV contained in the juice of diseased leaves. Three hours after the caterpillars began to feed on diseased leaves, TMV could be detected in the feces, and even 18 hrs later, although the caterpillars were maintained on healthy plants, TMV was still present in feces.

A plausible explanation for the inability to find an efficient natural vector of TMV can be provided on the basis of work with leafhopper-borne viruses. Black (26) found that several leafhopper-borne viruses lost affinity to their original insect vectors when they were carried artificially in plants for many years by means of grafting. Tobacco mosaic virus is so easily transmitted mechanically, and has for so many years been carried to plants by man, that it could have mutated and lost its affinity to the original arthropod vector.

CONCLUSIONS

Every year new virus vectors are being added to the long list of known virus transmitters. In the last decade, additions were made not only to previously known groups of arthropods, but several new and unexpected groups of vectors were discovered. The Membracidae and the Acarina have been discussed briefly in this review. The mystery of soil-borne virus transmission has been clarified in a number of instances, when vectors were found among the Nematoda (90), first known nonarthropod vectors of plant viruses. The transmission of viruses is a complex process, even in the "simple" stylet-borne category. We need new techniques to study and understand the basic mechanisms involved. One approach that seems very promising is through the development of insect tissue culture (133). It is hoped that the study of viruses in tissues and cells of vectors *in vitro* will eventually provide a new method for the investigation of arthropod-borne viruses and will permit accurate quantitative measurement of virus concentration by a plaque technique. Propagative viruses and even stylet-borne viruses could perhaps be adapted and cultivated in cells of higher, cold- and warm-blooded animals. Studies of the histology and fine structure of organs of arthropod vectors with the aid of the electron microscope may reveal changes caused by viruses and, in turn, may help in the understanding of virus-vector interactions.

LITERATURE CITED

1. Adams, J. B., and McAllan, J. W. Pectinase in the saliva of *Myzus persicae* (Sulz.). *Can. J. Zool.*, **34**, 541–43 (1956)
2. Allard, H. A. The mosaic disease of tobacco. *U. S. Dept. Agr. Bull. No. 40*, 1–33 (1914)
3. Amos, J., Hatton, R. G., Knight, R. C., and Massee, A. M. Experiments in the transmission of "reversion" in black currants. *Ann. Rept. East Malling Res. Sta., Kent, 1925*, Suppl. II, **13**, 126–50 (1927)
4. Anderson, C. W. The insect vector realtionships of the filaree red-leaf virus, with special reference to a latent-period difference between nymphs and adults in *Macrosiphum geranicola* (Lambers). *Phytopathology*, **41**, 699–708 (1951)
5. Badami, R. S. Changes in the transmissibility by aphids of a strain of cucumber mosaic virus. *Ann. Appl. Biol.*, **46**, 554–62 (1958)
6. Bald, J. G., and Samuel, G. Investigations on "spotted wilt" of tomatoes. II. *Australia, Council Sci. Ind. Research Bull. No. 54*, 1–24 (1931)
7. Bawden, F. C. The transmission of plant viruses by insects. *Biological Aspects of the Transmission of Disease*, 87–93 (Horton-Smith, C., Ed., Oliver and Boyd, Edinburgh, Scotland, 184 pp., 1957)
8. Bawden, F. C., and Kassanis, B. The behaviour of some naturally occurring strains of potato virus Y. *Ann. Appl. Biol.*, **34**, 503–16 (1947)
9. Bennett, C. W., and Wallace, H. E. Relation of the curly top virus to the vector, *Eutettix tenellus. J. Agr. Research*, **56**, 31–51 (1938)
10. Best, R. J. Cross protection by strains of tomato spotted wilt virus and a new theory to explain it. *Australian J. Biol. Sci.*, **7**, 415–24 (1954)
11. Best, R. J., and Gallus, H. P. C. Further evidence for the transfer of character-determinants (recombination) between strains of tomato spotted wilt virus. *Enzymologia*, **17**, 207–21 (1955)
12. Bils, R. F., and Hall, C. E. Electron microscopy of wound-tumor virus. *Virology*, **17**, 123–30 (1962)
13. Bird, J. Mealybug wilt of pineapple. *Ann. Rept. Dept. Plant Pathol., Agr. Expt. Sta., Univ. Puerto Rico*, 2–3 (1953–54)
14. Bird, J. Infectious chlorosis of *Sida carpinifolia* in Puerto Rico. *Puerto Rico, Univ. Agr. Expt. Sta. Tech. Paper No. 26*, 1–23 (1958)
15. Bird, J. A whitefly transmitted mosaic of *Rhynchosia minima* DC, and its relation to tobacco leaf curl and other virus diseases of plants in Puerto Rico. *Proc. Am. Soc. Hort. Sci., Carib. Region*, **5** (In press)
16. Björling, K., Lihnell, D., and Ossiannilsson, F. Marking viruliferous aphids with radioactive phosphorus. *Acta Agr. Scand.*, **1**, 301–17 (1951)
17. Björling, K., and Ossiannilsson, F. Investigations on individual variations in the virus-transmitting ability of different aphid species. *Socker Handl. II*, **14**, 1–13 (1958)
18. Black, L. M. Genetic variation in the clover leafhopper's ability to transmit potato yellow-dwarf virus. *Genetics*, **28**, 200–9 (1943)
19. Black, L. M. Some viruses transmitted by agallian leafhoppers. *Proc. Am. Phil. Soc.*, **88**, 132–44 (1944)
20. Black, L. M. A virus tumor disease of plants. *Am. J. Botany*, **32**, 408–15 (1945)
21. Black, L. M. Virus tumors in plants. *Growth*, **10** (Suppl. 6th Symposium), 79–84 (1947)
22. Black, L. M. A plant virus that multiplies in its insect vector. *Nature*, **166**, 852–53 (1950)
23. Black, L. M. Viruses that reproduce in plants and insects. *Ann. N. Y. Acad. Sci.*, **56**, 398–412 (1953)
24. Black, L. M. Transmission of plant viruses by cicadellids. *Advances in Virus Research*, **1**, 69–89 (1953)
25. Black, L. M. Occasional transmission of some plant viruses through the eggs of their insect vectors. *Phytopathology*, **43**, 9–10 (1953)
26. Black, L. M. Loss of vector transmissibility by viruses normally insect transmitted. *Phytopathology*, **43**, 466 (1953) (Abstr.)
27. Black, L. M. Parasitological Reviews. Arthropod transmission of plant viruses. *Exptl. Parasitol.*, **3**, 72–104 (1954)
28. Black, L. M. Concepts and problems concerning purification of labile

insect-transmitted plant viruses. *Phytopathology*, **45**, 208–16 (1955)

29. Black, L. M. Biological cycles of plant viruses in insect vectors. *The Viruses*, **2**, 157–85 (Burnet, F. M., and Stanley, W. M., Eds., Academic Press, Inc., New York, 3 vols., 1959)

30. Black, L. M. Some recent advances on leafhopper-borne viruses. *Biological Transmission of Disease Agents*, 1–9 (Maramorosch, K., Ed., Academic Press, Inc., New York, 192 pp., 1962)

31. Black, L. M., and Brakke, M. K. Multiplication of wound-tumor virus in an insect vector. *Phytopathology*, **42**, 269–73 (1952)

32. Black, L. M., Brakke, M. K., and Vatter, A. E. Partial purification and electron microscopy of tomato spotted-wilt virus. *Phytopathology*, **42**, 3 (1952) (Abstr.)

33. Blattný, C. Sen. Über das Schwanken des Virusniveaus der europäischen Sommer-Astern-Gelbsucht in den Pflanzen des *Allium ampeloprasum* L. subsp. *porrum* (L.) Regel. *Preslia*, **32**, 406–7 (1960) (Abstr.)

34. Bovey, R. Une anomalie des fleurs du trèfle causée par un virus transmis par des cicadelles. *Rev. Romande Agr. Viticult. Arboricult.*, **13**, 106–8 (1957)

35. Bradley, R. H. E. Studies on the aphid transmission of a strain of henbane mosaic virus. *Ann. Appl. Biol.*, **39**, 78–97 (1952)

36. Bradley, R. H. E. Effects of depth of stylet penetration on aphid transmission of potato virus Y. *Can. J. Microbiol.*, **2**, 539–47 (1956)

37. Bradley, R. H. E. Our concepts: on rock or sand? *Recent Advances in Botany*, 528–33 (Univ. of Toronto Press, Toronto, Canada, 1766 pp., 1961)

38. Bradley, R. H. E. Aphid transmission of potato virus Y diminished by electrostatic charge. *Virology*, **15**, 379 (1961)

39. Bradley, R. H. E. Response of the aphid *Myzus persicae* (Sulz.) to some fluids applied to the mouthparts. *Can. Entomologist*, **94**, 707–22 (1962)

40. Bradley, R. H. E., and Ganong, R. Y. Evidence that the potato virus Y is carried near the tip of the stylets of the aphid vector *Myzus*

persicae (Sulz.). *Can. J. Microbiol.*, **1**, 775–82 (1955)

41. Bradley, R. H. E., and Ganong, R. Y. Three more viruses borne at the stylet tips of the aphid *Myzus persicae* (Sulz.). *Can. J. Microbiol.*, **3**, 669–70 (1957)

41a. Bradley, R. H. E., and Sylvester, E. S. Do aphids carry transmissible sugar beet yellows virus via their stylets? Evidence from ultraviolet irradiation. *Virology*, **17**, 599–60 (1962)

42. Brakke, M. K., Black, L. M., and Wyckoff, R. W. G. The sedimentation rate of potato yellow-dwarf virus. *Am. J. Botany*, **38**, 332–42 (1951)

43. Brakke, M. K., Vatter, A. E., and Black, L. M. Size and shape of wound-tumor virus. *Brookhaven Symposia in Biology*, **6**, 137–56 (1954)

44. Brčák, J. K poznání kontaminativního přenosu viru mosaiky tabáku hmyzem a kousacím ústním ústrojím. (Concerning the contaminative transmission of the tobacco mosaic virus by insects with biting mouth parts). *Acta Soc. Entomol. Čechoslav.*, **52**, 107–12 (1955)

45. Brčák, J. Änderungen der Infektiosität des Tabakmosaikvirus während der Passage durch den Darm von *Barathra brassicae* L. *Phytopathol. Z.*, **30**, 415–28 (1957)

46. Brčák, J. Über die Möglichkeit der Übertragung des TMV durch Insekten. *Preslia*, **32**, 30 (1960) (Abstr.)

47. Broadbent L. Control by insecticides of the spread of plant viruses. *Rept. of the Commonwealth Entomol. Conf., 1960, London 7th*, 168–70 (1960)

48. Broadbent, L. The epidemiology of tomato mosaic: A review of the literature. *Rept. Glasshouse Crops Research Inst., 1960*, 96–116 (1961)

49. Broadbent, L., and Martini, C. The spread of plant viruses. *Advances in Virus Research*, **6**, 93–135 (1959)

50. Carter, W. **The feeding sequence of** *Pseudococcus brevipes* (Ckl.) in relation to mealybug wilt of pineapples in Hawaii. *Phytopathology*, **41**, 769–80 (1951)

51. Carter, W. Injuries to plants caused by insect toxins. II. *Botan. Rev.*, **18**, 680–721 (1952)

318

52. Carter, W. Ecological aspects of plant virus transmissions. *Ann. Rev. Entomol.*, **6**, 347–70 (1961)
53. Carter, W. Mealybug wilt of pineapple: a reappraisal. *Ann. N.Y. Acad. Sci.* (In press)
54. Chiykowski, L. N. Clover phyllody virus in Canada and its transmission. *Can. J. Botany*, **40**, 397–404 (1962)
55. Condit, I. J., and Horne, W. T. A mosaic of the fig in California. *Phytopathology*, **23**, 887–96 (1933)
55a. Cook, P. P., Jr. *Behavior as a factor in the transmission of cabbage viruses by aphids.* (Unpublished Doctoral thesis, University of California, Berkeley, 1962)
56. Cornuet, P., and Morand, J. C. Transmission du virus de la mosaïque du tabac par le puceron du fraisier, *Passerina fragaefolii* Cock. *Compt. rend.*, **250**, 1750–52 (1960)
57. Costa, A. S., and Bennett, C. W. White fly-transmitted mosaic of *Euphorbia prunifolia. Phytopathology*, **40**, 266–83 (1950)
58. Costa, A. S., de Silva, D. M., and Duffus, J. E. Plant virus transmission by a leaf-miner fly. *Virology*, **5**, 145–49 (1958)
59. Day, M. F. The mechanism of the transmission of potato leaf roll virus by aphids. *Australian J. Biol. Sci.*, **8**, 498–513 (1955)
60. Day, M. F., and Irzykiewicz, H. On the mechanism of transmission of non-persistent phytopathogenic viruses by aphids. *Australian J. Biol. Sci.*, **7**, 251–73 (1954)
60a. Day, M. F., and Venables, D. G. The transmission of cauliflower mosaic virus by aphids. *Australian J. Biol. Sci.*, **14**, 187–97 (1961)
61. de Fluiter, H. J., Evenhuis, H. H., and van der Meer, F. A. Observations on some leafhopper-borne virus diseases in the Netherlands. *Proc. Conf. Potato Virus Diseases, Lisse, Wageningen, 2nd Conf.*, 84–88 (H. Veenman & Zoner, Wageningen, 1955)
62. Ehrhardt, P. Zum Sauerstoffverbrauch von *Myzus persicae* (Sulz.) vor und nach Aufnahme des Blattrollvirus. *Entomol. Exptl. et Appl.*, **3**, 114–17 (1960)
63. Esau, K. *Plants, Viruses, and Insects.* (Harvard University Press, Cambridge, Mass., 110 pp., 1961)
64. Evenhuis, H. H. De vectoren van het bloemvergroeningsvirus van klaver.

Tijdschr. Plantenziekten, 64, 335–36 (1958)
65. Flock, R. A., and Wallace, J. M. Transmission of fig mosaic by the eriophyid mite *Aceria ficus. Phytopathology*, **45**, 52–54 (1955)
66. Flores, E., and Silberschmidt, K. Observations on a mosaic disease of *Leonurus sibiricus* occurring spontaneously in São Paulo. *Phytopathol. Z., 43*, 221–33 (1962)
67. Fraser, L. Virus diseases of citrus in Australia. *Proc. Linnean Soc. N. S. Wales, 83* (Pt. I), 9–19 (1958)
68. Frazier, N. W., and Posnette, A. F. Leafhopper transmission of a clover virus causing green petal disease in strawberry. *Nature, 177*, 1040–41 (1956)
69. Frazier, N. W., and Posnette, A. F. Transmission and host-range studies of strawberry green-petal virus. *Ann. Appl. Biol., 45*, 580–88 (1957)
70. Freitag, J. H. Negative evidence on multiplication of curly-top virus in the beet leafhopper, *Eutettix tenellus. Hilgardia, 10*, 305–42 (1936)
71. Fukushi, T. Aster yellows in Japan. (In Japanese) *Nogyo Oyobi Engei, 5*, 577–84 (1930)
72. Fukushi, T. Multiplication of virus in its insect vector. *Proc. Imp. Acad. (Tokyo)*, **11**, 301–3 (1935)
73. Fukushi, T. Further studies on the dwarf disease of rice plant. *J. Fac. Agr. Hokkaido Univ., 45*, 83–154 (1940)
74. Fukushi, T., and Kimura, I. Mechanical transmission of rice dwarf virus to *Nephotettix cincticeps* (In Japanese). *Nippon Shokubutsu Byori Gakkaiho, 23*, 54 (1958) (Abstr.)
75. Fukushi, T., and Nemoto, M. Insect vector of aster yellows. *Virus, 3*, 208 (1953) (Abstr.)
76. Fukushi, T., and Nemoto, M. Insect vector of aster yellows (In Japanese). *Nippon Shokubutsu Byori Gakkaiho, 18*, 146 (1954) (Abstr.)
77. Fukushi, T., and Shikata, E. Japanese aster yellows (In Japanese). *Nippon Shokubutsu Byori Gakkaiho*, (Abstr.)
78. Fukushi, T., Shikata, E., Kimura, I., and Nemoto, M. Electron microscopic studies on the rice-dwarf virus. *Proc. Japan. Acad., 36*, 352–57 (1960)
79. Galvez, G. E., Thurston, H. D., and Jennings, P. R. Transmission of

hoja blanca of rice by the plant-hopper, *Sogata cubana. Plant Disease Reptr.*, **44**, 394 (1960)

80. Galvez, G. E., Thurston, H. D., and Jennings, P. R. Host range and insect transmission of the hoja blanca disease of rice. *Plant Disease Reptr.*, **45**, 949–53 (1961)

81. Gardner, M. W., Tomkins, C. M., and Whipple, O. C. Spotted wilt of truck crops and ornamental plants. *Phytopathology*, **25**, 17 (1935) (Abstr.)

82. Grylls, N. E. Rugose leaf curl—a new virus disease transovarially transmitted by the leafhopper *Austroagallia torrida. Australian J. Biol. Sci.*, **7**, 47–58 (1954)

83. Harpaz, I. *Calligypona marginata,* the vector of maize rough dwarf virus. *Food and Agr. Organization U.N., Plant Protection Bull.*, **9**, 144–47 (1961)

84. Harrison, B. D. Studies on the behavior of potato leaf roll and other viruses in the body of their aphid vector *Myzus persicae* (Sulz.). *Virology*, **6**, 265–77 (1958)

85. Heinze, K. Survival of aphids after injection. *J. Econ. Entomol.*, **48**, 751 (1955)

86. Heinze, K. *Phytopathogene Viren und ihre Überträger* (Duncker & Humblot, Berlin, 290 pp., 1959)

87. Heinze, K. Versuche zur Ermittlung der Haltbarkeit des Blattroll-Virus der Kartoffel und des Virus der Vergilbungskrankheit der Rübe im Überträger. *Arch. ges. Virusforsch.*, **9**, 396–410 (1959)

88. Heinze, K., and Kunze, L. Die europäische Asterngelbsucht und ihre Übertragung durch Zwergzikaden. *Nachr. deut. Pflanzenschutzdienstes, (Stuttgart)*, **7**, 161–64 (1955)

89. Herold, F., Bergold, G. H., and Weibel, J. Isolation and electron microscopic demonstration of a virus infecting corn (*Zea mays* L.). *Virology*, **12**, 335–47 (1960)

90. Hewitt, W. B., and Raski, D. J. Nematode vectors of plant viruses. *Biological Transmission of Disease Agents*, 63–72 (Maramorosch, K., Ed., Academic Press, Inc., New York, 192 pp., 1962)

91. Hoggan, I. A. Transmissibility by aphids of the tobacco mosaic virus from different hosts. *J. Agr. Research*, **49**, 1135–42 (1934)

91a. Hoof, H. A. van. Verschillen in de overdracht van het bloemkoolmozaiekvirus bij *Myzus persicae* Sulzer en *Brevicoryne brassicae* L. *Tijdschr. Plantenziekten*, **60**, 267–72 (1960)

92. Hoof, H. A. van. *Onderzoekingen over de biologische overdracht van een nonpersistent virus.* (Doctoral thesis, Wageningen Agr. Univ., Van Putten & Oortmeijer, Alkmaar, The Netherlands, 96 pp., 1958)

93. Jensen, D. D. Insect transmission of virus between tree and herbaceous plants. *Virology*, **2**, 249–60 (1956)

94. Jensen, D. D. Reduction in longevity of leafhoppers carrying peach yellow leaf roll virus. *Phytopathology*, **48**, 394 (1958) (Abstr.)

95. Jensen, D. D. A plant virus lethal to its insect vector. *Virology*, **8**, 164–75 (1959)

96. Jensen, D. D. Effects of plant viruses on insects. *Ann. N. Y. Acad. Sci.* (In press)

97. Kelly, S. M., and Black, L. M. The origin, development and cell structure of a virus tumor in plants. *Am. J. Botany*, **36**, 65–73 (1949)

98. Kennedy, J. S. The behavioural fitness of aphids as field vectors of viruses. *Rept. Commonwealth Entomol. Conf., 1960, London, 7th Conf.*, 165–68 (1960)

99. Kennedy, J. S., Booth, C. O., and Kershaw, W. J. S. Host finding by aphids in the field. II. *Aphis fabae* Scop. (Gynoparae) and *Brevicoryne brassicae* L.; with a reappraisal of the role of host-finding behaviour in virus spread. *Ann. Appl. Biol.*, **47**, 424–44 (1959)

100. Kennedy, J. S., Day, M. F., and Eastop, V. F. *A Conspectus of Aphids as Vectors of Plant Viruses.* (Commonwealth Inst. Entomol., London, 114 pp., 1962)

101. Kimura, I., and Fukushi, T. Studies on the rice-dwarf virus (In Japanese). *Nippon Shokubutsu Byori Gakkaiho*, **25**, 131–35 (1960)

102. Kirkpatrick, H. C., and Ross, A. F. Aphid-transmission of potato leafroll virus to solanaceous species. *Phytopathology*, **42**, 540–46 (1952)

103. Klostermeyer, E. C. Entomological aspects of the potato leaf roll problem in central Washington. *Washington State Coll. Agr. Expt. Sta., Tech. Bull.*, **9**, 1–42 (1953)

104. Köhler, E., and Klinkowski, M.

Viruskrankheiten. (Sorauer's *Handbuch der Pflanzenkrankheiten.* 6th ed., **2** (Pt. I), 1–770, (Paul Parey, Berlin, Germany, 1954)

105. Kovachevski, I., and Markov, M. Bronzing of tomatoes (In Bulgarian). *Gradinarstvo,* **1,** 26–29 (1959)

106. Kunkel, L. O. Effect of heat on ability of *Cicadula sexnotata* (Fall.) to transmit aster yellows. *Am. J. Botany,* **24,** 316–27 (1937)

107. Kunkel, L. O. Maintenance of yellows-type viruses in plant and insect reservoirs. *The Dynamics of Virus and Rickettsial Infections,* 150–63 (Hartman, F. W., Horsfall, F. L., Jr., and Kidd, J. G., Eds., The Blakiston Co., New York, 461 pp., 1954)

108. Kunkel, L. O. Cross protection between strains of yellows-type viruses. *Advances in Virus Research,* **3,** 251–73 (1955)

109. Kunkel, L. O. Acquired immunity from infection by strains of aster-yellows virus in aster leafhopper. *Science,* **126,** 1233 (1957) (Abstr.)

110. Lindsten, K. Studies on virus diseases of cereals in Sweden. II. On virus diseases transmitted by the leafhopper, *Calligypona pellucida* (F.). *Kgl. Lantbruks-Högskol. Ann.,* **27,** 199–271 (1961)

111. Littau, V. C., and Maramorosch, K. Cytological effects of aster-yellows virus on its insect vector. *Virology,* **2,** 128–30 (1956)

112. Littau, V. C., and Maramorosch, K. A study of the cytological effects of aster yellows virus on its insect vector. *Virology,* **10,** 483–500 (1960)

113. Luria, S. E. The multiplication of viruses. *Protoplasmatologia,* **4,** 1–63 (1958)

114. MacCarthy, H. R. Aphid transmission of potato leafroll virus. *Phytopathology,* **44,** 167–74 (1954)

115. McClean, A. P. D. Citrus vein-enation virus. *S. African J. Sci.,* **50,** 147–51 (1954)

116. Magie, R. O., Smith, F. F., and Brierley, P. Occurrence of western aster yellows virus infection in gladiolus in eastern United States. *Gladiolus,* **28,** 93–99 (1953)

117. Maramorosch, K. Direct evidence for the multiplication of aster-yellows virus in its insect vector. *Phytopathology,* **42,** 59–64 (1952)

118. Maramorosch, K. Incubation period of aster-yellows virus. *Am. J. Botany,* **40,** 797–809 (1953)

119. Maramorosch, K. A new leafhopper-borne plant disease from western Europe. *Plant Disease Reptr.,* **37,** 612–13 (1953)

120. Maramorosch, K. Do developmental stages occur in the reproductive cycle of aster-yellows virus? *Cold Spring Harbor Symposia Quant. Biol.,* **18,** 51–54 (1953)

121. Maramorosch, K. Biological transmission of plant viruses by animal vectors. *Trans. N. Y. Acad. Sci., Ser. 2,* **16,** 189–95 (1954)

122. Maramorosch, K. Multiplication of plant viruses in insect vectors. *Advances in Virus Research,* **3,** 221–49 (1955)

123. Maramorosch, K. Mechanical transmission of clover club-leaf virus to its insect vector. *Bull. Torrey Botan. Club,* **82,** 339–42 (1955)

124. Maramorosch, K. Cross protection between two strains of corn stunt virus in an insect vector. *Virology,* **6,** 448–59 (1958)

125. Maramorosch, K. Studies of aster yellows virus transmission by the leafhopper species *Macrosteles fascifrons* Stål. and *M. laevis* Ribaut. *Proc. Intern. Congr. of Entomol., Montreal, 1956, 10th,* **3,** 221–27 (1958)

126. Maramorosch, K. Beneficial effect of virus-diseased plants on non-vector insects. *Tijdschr. Plantenziekten,* **64,** 383–91 (1958)

127. Maramorosch, K. An ephemeral disease of maize transmitted by *Dalbulus elimatus. Entomol. Exptl. et Appl.,* **2,** 169–70 (1959)

128. Maramorosch, K. Leafhoppers (Cicadellidae) as vectors and reservoirs of phytopathogenic viruses. *Homm. Vol. Savulescu Annivers.,* 421–42 (1959)

129. Maramorosch, K. Leafhopper-transmitted plant viruses. *Protoplasma,* **52,** 457–66 (1960)

130. Maramorosch, K. The occurrence on Long Island, N. Y. of *Micrutalis calva,* a close relative of the vector of pseudo-curly-top virus. *Phytopathology,* **50,** 241 (1960) (Abstr.)

131. Maramorosch, K. Acquisition and transmission of aster yellow virus. *Phytopathology,* **52** (In press) (Abstr.)

132. Maramorosch, K. Differences in incubation periods of aster yellows

virus strains. *Phytopathology,* **52,** 925 (1962) (Abstr.)

133. Maramorosch, K. Present status of insect tissue culture. *Proc. Intern. Congr. Entomol., Vienna, 1961, 11th,* **2,** 801–7 (1962)

134. Maramorosch, K. Relation of plant viruses to their insect vectors. *Ann. Rev. Microbiol.,* **17** (In press)

135. Maramorosch, K., Calica, C. A., Agati, J. A., and Pableo, G. Further studies on the maize and rice leaf galls induced by *Cicadulina bipunctella. Entomol. Exptl. et Appl.,* **4,** 86–89 (1961)

136. Massee, A. M. Transmission of reversion of black currants. *Adm. Rept. East Malling Research Sta., Kent, 1951,* 162–65 (1952)

137. Meester-Manger Cats, V. de. Korte over drachttijd van bladrolvirus. *Tijdschr. Plantkenziekten,* **62,** 174–76 (1956)

138. Mueller, W. C., and Rochow, W. F. An aphid-injection method for the transmission of barley yellow dwarf virus. *Virology,* **14,** 253–58 (1961)

139. Musil, M. Transmission of the clover phyllody virus by means of the leafhopper *Euscelis plebejus* (Fallen). *Biol. Plantarum,* **3,** 29–33 (1961)

140. Nagaraj, A. N., and Black, L. M. Hereditary variation in the ability of a leafhopper to transmit two unrelated plant viruses. *Virology,* **16,** 152–62 (1962)

141. Nagaraj, A. N., Sinha, R. C., and Black, L. M. A smear technique for detecting virus antigen in individual vectors by the use of fluorescent antibodies. *Virology,* **15,** 205–8 (1961)

142. Nasu, S. Studies on some leafhoppers and planthoppers which transmit virus diseases of rice plant in Japan (In Japanese). *Kyushu Agr. Exp. Sta. Bull.* (In press)

143. Newton, W. Transmission of tobacco mosaic by citurs mealybug. *Food and Agr. Organization, U.N., Plant Protection Bull.,* **2,** 40 (1953)

144. Nishi, Y. Inhibitory action of the sap from aphid-infested plants against the infectivity of tobacco mosaic virus. *Nippon Shokubutsu Byori Gakkaiho,* **23,** 185–88 (1958)

145. Nishizawa, T., Nishi, Y., and Kimura, T. Studies on the mechanism of aphid transmission of Japanese radish mosaic by means of P^{32} (In Japanese). *Virus,* **9,** 130–33 (1959)

146. Nishizawa, T., Nishi, Y., and Yoshii, H. Studies on the varietal resistance of garden crops to virus disease. V. On the process of aphid transmission of Japanese radish mosaic investigated by P^{32} or S^{35} (In Japanese). *Kyushu Agr. Expt. Sta. Bull.,* **5,** 35–40 (1958)

147. Olitsky, P. K. The transfer of tobacco and tomato mosaic disease by the *Pseudococcus citri. Science,* **62,** 442 (1925)

148. Orenski, S. W., and Maramorosch, K. The feeding of normal and aster yellows inoculated leafhoppers. *Phytopathology,* **52** (In press) (Abstr.)

149. Orenski, S. W., Staples, R. C., and Maramorosch, K. The uptake of C^{14} and P^{32} from labeled leaves by two species of leafhopper vectors. *Phytopathology,* **52** (In press) (Abstr.)

150. Orlando, A., and Silberschmidt, K. Estudes sôbre a disseminação natural do virus da "clorose infecciosa" das Malváceas (Abutilon virus) 1. Baur) e sua relação com o inset-vetor *"Bemisia tabaci* (Genn.)." *Arquiv, inst. biol. (São Paulo),* **17,** 1–36 (1946)

151. Orlob, G. B. Further studies on the transmission of plant viruses by different forms of aphids. *Virology,* **16,** 301–4 (1962)

152. Orlob, G. B., and Arny, D. C. Transmission of barley yellow dwarf virus by different forms of the apple grain aphid, *Rhopalosiphum fitchii* (Sand.). *Virology,* **10,** 273–74 (1960)

152a. Orlob, G. B., and Bradley, R. H. E. Where cabbage aphids carry transmissible virus B. *Phytopathology,* **51,** 397–99 (1961)

153. Oshima, N., and Goto, T. The two diseases of yellows-type naturally occurring in Hokkaido (In Japanese). *Research Bull. Hokkaido Natl. Agr. Expt. Sta.,* **71,** 56–66 (1956)

154. Ossiannilsson, F. Is tobacco mosaic not imbibed by aphids and leafhoppers? *Kgl. Lantbruks-Högskol. Ann.* **24,** 369–74 (1958)

155. Oswald, J. W., and Houston, B. R. The yellow-dwarf virus disease of

cereal crops. *Phytopathology, 43,* 128–36 (1953)

156. Paine, J., and Legg, J. T. Transmission of hop mosaic by *Phorodon humuli* (Schrank). *Nature, 171,* 263–64 (1953)

157. Pittman, H. A. Spotted wilt of tomatoes. Preliminary note concerning the transmission of the "spotted wilt" of tomatoes by an insect vector (*Thrips tabaci* Lind.). *J. Council Sci. Ind. Research, 1,* 74–77 (1927)

158. Posnette, A. F. Virus diseases of cacao in West Africa: The present position. *Rept. Intern. Horticult. Congr. 1952, 13th Congr.,* 2, 1224–30 (1953)

159. Posnette, A. F. Some aspects of virus spread among plants by vectors. *Rept. Commonwealth Entomol. Conf., 1960, London, 7th Conf.,* 162–65 (1960)

160. Posnette, A. F., and Robertson, N. F. Virus diseases of cacao in West Africa. VI. Vector investigations. *Ann. Appl. Biol.,* 37, 363–77 (1950)

161. Posnette, A. F., and Strickland, A. H. Virus diseases of cacao in West Africa. III. Technique of insect transmission. *Ann. Appl. Biol.,* 35, 53–63 (1948)

162. Prusa, V., Jermoljev, E., and Vacke, J. Oat sterile-dwarf virus disease. *Biol. Plantarum,* 1, 223–34 (1959)

163. Razvyazkina, G. M. The importance of the tobacco thrips in the development of outbreaks of tip chlorosis of Makhorka (In Russian). *Doklady Vsesoyuz. Akad. Sel' skokhoz. Nauk im. V. I. Lenina,* 18, 27–31 (1953)

164. Richter, H. Die Gelbsucht der Sommerastern. *Nachr. deut. Pflanzenschutzdienst (Berlin),* 16, 66–67 (1936)

165. Rochow, W. F. Barley yellow dwarf virus disease of oats in New York. *Plant Disease Reptr.,* 42, 36–41 (1958)

166. Rochow, W. F. Transmission of strains of barely yellow dwarf virus by two aphid species. *Phytopathology,* 49, 744-48 (1959)

167. Rochow, W. F. Specialization among greenbugs in the transmission of barley yellow dwarf virus. *Phytopathology,* 50, 881–84 (1960)

168. Rochow, W. F. Transmission of barley yellow dwarf virus acquired from liquid extracts by aphids feeding through membranes. *Virology,* 12, 223–32 (1960)

169. Rochow, W. F. A strain of barley yellow dwarf virus transmitted specifically by the corn leaf aphid. *Phytopathology,* 51, 809–10 (1961)

170. Rochow, W. F. Variation within and among aphid vectors of plant viruses. *Ann. N.Y. Acad. Sci.* (In press)

171. Rochow, W. F., and Pang, E-Wa. Aphids can acquire strains of barley yellow dwarf virus they do not transmit. *Virology,* 15, 382–84 (1961)

172. Ruppel, R. F. A review of the genus *Cicadulina* (Hemiptera, Cicadellidae). *Agr. J. Series Rockefeller Found.* (In press)

173. Rutschky, C. W., and Campbell, R. L. Fat body morphology of English grain aphids infected with barley yellow dwarf virus. *Ann. Entomol.* (In press)

174. Ryshkow, V. A mass-infection with a flower phyllody (In Russian). *Sbornik Akad. V. L. Kotarov,* 696-706 (1940)

175. Ryshkow, V. Kok-saghyz yellows. *Compt. rend acad. sci. U.R.S.S.,* 41, 90–92 (1943)

176. Ryshkow, V. Fortschritte in der Systematik der Viren. *Tagungsber. deut. Akad. Landwirsch. Berlin,* No. 33, 17–32 (1961)

177. Sakimura, K. Thrips in relation to gall-forming and plant disease transmission: a review. *Proc. Hawaiian Entomol. Soc.,* 13, 59–95 (1947)

178. Sakimura, K. The present status of thrips-borne viruses. *Biological Transmission of Disease Agents,* 33-40 (Maramorosch, K., Ed., Academic Press, Inc., New York, 192 pp., 1962)

179. Samuel, G., Bald, J. G., and Pittman, H. A. Investigations on "spotted wilt" of tomatoes. *Australia, Council Sci. Ind. Research, Bull. No. 44,* 1–64 (1930)

180. Schmidt, H. B. Die Übertragung Pflanzlicher Viren durch Insekten. *Monatsber. Dent. Akad. Wiss. Berlin,* 2, 214–23 (1960)

180a. Schmidt, H. B. Beiträge zur Kenntnis der Übertragung pflanzlicher Viren durch Aphiden. *Biol. Zentr.,* 78, 889–936 (1959)

181. Severin, H. H. P. Yellows disease of celery, lettuce, and other plants, transmitted by *Cicadula sexnotata*

(Fall.). *Hilgardia*, **3**, 543-71 (1929)

182. Shinkai, A. The relation between *Delphacodes striatella* and rice stripe disease (In Japanese). *Ann. Rept. Kanto and Tosan Phytopathol. Entomol. Soc. 1955, 5–6* (1955)

183. Shinkai, A. Epidemics of rice dwarf and yellows with special reference to the infectivity of *Nephotettix cincticeps* (In Japanese). *Plant Protection*, **14**, 146–50 (1960)

184. Shinkai, A. Studies on insect transmissions of rice virus diseases in Japan. *Nôgyô Gijutsu Kenkyûjo Hôkoku, C, No. 14*, 1–112 (1962) (In Japanese with English summary, 108–12)

185. Shirahama, K. Relation between the population of winged aphids infesting radish seedlings and infection by mosaic viruses. I (In Japanese). *Nippon Shokubutsu Byori Gakkaiho*, **14**, 79–80 (1950)

186. Silberschmidt, K., Flores, E., and Tommasi, L. R. Further studies on the experimental transmission of "infectious chlorosis" of *Malvaceae. Phytopathol. Z.*, **30**, 387–414 (1957)

186a. Simons, J. N. Vector-virus relationships of pea-enation mosaic and the pea aphid *Macrosiphum pisi* (Kalt.). *Phytopathology*, **44**, 283–89 (1954)

187. Simons, J. N. Variation in efficiency of aphid transmission of southern cucumber mosaic virus and potato virus Y in pepper. *Virology*, **9**, 612–23 (1959)

188. Simons, J. N. The pseudo-curly top disease in South Florida. *J. Econ. Entomol.*, **55**, 358–63 (1962)

189. Simons, J. N., and Coe, D. M. Transmission of pseudo-curly top virus in Florida by a treehopper. *Virology*, **6**, 43–48 (1958)

190. Sinha, R. C. Comparison of the ability of nymph and adult *Delphacodes pellucida* Fabricius, to transmit European wheat striate mosaic virus. *Virology*, **10**, 344–52 (1960)

191. Slykhuis, J. T. *Aceria tulipae* Keifer in relation to the spread of wheat streak mosaic. *Phytopathology*, **45**, 116–28 (1955)

192. Slykhuis, J. T. Current status of mite-transmitted plant viruses. *Proc. Entomol. Soc. Ontario*, **90**, 22–30 (1960)

193. Slykhuis, J. T. Mite transmission of plant viruses. *Biological Transmission of Disease Agents*, 41–61 (Maramorosch, K., Ed., Academic Press, Inc., New York, 192 pp., 1962)

194. Slykhuis, J. T., Zillinsky, F. J., Hannah, A. E., and Richards, W. R. Barley yellow dwarf virus on cereals in Ontario. *Plant Disease Reptr.*, **43**, 849–5 (1959)

195. Smith, F. F. The need of permanent reference collections of insect vectors of plant diseases. *Phytopathology*, **27**, 198–202 (1937)

196. Smith, F. F., and Brierley, P. Insect transmission of plant viruses. *Ann. Rev. Entomol.*, **1**, 299–322 (1956)

197. Smith, H. C. Barley yellow dwarf virus survey in Canada, 1961. *Can. Plant Disease Survey*, **41**, 344–52 (1961)

198. Smith, K. M. Arthropods as vectors and reservoirs of phytopathogenic viruses. *Handb. Virusforsch.*, **4**, 143–76 (1957)

199. Smith, K. M. Transmission of plant viruses by anthropods. *Ann. Rev. Entomol.*, **3**, 469–82 (1958)

200. Stegwee, D. Further investigations on the relation between *Myzus persicae* and the potato leaf-roll virus. *Proc. Conf. Potato Virus Diseases, 4th Conf., Braunschweig, 1960*, 106–10 (1960)

201. Stegwee, D. Multiplication of plant viruses in their aphid vectors. *Recent Advances in Botany*, 533-35 (Univ. of Toronto Press, Toronto, Canada, 1766 pp., 1961)

202. Stegwee, D., and Ponsen, M. B. Multiplication of potato leaf roll virus in the aphid *Myzus persicae* (Sulz.). *Entomol. Expt. et Appl.*, **1**, 291–300 (1958)

203. Storey, H. H. The inheritance by an insect vector of the ability to transmit a plant virus. *Proc. Roy. Soc. (London)*, **112 [B]**, 46–60 (1932)

204. Storey, H. H. Investigations of the mechanism of the transmission of plant viruses by insect vectors. -I. *Proc. Roy. Soc. (London)*, **113[B]**, 463–85 (1933)

205. Stubbs, L. L. Strains of *Myzus persicae* (Sulz.) active and inactive with respect to virus transmission. *Australian J. Biol. Sci.*, **8**, 68–74 (1955)

206. Sugiura, M., and Hirayama, S. Transmission of tobacco mosaic virus

by the larvae of *Barathra (Mamestra) brassicae* L. (In Japanese). *Mie Daigaku Nôgakubu Gakujutsu Hôkoku,* **16,** 47–63 (1958)

207. Sukhov, K. S. X-bodies in salivary glands of *Delphax striatella* Fallen, the carrier of zakuklivanie. *Compt. rend. acad. sci. U.R.S.S.,* **27,** 377–79 (1940)

208. Sukhov, K. S. Intracellular protein inclusions in cereals affected with the mosaic disease "zakuklivanie" (In Russian). *Mikrobiologia,* **9,** 188–95 (1940)

209. Sukhov, K. S. *Viruses* (In Russian). (Acad. Sci. USSR, Moscow, U.S.S.R., 370 pp., 1956)

210. Sukhov, K. S., and Vovk, A. M. Transmission of the mosaic virus of tobacco through larvae of *Plusia gamma* L. *Compt. rend. acad. sci. U.S.S.R.,* **49,** 146–47 (1945)

211. Sukhov, K. S., and Vovk, A. M. On the identity between yellow of koksaghyz and yellow of aster and its possible relation to big bud in tomato. *Compt. rend. acad. sci. U.S.S.R.,* **48,** 365–68 (1945)

212. Swenson, K. G. Effects of insect and virus host plants on transmission of viruses by insects. *Ann. N.Y. Acad. Sci.* (In press)

213. Sylvester, E. S. Beet-mosaic virus-green peach aphid relationships. *Phytopathology,* **39,** 417–24 (1949)

213a. Sylvester, E. S. Aphid transmission of nonpersistent plant viruses with special reference to the *Brassica nigra* virus. *Hilgardia,* **23,** 53–98 (1954)

214. Sylvester, E. S. Aphid transmission of plant viruses. *Proc. Intern. Congr. Entomol., Montreal, 1956, 10th,* **3,** 195-200 (1958)

215. Sylvester, E. S. Problems in the classification of plant virus transmission by aphids. *Recent Advances in Botany,* 517–22 (Univ. of Toronto Press, Toronto, Canada, 1766 pp., 1961)

216. Sylvester, E. S. Mechanisms of plant virus transmission by aphids. *Biological Transmission of Disease Agents,* 11–31 (Maramorosch, K., Ed., Academic Press, Inc., New York, 192 pp., 1962)

216a. Sylvester, E. S., and Bradley, R. H. E. Effect of treating stylets of aphids with formalin on the transmission of sugar beet yellow virus. *Virology,* **17,** 381–86 (1962)

217. Takahashi, Y., and Sekiya, I. Adipose tissue of the green rice leafhopper, *Nephotettix cincticeps* Uhler, infected with the virus of the yellow dwarf disease of the rice plant. *Japan. J. Appl. Entomol. Zool.,* **7** (In press)

217a. Teakle, D. S., and Sylvester, E. S. Infection of plants by the feeding of aphids on leaves sprayed with tobacco mosaic virus. *Virology,* **16,** 363–65 (1962)

218. Toko, H. V., and Bruehl, G. W. Strains of the cereal yellow-dwarf virus differentiated by means of the apple-grain and the English grain aphids. *Phytopathology,* **47,** 536 (1957) (Abstr.)

219. Toko, H. V., and Bruehl, G. W. Some host and vector relationships of strains of the barley yellow-dwarf virus. *Phytopathology.* **49,** 343-47 (1959)

220. Valenta, V. Potato witches' broom virus in Czechoslovakia. *Proc. Conf. Potato Virus Diseases, Lisse, Wageningen, 1957, 3rd Conf.,* 246–50 (1958)

221. Valenta, V. Interference studies with yellows-type plant viruses. I. Cross protection tests with European viruses. II. Cross protection tests with European and American Viruses. *Acta Virol.,* **3,** 65–72, 145-52 (1959)

222. Valenta, V. Untersuchungen über Stolbur und verwandte Viren. *Proc. Conf. Potato Virus Dis., Braunschweig, 1960, 4th Conf.,* 141–45 (1960)

223. Valenta, V. Rozšírenie a hospodársky význam metlovitosti zemiakov na Slovensku. *Sborník Ceskoslov. akad. zemědělských věd,* **7,** 967–78 (1961)

224. Valenta, V., Musil, M., and Mišiga, S. Investigations on European yellows-type viruses. *Phytopathol. Z.,* **42,** 1–38 (1962)

225. van Soest, W., and Meester-Manger Cats, V. de. Does the aphid *Myzus persicae* (Sulz.) imbibe tobacco mosaic virus? *Virology,* **2,** 411–14 (1956)

226. Varma, P. M. Ability of the whitefly to carry more than one virus simultaneously. *Current Sci.,* **24,** 317–18 (1955)

227. Völk, J. Übertragung durch Insekten und das Virus-Insekt Verhältnis. *Pflanzliche Virologie,* **1,** 63–102 (Klinkowski, M., Ed., Akademie Verlag, Berlin, 279 pp., 1958)

325

228. Wallace, J. M., and Drake, R. J. A virus-induced vein enation in citrus. *Citrus Leaves,* **33,** 22–24 (1953)

229. Wallace, J. M., and Drake, R. J. Induction of woody galls by wounding of citrus infected with vein-enation virus. *Plant Disease Reptr.,* **45,** 682–86 (1961)

230. Walters, H. J. Some relationships of three plant viruses to the differential grasshopper, *Melanoplus differentialis* (Thos.). *Phytopathology,* **42,** 355–62 (1952)

231. Want, J. P. H. van der. Onderzoekingen over Virusziekten van de Boon (*Phaseolus vulgaris* L.). (H. Veenman & Zonen, Wageningen, Netherlands, 84 pp., 1954)

232. Watson, M. A. Further studies on the relationships between Hyoscyamus virus 3 and the aphis *Myzus persicae* (Sulz.) with special reference to the effects of fasting. *Proc. Roy. Soc. (London),* **125 B,** 144–70 (1938)

233. Watson, M. A. The ways in which plant viruses are transmitted by vectors. *Rept. Commonwealth Entomol. Conf., 1960, London, 7th Conf.,* 157–61 (1960)

234. Watson, M. A., and Mulligan, T. The manner of transmission of some barley yellow-dwarf viruses by different aphid species. *Ann. Appl. Biol.,* **48,** 711–20 (1960)

235. Watson, M. A., and Sinha, R. C. Studies on the transmission of European wheat striate mosaic virus by *Delphacodes pellucida* Fabricius. *Virology,* **8,** 139–63 (1959)

236. Weathers, L. G., and Laird, E. F.

Aphis gossypii Glover found as a vector of vein-enation virus. (In press)

237. Whitcomb, R. F., and Black, L. M. Synthesis and assay of wound-tumor soluble antigen in an insect vector. *Virology,* **15,** 136–45 (1961)

238. Williams, W. L., and Ross, A. F. Aphid transmission of potato leafroll virus as affected by the feeding of nonviruliferous aphids on the test plants and by vector variability. *Phytopathology,* **47,** 538 (1957) (Abstr.)

239. Wilson, N. S., Jones, L. S., and Cochran, L. C. An eriophyid mite vector of the peach-mosaic virus. *Plant Disease Reptr.,* **39,** 889–92 (1955)

240. Yamada, W., and Yamamoto, Y. Studies on the stripe disease of rice plant. I. (In Japanese). *Okayama Pref. Agr. Expt. Sta. Special Bull.,* **52,** 93–112 (1955)

241. Yamada, W., and Yamamoto, Y. Studies on the stripe disease of rice plant. III. (In Japanese). *Okayama Pref. Agr. Expt. Sta. Special Bull.,* **55,** 35–56 (1956)

242. Yoshii, H. Studies on the nature of insect-transmission in plant viruses (V). On the abnormal metabolism of the virus-transmitting green rice leafhopper, *Nephotettix bipunctatus cincticeps* Uhler, as affected with the rice stunt virus (In Japanese). *Virus,* **9,** 415-22 (1959)

243. Yoshii, H., and Kiso, A. IX. On the biological activity of ribonucleic acid from stunt virus infected rice plant. *Virus,* **9,** 582-89 (1959)

SOME RELATIONSHIPS OF THREE PLANT VIRUSES TO THE DIFFERENTIAL GRASSHOPPER, *MELANOPLUS DIFFERENTIALIS* (THOS.)

H. J. Walters

It is generally believed that most of the known insect-transmitted viruses are carried by sucking insects and that chewing insects play a relatively small part in virus transmission. The fact that certain sap-transmissible viruses are spread so rapidly without the aid of a known vector indicates that something more than purely mechanical transmission might occur. The possible relations of these viruses to insect vectors have been comparatively neglected, since they can be easily propagated and their properties determined without use of vectors.

There are only a few authentic records of insects with chewing mouth parts acting as vectors. The viruses of cucumber mosaic, spindle tuber and unmottled curly dwarf of potato, turnip yellow mosaic, and cowpea mosaic have been transmitted by chewing insects (9, 13, 25, 30).

Insect transmission of tobacco mosaic virus has been investigated by several workers whose studies have shown conflicting results. Allard (1, 2) was the first to report transmission of a virus, thought to be tobacco mosaic, from tobacco to tobacco with aphids. Later Hoggan (16) suggested that Allard was working with cucumber mosaic virus. Hoggan (17, 18, 20) failed to transmit tobacco mosaic virus from tobacco to tobacco with aphids, but did transmit it from tomato to tobacco and other solanaceous hosts. Gigante (12) also reported aphid transmission of the virus. Elmer (10), Olitsky (27) and Sulkov and Vovk (36) reported transmission of tobacco mosaic virus with other insects. Attempts to transmit the virus with *Angytatus volucer* Kirk and *Thrips tobaci* Lindeman were unsuccessful (21, 29).

Smith (32) and Koch (23) were unable to transmit potato virus X with *Myzus persicae* (Sulz.). Smith (32) states that none of the common sap-sucking insect fauna of the potato plant is able to act as a vector, but suggests that the virus may be transmitted by

PHYTOPATHOLOGY, 1952, Vol. 42, pp. 355-362.

a flower-feeding species of thrips. Cockerham (8) found no correlation between the flowering habit of potatoes and the presence of X virus.

Fenne (11) was unable to transmit tobacco ringspot virus with several insects frequenting tobacco. Hoggan (19) failed to transmit the virus to spinach with aphids. Pound (28) was unable to transmit a yellow strain of tobacco ringspot virus responsible for a mosaic disease of watermelons from tobacco to other hosts with *Myzus persicae*.

Earlier studies on the relationships of viruses to insect vectors showed that juices of macerated insects usually inhibit the infectivity of viruses (5, 14, 31). McClintock and Smith (26) reported that inoculations with juice of virus-bearing aphids produced infection with the virus causing spinach blight. Smith (34) reported that blood of *Protoparce sexta* (Johan.) inhibited the infective power of tobacco mosaic and tobacco necrosis viruses, and that certain viruses were destroyed within the digestive tract of the caterpillar.

Grasshopper transmission of plant viruses has been reported only twice previously (13, 25). Transmission of the viruses of tobacco mosaic, potato X and tobacco ringspot by grasshoppers discussed in this paper was published earlier in a preliminary report by the author (37). It was hoped that the present investigation might yield additional information concerning certain relations of insects with chewing mouth parts to the viruses they transmit.

MATERIALS AND METHODS.—The original stock of the differential grasshopper, *Melanoplus differentialis* (Thos.), was obtained from eggs taken from fields, and incubated until hatched at 80° F. in small containers partly filled with moist soil. To maintain the supply eggs were taken from soil, incubated approximately 7 wk. at 70° to 80° F. for embryo development, and stored at 40° F. The insects, kept in plastic screened cages at 90° F., were fed alfalfa and young corn while immature. As adults, the stage used for all tests, they were fed only corn.

For transmission experiments grasshoppers were starved from 4 to 6 hr. before an infection feeding, transferred by hand, 1 to each test plant, and released. Precautions were taken to prevent contamination in transferring insects and to avoid infection from other sources. For tobacco mosaic virus, the hybrid plant, *Nicotiana tabacum* L. x *N. glutinosa* L., was usually used (22), but a few tests were made with tobacco, *N. tabacum*. Tobacco was also used as test plant for potato virus X and tobacco ringspot virus. Unless otherwise stated, each grasshopper was moved to a new location on the test plant after taking a few bites

328

or making a hole in the leaf about 1 to 6 mm. in diameter.

The dark brown fluid emitted from grasshopper mouths, referred to in this report as buccal fluid, is undoubtedly made up of regurgitated substances from the insect's crop as well as salivary secretions (6). The fluid was collected with a tapered blood pipette, inserted between the insect's mandibles, and sucked into the pipette through a piece of small rubber tubing attached to its basal end. A composite sample of fluid from several insects was used for each experiment. Grasshoppers were starved 3 to 4 hr. prior to collecting the fluid to avoid an admixture of plant extracts. The pH of buccal fluid was found to be about 5.6.

Blood was extracted in a similar manner by inserting a fine glass capillary between the hind leg and the abdomen of a grasshopper. A composite sample of blood from several insects was used in most tests, but blood of several individual grasshoppers was tested separately. The pH of blood was near 6.8. Where virus was injected into the bloodstream of insects, the method described by Heal and Menusan (15) was employed.

Inoculum was prepared from leaf tissue of tobacco infected with the virus of tobacco mosaic, potato X (ringspot strain), or tobacco ringspot. The leaves were ground up and the juice expressed through cheese cloth. Dilutions were made with distilled water.

Experimental plants were grown in composted soil at greenhouse temperatures of 75° to 80° F. Quantitative tests with tobacco mosaic virus were made using the local lesion reaction on *N. glutinosa*. Tobacco was used for potato ringspot virus, and the primary leaves of cowpea (*Vigna sinensis* Endl. var. Blackeye) usually were used with tobacco ringspot virus.

A Latin square design of half-leaf units was used in most infectivity comparisons of tobacco mosaic virus; in most tests with the other 2 viruses half-leaf comparisons were made on 1 or 2 leaves on 4 suitable plants. Inoculations were made by dipping the forefinger in the inoculum, rubbing the leaves dusted with 600 mesh carborundum, and then rinsing with tapwater. Except as noted, inoculations were completed within 2 or 3 min. after mixing virus and buccal fluid or blood of grasshoppers; each experiment was completed in 20-30 min.

EXPERIMENTAL WORK.—*Transmission Experiments.* —a) *Tobacco mosaic virus.*—Preliminary tests showed that 29 per cent of grasshoppers tested immediately after an infection feeding transmitted tobacco mosaic virus and that successful transmission occurred after 12 hr. of starvation following an infection feeding.

To ascertain how long grasshoppers remain infective, they were tested immediately, and after starvation periods of 2, 4, 8, 12, 16, 20 and 24 hr. following an infection feeding of 20 to 30 min. Twelve insects were used for each test and each insect was allowed to feed at approximately 10 different locations on individual test plants. Transmission of virus occurred in all tests (Table 1). The percentage of transmission did not vary to a great extent in tests made immediately after an infection feeding through the 12-hr. tests. Only 1 plant became infected in the 24-hr. test.

To determine if grasshoppers could transmit virus over a series of feedings on healthy plants, they were transferred to hybrid plants immediately after an infection feeding of approximately 2 min. Each insect was allowed to feed in 1 location on each half of 3 leaves on 3 plants, a total of 18 feeding areas on 9 leaves. Forty of the 48 grasshoppers tested transmitted the virus. The greatest number of lesions occurred adjacent to the first 6 feeding areas. In some cases lesions were consecutive, and in others there was lack of infection in as many as 16 feeding areas with infection occurring with subsequent feedings (Table 2).

When undisturbed, grasshoppers may feed for a short time in a location or may completely consume an entire leaf or plant. To make sure that under natural conditions these insects did not always consume tissue already inoculated, they were transferred to hybrid plants immediately after a 5-min. infection feeding and each insect was allowed to feed at will on individual plants from 4:00 P. M. to 9:00 A. M. the following day, a period of 17 hr. Feeding ranged from single penetrations of the leaf tissue with the mandibles to almost complete consumption of nearly all leaves on a plant (Fig. 1). Ten of 20 grasshoppers tested transmitted the virus. In a similar test with tobacco as the test plant, 9 of 20 insects transmitted tobacco mosaic virus. These results demonstrate transmission of tobacco mosaic virus by *Melanoplus differentialis* under conditions such as might occur in the field.

Local infection caused by tobacco mosaic virus on hybrid plants was not always adjacent to apparent feeding areas. Approximately 3 per cent of the total lesions occurred elsewhere. In most cases, a single lesion occurred adjacent to a feeding area, but in others as many as 3 lesions were evident. Feeding on a vein, or development of a lesion adjacent to a vein,

330

TABLE 1.—*Transmission obtained with 12 grasshoppers tested at various intervals after an infection feeding on tobacco plants infected with tobacco mosaic virus*[a]

| | Hours after feeding on the virus source | | | | | | | |
	0	2	4	8	12	16	20	24
No. insects transmitting	10	8	9	8	7	6	2	1
Percentage of insects transmitting	83.3	66.6	75.0	66.6	58.3	50.0	16.6	8.3
No. lesions produced from 120 feeding areas[b]	5/17	5/16	6/19	4/13	5/9	4/7	1/2	0/1

[a] Grasshoppers were allowed an infection feeding time of 20 to 30 min. and 10 feeding areas on hybrid test plants.
[b] The numerator indicates the number of lesions that were not adjacent to known feeding areas, while the denominator shows the total number of lesions produced.

TABLE 2.—*Number of local lesions of tobacco mosaic virus produced on hybrid plants as a result of the feeding of 40 individual grasshoppers in a series of 18 feedings*[a]

| Location of lesions | Feeding Number | | | | | | | | | | | | | | | | | |
	1	2	3	4	5	6	7	8	9	10	11	12	13	14	15	16	17	18
Adjacent to feeding areas	11	9	7	11	10	9	4	0	5	0	3	0	5	1	1	1	5	2
Away from feeding areas	2	0	3	0	4	2	0	0	0	0	0	0	1	0	0	0	0	0
Total lesions	13	9	10	11	14	11	4	0	5	0	3	0	6	1	1	1	5	2

[a] 48 grasshoppers were tested of which 40 transmitted tobacco mosaic virus.

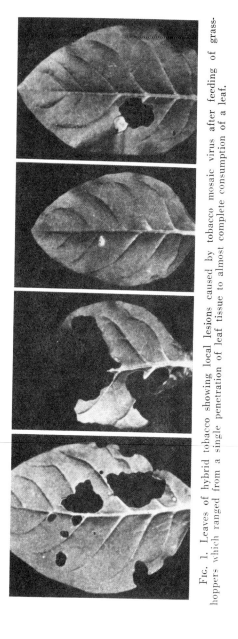

Fig. 1. Leaves of hybrid tobacco showing local lesions caused by tobacco mosaic virus after feeding of grasshoppers which ranged from a single penetration of leaf tissue to almost complete consumption of a leaf.

brought about systemic infection of hybrid plants in several instances.

b) *Potato X and tobacco ringspot viruses.*—Grasshoppers were transferred to healthy tobacco plants immediately after an infection feeding of approximately 2 min. on tobacco infected with either the virus of potato X (ringspot strain) or tobacco ringspot virus. The insects were allowed to feed at 6 to 8 different locations on the test plants. Primary symptoms were evident on the test plants within 5 to 7 days. Later the plants became systemically infected. Eighteen of 100 grasshoppers tested transmitted potato virus X and 6 of 100 insects transmitted tobacco ringspot virus. With potato virus X 4 of the initial infections occurred away from apparent feeding areas. while with tobacco ringspot virus only 1 initial infection occurred away from a known feeding area. In a majority of cases, with both viruses, initial infection developed adjacent to feeding areas near 1 of the larger veins.

Effect of Buccal Fluid on Viruses.—Smith (30) obtained some infection with cowpea mosaic virus by inoculations with regurgitated juice from *Cerotoma trifurcata* Forst. which had previously fed on diseased plants. Markham and Smith (25) stated that there appears to be a correlation between the ability of the larva of *Phaedon cochleariae* F. to transmit turnip yellow mosaic virus and its regurgitation of some of the contents of the foregut. Results of the present investigation demonstrated that regurgitated substances (buccal fluid) of grasshoppers do not completely inhibit infectivity of tobacco mosaic, potato ringspot, and tobacco ringspot viruses.

Preliminary tests using equal amounts of each of the 3 virus extracts and buccal fluid inoculated to leaves of suitable plants showed that none of the viruses were completely inhibited. Buccal fluid was most inhibitive for tobacco ringspot virus. least for tobacco mosaic virus, and intermediate for potato ringspot virus.

a) *Effect of concentration of buccal fluid on viruses.*—Extracts of tobacco mosaic virus were diluted 1:1, 1:10, 1:50, and 1:100 with buccal fluid and compared with similar virus-water dilutions. Inoculations were made on leaves of *Nicotiana glutinosa*. Results of 5 tests are in Table 3. Infectivity of virus was decreased with increased concentration of buccal fluid. Almost complete inhibition of virus occurred at the 1:100 dilution. Potato ringspot and tobacco ringspot viruses were completely inhibited at dilutions greater than 1:1 with buccal fluid.

b) *Effect of dilution of the inhibitor.*—To test the

TABLE 3.—*Effect of concentration of buccal fluid on infectivity of tobacco mosaic virus*

Tests	1 part buccal fluid		10 parts buccal fluid		50 parts buccal fluid		100 parts buccal fluid	
	Treated	Control[b]	Treated	Control[b]	Treated	Control[b]	Treated	Control[b]
1	36.0	248.3	10.0	171.0	1.8	130.3	0.8	89.8
2	34.0	269.3	4.5	160.8	1.8	95.8	0.3	67.0
3	20.8	179.8	3.0	106.8	0.0	70.3	0.0	47.3
4	31.0	218.0	4.3	149.5	0.8	123.5	0.0	60.0
5	17.0	181.8	2.0	84.5	0.3	61.0	0.3	34.5

Average[a] *number lesions per half-leaf on N. glutinosa produced by 1 part virus in*

[a] Average of 4 half-leaves for each test.
[b] Controls consisted of similar dilutions of virus and water.

effect of dilution of the inhibitor in buccal fluid a basic mixture of the fluid and extracts of each of the 3 viruses was prepared. For tobacco mosaic virus the basic mixture consisted of 1:10 virus extracts in buccal fluid, while for potato ringspot and tobacco ringspot viruses a mixture consisting of equal parts of the desired virus extract and fluid was used. These mixtures were diluted 1:10, 1:100, and 1:1000 with water and the 4 mixtures were compared with similar virus-water dilutions. The tobacco mosaic virus-buccal fluid mixtures were inoculated in a Latin square design to *N. glutinosa* and the mixtures of potato ringspot and tobacco ringspot viruses to 8 half-leaves of tobacco and cowpea respectively. Results of these tests are in Table 4. With tobacco mosaic virus and tobacco ringspot virus a definite increase over the infectivity of the original mixture in number of lesions occurred with dilution up to 1:100, but infectivity was greatest at dilution of 1:10. With potato ringspot virus, all dilutions increased infectivity but the greatest infectivity occurred at dilution of 1:100.

c) *Effect of heat on the inhibitor.*—Temperature treatments were carried out on mixtures of virus extracts and buccal fluid and compared with similar virus-water mixtures. For tobacco mosaic virus, a mixture of 1 part infectious plant extracts in 10 parts buccal fluid was diluted 1:10 with water. A mixture of equal amounts of buccal fluid and virus extracts was diluted 1:10 with water for potato ringspot virus, while the mixture for tobacco ringspot virus was 1 part buccal fluid in 100 parts virus extracts diluted 1:10 with water. Treatments were made by immersing 75 x 10 mm. test tubes, containing 1 cc. of mixture, in a water bath held within 0.1° C. of the desired temperature for 10 min. The preparations for tobacco mosaic virus were treated at 60°, 65°, 70°, 75°, and 80° C. and compared with a preparation kept at room temperature (23° C.), while those for both potato ringspot and tobacco ringspot viruses were treated at 55°, 60°, and 65° C. At the end of the 10-min. treatment, the tubes were immersed in cold water. Inoculations were made to suitable host plants after each series of temperature treatments was completed. Infectivity of the mixture of tobacco mosaic virus extracts and buccal fluid increased with rising temperature with highest infectivity at 70° C. A greater number of lesions occurred at 75° C. than with the preparation kept at room temperature, but infectivity of the suspension treated at 80° C. was markedly lower.

Infectivity of the 55° C. treatment of both the

TABLE 4.—*Effect of dilution on mixtures[a] of buccal fluid and each of 3 viruses.*

	Average[b] number of lesions per half-leaf produced on suitable hosts[c] by virus-buccal fluid mixtures at the following dilutions							
	No dilution		1:10		1:100		1:1000	
Virus	Treated[d]	Control[d]	Treated[d]	Control[d]	Treated[d]	Control[d]	Treated[d]	Control[d]
Tobacco mosaic	13.6	186.9	24.0	95.4	16.3	27.0	5.4	3.8
Potato ringspot	2.8	295.7	8.0	172.6	12.4	84.1	8.1	24.8
Tobacco ringspot	13.8	117.4	41.7	91.8	33.0	59.7	4.9	2.6

[a] Mixtures of buccal fluid and tobacco mosaic virus consisted of 1 part virus to 10 parts buccal fluid, while mixtures of potato ringspot virus and tobacco ringspot virus and buccal fluid consisted of equal amounts of virus extracts and buccal fluid.

[b] Average of 20 half-leaves for tobacco mosaic virus and 40 half-leaves for potato ringspot and tobacco ringspot viruses in 5 experiments.

[c] *Nicotiana glutinosa* was host for tobacco mosaic virus, tobacco for potato ringspot virus, and cowpea for tobacco ringspot virus.

[d] Control consisted of similar dilutions of virus and water.

buccal fluid-virus mixtures and control for potato ringspot and tobacco ringspot viruses was below that kept at room temperature with infectivity completely suppressed at 60° C. There was no indication of the effect of heat on the inhibitor in preparations of potato ringspot and tobacco ringspot viruses since infectivity of the 2 viruses was destroyed at 60° C.

d) *Effect of dialysis.*—Attempts were made to separate the buccal-fluid inhibitor from a mixture of tobacco mosaic virus extracts and buccal fluid by dialysis through a cellophane membrane. A mixture of 1 part virus extracts to 10 parts buccal fluid was diluted 1:50 with water and dialyzed against running tap water, along with a similar virus and water preparation, for 48 hours. A nondialyzed sample of both preparations was stored at 2° C. for the same period of time and the materials compared on half-leaves of *N. glutinosa.* Results of 3 trials showed no increase in number of lesions produced by the buccal fluid-virus mixture which was dialyzed over that not dialyzed. The inhibitor in buccal fluid is not readily dialyzable through a cellophane membrane. There was a slight increase in number of lesions produced with the dialyzed virus-water preparation over that not dialyzed. This was probably due to dialysis of some inhibitive agent present in plant extracts.

Recovery of Virus after Ingestion by Grasshoppers.—Markham and Smith (25) found that turnip yellow mosaic virus was retained in an infective condition for 4 days in larvae of *Phaedon cochleariae.* Viruses of tobacco mosaic, potato ringspot, and tobacco ringspot were found to remain infective in buccal fluid within grasshoppers for several hours. A sample of buccal fluid was extracted from each of 12 insects at different time intervals, following a 30-min. infection feeding on tobacco infected with the desired virus, and inoculated to suitable hosts for each virus. *Nicotiana glutinosa* was used for tobacco mosaic virus and tobacco for the other 2 viruses. All samples were infective immediately after the insects fed, but their infectivity decreased as the interval between feeding and extraction of buccal fluid increased. Tobacco mosaic virus remained infective in 3 insects for 12 hr., while potato ringspot virus remained infective in 5 insects for 6 hr. and tobacco ringspot virus in 3 insects for 4 hr.

Negative results were obtained in an effort to ascertain whether the virus of tobacco mosaic entered the blood of grasshoppers after they had fed on virus-infected plants. At 24-hr. intervals, up to 10 days, after feeding for an hour on infected tobacco, a

337

sample of blood was extracted from each of 20 grasshoppers and inoculated to 1 leaf of *N. glutinosa.* All attempts to demonstrate the presence of virus in the blood were unsuccessful.

Tobacco mosaic virus has been shown to pass through the digestive tract of *Protoparce sexta* unchanged though greatly reduced in concentration (34). To ascertain whether this virus is inactivated within the digestive tract of grasshoppers, 12 insects were starved for 24 hr. and then allowed to feed on mosaic-infected tobacco over a period of 3 days. Fresh feces were collected at different intervals of time during the feeding period, suspended in water, and inoculated to 8 *Nicotiana glutinosa* leaves. An average of 189, 275, 222, 292, and 202 local lesions per leaf was produced by collections made at 5, 20, 24, 48, and 72 hr. respectively. Similar tests were conducted with grasshoppers fed on plants infected with either potato ringspot virus or tobacco ringspot virus and the fecal suspension inoculated to 6 leaves of healthy tobacco. An average of 17, 24, and 19 lesions were produced by fecal suspensions of potato ringspot virus collected 24, 48, and 72 hr. respectively. Lesions did not occur on all leaves inoculated with fecal suspensions of tobacco ringspot virus. Only 2 lesions occurred on 1 of 6 leaves inoculated with the 24-hr. collection. Negative results were obtained with the 48-hr. collection and only 1 lesion was produced on 1 of 6 leaves inoculated with the 72-hr. collection.

To determine concentration of tobacco mosaic virus present in naturally voided feces a suspension consisting of equal amounts by weight of feces and water was inoculated to 5 half-leaves of *N. glutinosa* and compared with a 1:10 dilution of extracts from plants on which the grasshoppers had fed. Suspensions of fecal collections made at 24, 48, and 72 hr. produced an average of 221, 239, and 137 lesions per half-leaf respectively, as compared with 157, 243, and 143 lesions produced by diluted plant extracts. Tobacco mosaic virus passing through grasshoppers was not greatly reduced in concentration, but was comparable to that of a 1:5 dilution of infectious plant extracts.

Injection of Tobacco Mosaic Virus into Blood of Grasshoppers.—Injection of tobacco mosaic virus into the blood of living insects has been reported to inhibit the infectivity of the virus (34). To study the effect of blood on tobacco mosaic virus, 0.02 cc. of infective plant extracts were injected into the blood stream of each of 12 grasshoppers between the third and fourth abdominal segments, 0.01 cc. on each side. The hypodermic needle was inserted just beneath the integument

338

to prevent entry of virus into the alimentary tract. A blood sample was extracted from each insect at 24-hr. intervals for 7 days and on the tenth and fifteenth day after injection and inoculated to 1 *N. glutinosa* leaf. Results of these tests are in Table 5. At least 91 per cent of the blood samples taken up to 120 hr. after injection were infective and 50 per cent after 10 days, but after 15 days virus was detected in blood of only 1 sample.

To determine whether tobacco mosaic injected into the blood of living grasshoppers would enter the buccal cavity, a sample of buccal fluid collected from each of 12 insects was inoculated to 1 leaf of *N. glutinosa*. A total of 5 lesions was produced from 3 of 12 samples taken 4 hr. after injection and a total of 7 lesions from 3 samples was produced after 8 hr. Negative results were obtained with samples collected 12, 24, 48, 72, and 96 hr. after injection. Apparently

TABLE 5.—*Infectious nature of individual blood samples of 12 grasshoppers taken at different intervals after an injection of tobacco mosaic virus into the blood stream*[a]

Time blood sample was taken after injection (hours)	Number samples infective	Average [b] number lesions produced on 1 *N. glutinosa* leaf per infective sample
24	12	36.0
48	11	18.0
72	12	8.8
96	12	27.0
120	11	13.8
144	9	4.7
168	7	2.1
240	6	3.8
360	1	1.0

[a] 0.02 cc. of infectious plant extracts was injected into each of 12 insects, 0.01 cc. on either side.
[b] An average of 1 *N. glutinosa* leaf in 1 trial.

some virus passed from the blood into the buccal cavity up to 8 hr. after the virus injection.

Effect of Extracted Blood on Viruses.—Smith (34) found that blood from *Protoparce sexta* when mixed with "fairly concentrated samples" of tobacco necrosis virus completely inhibited infection on *Phaseolus vulgaris* L. Preliminary results with extracted grasshopper blood showed that mixtures consisting of equal amounts of blood and virus extracts of tobacco mosaic, potato ringspot, or tobacco ringspot were not completely inhibited when inoculated to suitable hosts. Blood had the greatest inhibitive effect on tobacco ringspot virus, and had the least effect on tobacco mosaic virus. Infectivity of tobacco ringspot virus was almost completely inhibited on cowpea.

To study the effect of dilution, a basic mixture consisting of equal amounts of blood and extracts of tobacco infected with tobacco mosaic, potato ringspot, or tobacco ringspot virus was prepared and diluted 1:10, 1:100, and 1:1000. The basic mixtures and dilutions were compared with similar virus-water preparations on half-leaves of test plants. Results of these tests are in Table 6. Infectivity of the virus-blood mixtures of tobacco mosaic and potato ringspot viruses were highest at the 1:10 dilution. Only a slight increase in infectivity occurred with dilution up to 1:100 with tobacco ringspot virus.

Discussion.—Results of this investigation showed that such highly infectious viruses as tobacco mosaic, potato ringspot, and tobacco ringspot may be transmitted by insects with chewing mouth parts. The general lack of information concerning the relationships of highly infectious sap-transmissible viruses to insects is understandable. Since such viruses are easy to transmit mechanically, less effort has been made to establish their insect vectors. A greater percentage of the sap-transmissible viruses having vectors are transmitted by insects which lose their infectivity in a relatively short period of time. In this group of vectors are found insects with sucking mouth parts as well as those with chewing mouth parts. Undoubtedly more of the sap-transmissible viruses will be found to be transmitted by chewing insects.

In considering the mode of transmission of the viruses of tobacco mosaic, potato ringspot, or tobacco ringspot by grasshoppers, the most likely assumption is that the viruses are carried mechanically on the insects' mandibles. Markham and Smith (25) have suggested a correlation between the ability of the larva of *Phaedon cochleariae*, vector of turnip yellow mosaic virus, to transmit the virus and the regurgitation of some of the contents of the foregut. A similar phenomenon may occur with grasshoppers and the viruses studied, for the viruses were detected in buccal fluid extracted from grasshoppers several hours after an infection feeding.

The occurrence of local infection away from apparent feeding areas could be assumed to be due to transfer of virus on the feet of grasshoppers. However, grasshoppers may scar or make depressions in leaf tissue with their mandibles while in search of a suitable feeding location; this seems to be the more plausible explanation.

Previous studies show that the juice of macerated insects usually inhibits infectivity of viruses (5, 14, 31). A satisfactory explanation has not appeared for

TABLE 6.—*Effect of dilution on mixtures each of which contained equal volumes of grasshopper blood and an extract from virus-injected plants*

Virus	Average[a] number of lesions per half-leaf produced with virus-blood mixtures at the following dilutions							
	No dilution		1:10		1:100		1:1000	
	Treated	Control[b]	Treated	Control[b]	Treated	Control[b]	Treated	Control[b]
Tobacco mosaic	99.5	218.0	144.4	181.4	79.0	74.6	11.3	21.4
Potato ringspot	94.5	315.0	213.5	215.9	129.2	137.1	31.7	36.3
Tobacco ringspot	0.3	66.6	3.2	80.1	3.4	0.6	0.0	0.0

[a] Average of 20 half-leaves of *N. glutinosa* for tobacco mosaic, 20 half-leaves of tobacco for potato ringspot virus, and 40 half-leaves of cowpea for tobacco ringspot virus in five tests.
[b] Controls consisted of similar dilutions of virus and water.

the loss in infectivity of viruses that are easily sap-transmissible when mixed with juices of certain insects. The majority of investigations of this nature have been conducted with juices of macerated insects with little attention directed to the importance of body contents from definite regions of the insect. The effect of buccal fluid and blood of grasshoppers on the infectivity of the viruses studied revealed an inhibitive action, although certain mixtures of virus extracts and buccal fluid or blood did not completely inhibit the infectivity of tobacco mosaic, potato ringspot, or tobacco ringspot viruses. Dilution studies with the 3 viruses and the heat treatments on tobacco mosaic virus indicated that the inhibitive action of buccal fluid was reversible. In dilution studies, extracted blood with virus reacted in a manner similar to buccal fluid with virus, indicating that the inhibitive action of blood was also reversible.

None of the viruses were completely inactivated within the digestive tract of the grasshopper; however, their infectivity was decreased, though only slightly in the case of tobacco mosaic virus. The regurgitated substances present in buccal fluid are composed of secretions passed forward from the mid-gut into the crop and carry with them enzymes present in the mid-gut. Wigglesworth (38) states that the proteinase present in the mid-gut of insects is always of tryptic type. Lojkin and Vinson (24), Caldwell (7), Stanley (35), and Bawden and Pirie (3) have shown that trypsin can inhibit the infectivity of certain plant viruses. Trypsin might aid in the reduction of infectivity of virus in the buccal fluid and naturally voided feces. Failure to obtain tobacco mosaic virus in blood of grasshoppers previously fed on virus-infected plants cannot be explained at this time, unless the intestinal wall acts as a mechanical barrier.

Although the concentration of tobacco mosaic virus was somewhat reduced after being injected into the blood of living grasshoppers, it appears that the blood was a more favorable medium for the virus than buccal fluid. Bennett and Wallace (4) suggested that blood of *Eutettix tenellus* Baker appears to be a favorable medium for preserving curly top virus, for the reaction of the leafhopper blood is slightly alkaline. Since grasshopper blood is only slightly acid, it should not cause any considerable loss of infectivity for tobacco mosaic.

The appearance of tobacco mosaic virus in the buccal fluid after it was injected into the blood of the insects indicates that some virus may pass through the salivary glands. The concentration of virus detected in the buccal fluid was considerably lower than that in blood extracted at the same time. It is possible that only a very small quantity of virus may enter the salivary glands or that conditions in the salivary glands may be somewhat unfavorable for the virus. It is possible that the infection obtained with buccal fluid of grasshoppers whose blood had been injected with tobacco mosaic virus was due to contamination. This appears unlikely since care was taken to prevent entry of the virus into the alimentary tract during injection and to avoid contamination during extraction of the buccal fluid and inoculation of plants.

SUMMARY

The relationships of the differential grasshopper, *Melanoplus differentialis*, to 3 plant viruses were studied. This grasshopper was found to transmit tobacco mosaic, potato ringspot, and tobacco ringspot viruses from tobacco to tobacco. Primary symptoms occurred, in the majority of cases, adjacent to a known feeding area although a very small percentage occurred elsewhere.

Transmission of tobacco mosaic virus by grasshoppers such as might occur in the field was demonstrated. Insects were transferred to healthy tobacco immediately after a 5-min. infection feeding and allowed to feed at will for 17 hr.

Buccal fluid of the grasshopper inhibited the infectivity of plant extracts containing the viruses of tobacco mosaic, potato ringspot, or tobacco ringspot when mixtures of the buccal fluid and virus extracts were inoculated to suitable host plants. Similar results were obtained with mixtures of blood and virus. The buccal fluid decreased the infectivity of the viruses in the following order: tobacco mosaic, potato ringspot, and tobacco ringspot. Blood affected the infectivity of the viruses in the same order.

The inhibitive action of both the buccal fluid and the blood was found to be reversible. The infectivity of certain mixtures of tobacco mosaic virus and buccal fluid was increased by dilution or by heat treatment. Dilution increased the infectivity of mixtures of potato ringspot or tobacco ringspot viruses and buccal fluid. The infectivity of mixtures of viruses of tobacco mosaic, potato ringspot, or tobacco ringspot and blood was increased by dilution.

The inhibitor in the buccal fluid was thermolabile and not readily dialyzable.

Infectivity of the 3 viruses was decreased within the

digestive tract of grasshoppers though only slightly in the case of tobacco mosaic virus. Virus was detected in the naturally voided feces of grasshoppers previously fed on plants infected with tobacco mosaic, potato ringspot, or tobacco ringspot viruses. The concentration of tobacco mosaic virus in the feces was comparable to that of a 1:5 dilution of extracts from the plants on which the insects had fed. The infectivity of the potato ringspot virus that passed through the grasshoppers was considerably reduced, and the infectivity of the tobacco ringspot virus was almost completely suppressed.

The viruses of tobacco mosaic, potato ringspot, and tobacco ringspot remained infective for several hours in buccal fluid within grasshoppers. Buccal fluid extracted from grasshoppers showed that tobacco mosaic virus remained infective within the insects for 12 hr., while potato ringspot virus remained infective for 6 hr. and tobacco ringspot virus for 4 hr.

Tobacco mosaic virus was inactivated when injected into the blood of living grasshoppers, however, inactivation was not completed immediately. The blood of 6 of the 12 injected insects remained infective for 10 days, but after 15 days virus was detected in the blood of only 1 insect. After injection of the virus into the blood, only a very small quantity of virus was detected in the buccal fluid.

LITERATURE CITED

1. ALLARD, H. A. The mosaic disease of tobacco. U. S. Dept. Agr. Bul. 40. 1914.
2. ———. Further studies on the mosaic disease of tobacco. Jour. Agr. Res. (U. S.) **10**: 615-632. 1917.
3. BAWDEN, F. C., AND N. W. PIRIE. Experiments on the chemical behaviour of potato virus 'X'. Brit. Jour. Exp. Path. **17**: 64-74. 1936.
4. BENNETT, C. W., AND H. E. WALLACE. Relation of the curly top virus to the vector *Eutettix tenellus.* Jour. Agr. Res. (U. S.) **56**: 31-51. 1938.
5. BLACK, L. M. Inhibition of virus activity by insect juices. Phytopath. **29**: 321-337. 1939.
6. BODINE, J. H. Physiology of the Orthoptera. Biol. Bul. **48**: 79-82. 1925.
7. CALDWELL, J. The physiology of virus diseases in plants. IV. The nature of the virus agent of aucuba or yellow mosaic of tomato. Ann. Appl. Biol. **20**: 100-116. 1933.
8. COCKERHAM, G. Potato flowers and dissemination of potato viruses. Nature (London) **140**: 1100-1101. 1937.
9. DOOLITTLE, S. P. The mosaic disease of cucurbits. U. S. Dept. Agr. Bul. 879. 1920.
10. ELMER, O. H. Transmissibility and pathological effects

of the mosaic disease. Iowa Agr. Exp. Sta. Bul. **82**: 39-91. 1925.

11. FENNE, S. B. Field studies on the ring-spot disease of burley tobacco in Washington County, Virginia. Phytopath. **21**: 891-899. 1931.

12. GIGANTE, R. Il mosaico del tabacco. Boll. Staz. Pat. Veg. Roma, N. S. **18**: 93-130. 1938.

13. GOSS, R. W. Infection experiments with spindle tuber and unmottled curly dwarf of the potato. Nebraska Agr. Exp. Sta. Res. Bul. **53**. 1931.

14. HAMILTON, M. A. Further experiments on the artificial feeding of *Myzus persicae* (Sulz.). Ann. Appl. Biol. **22**: 243-258. 1934.

15. HEAL, R. E. AND H. MENUSAN, JR. A technique for bloodstream injection of insects and its application in tests of certain insecticides. Jour. Econ. Entom. **41**: 535-543. 1948.

16. HOGGAN, ISME A. The peach aphid (Myzus persicae Sulz.) as an agent in virus transmission. Phytopath. **19**: 109-123. 1929.

17. ————. Studies on aphid transmission of plant viruses. Jour. Bact. **19**: 21-22. 1930.

18. ————. Further studies on aphid transmission of plant viruses. Phytopath. **21**: 199-212. 1931.

19. ————. Some viruses affecting spinach, and certain aspects of insect transmission. Phytopath. **23**: 446-474. 1933.

20. ————. Transmissibility by aphids of the tobacco mosaic virus from different hosts. Jour. Agr. Res. (U. S.) **49**: 1135-1142. 1934.

21. JARRETT, P. J. The role of Thrips tabaci Lindeman in the transmission of virus diseases of tomato. Ann. Appl. Biol. **17**: 444-451. 1930.

22. JOHNSON, J. A tobacco hybrid useful for virus studies. Amer. Jour. Bot. **23**: 40-46. 1936.

23. KOCH, K. L. The nature of potato rugose mosaic. Phytopath. **23**: 319-342. 1933.

24. LOJKIN, MARY, AND C. G. VINSON. Effect of enzymes upon the infectivity of the virus of tobacco mosaic. Contrib. Boyce Thompson Inst. **3**: 147-162. 1931.

25. MARKHAM, R., AND K. M. SMITH. Studies on the virus of turnip yellow mosaic. Parasitology **39**: 330-332. 1949.

26. McCLINTOCK, J. A., AND L. B. SMITH. True nature of spinach blight and relation of insects to its transmission. Jour. Agr. Res. (U. S.) **14**: 1-60. 1918.

27. OLITSKY, P. K. The transfer of tobacco and tomato mosaic diseases by the Pseudococcus citri. Science **62**: 442. 1925.

28. POUND, G. S. A virus disease of watermelon in Wisconsin incited by the tobacco ringspot virus. Jour. Agr. Res. (U. S.) **78**: 647-658. 1949.

29. ROBERTS, J. I. The tobacco caspid, Engytatus volucer Kirk., in Rhodesia. Bul. Entom. Res. **21**: 169-183. 1930.

30. SMITH, C. E. Transmission of cowpea mosaic by the bean leaf beetle. Science **60**: 268. 1924.

31. SMITH, K. M. Studies on potato virus diseases. IV. Further experiments with potato mosaic. Ann. Appl. Biol. **16**: 1-33. 1929.

32. ————. On the composite nature of certain potato virus diseases of the mosaic group as revealed by the use of plant indicators and selective methods of

transmission. Proc. Roy. Soc. (London), Ser. B. **109**: 251-266. 1931.

33. ————. A textbook of plant virus diseases. P. Blakiston's Son & Company, Philadelphia. 1937.

34. ————. Some notes on the relationship of plant viruses with vector and non-vector insects. Parasitology **33**: 110-116. 1941.

35. STANLEY, W. M. Chemical studies on the virus of tobacco mosaic. I. Some effects of trypsin. Phytopath. **24**: 1055-1085. 1934.

36. SULKHOV, K. S., AND A. M. VOVK. Transmission of the mosaic virus of tobacco through larvae of Plusia gamma L. Comptes Rendus (Doklay) de l 'Academie des Sciences de l 'USSR. **49**: 146-147. 1945.

37. WALTERS, H. J. Grasshopper transmission of three plant viruses. Science **113**: 36-37. 1951.

38. WIGGLESWORTH, V. B. The principles of insect physiology. 3 ed., Methuen & Company Ltd., London. 1947.

Evidence of Transovarial Passage of the Sowthistle Yellow Vein Virus in the Aphid *Hyperomyzus lactucae*[1]

EDWARD S. SYLVESTER

INTRODUCTION

Transovarial passage of plant viruses has been well documented in several cases of leafhopper or planthopper vectors (Fukushi, 1933; Black, 1950, 1953; Grylls, 1954; Yamada and Yamamoto, 1955; Watson and Sinha, 1959; Lindsten, 1961). Evidence of the phenomenon in aphid vectors has been meager. Recently Miyamoto and Miyamoto (1966) reported that the potato leafroll virus (PLRV) was occasionally transmitted from viruliferous apterae to their offspring in tests made with *Myzus persicae* (Sulz.) during the winter months.

It is usual practice, because of the rarity of transovarial passage of plant viruses among aphids, to establish virus-free clones of aphid vectors by letting viviparae deposit nymphs during a 24-hour period on a virus-free host plant, after which time the larvae produced are put on another virus-free host and allowed to mature. The assumptions underlying this method are two, *viz.* (1) that transovarial passage does not occur, and (2) a near-zero probability exists that the

larvae will acquire virus from that introduced by the viviparae into the host plants during the period of larviposition. This latter assumption exists whether or not the virus-free host is immune to the test virus.

The following report concerns observational and experimental results that indicate that the first of these assumptions is not true in the case of sowthistle yellow vein virus (SYVV).

MATERIALS AND METHODS

The SYVV used was derived from the isolate previously reported (Richardson and Sylvester, 1968). The vector, in the main, was a clonal line of *Hyperomyzus lactucae* (L.) originally isolated by the author in 1967. The virus was maintained in sowthistle, *Sonchus oleraceus* (L.) by aphid transmission. The test plants were seedlings of sowthistle that had been reared in the greenhouse. The acquisition and test access periods were done in plant growth chambers. The aphids were transferred with micropipettes and confined to test plants by caging with cellulose nitrate cages capped with nylon mesh. After the test access periods, pertinent vector data were taken and the plants were

[1] Supported in part by a grant from the U. S. Public Health Service, AI-07255.

347

fumigated with nicotine before being incubated in the greenhouse. Plants were observed for at least 30 days; after this time those without symptoms were discarded. Some plants, suspected of being infected, were kept for an additional period until definitive symptoms did or did not develop.

In one experiment, on transovarial passage in the absence of maternal feeding, an attempt was made to stimulate larviposition by amputation of the stylets (Bradley, 1960). Test aphids were anesthetized with CO_2, mounted on a moistened brush; while viewed under a stereomicroscope, the tip of the labium was cut off with microdissecting scissors. After the operation the aphids were individually put in small plastic boxes. A set of 9–12 boxes was wrapped with Parafilm® to lessen desiccation and put into a growth chamber at 25° and constant light for a period of 24 hours. The temperature of the 25° growth chamber averaged 24.5 ± 1.1°.

RESULTS

When the work with SYVV was being developed in 1967, a clonal line of noninoculative aphids was established by the following procedure. Ten apterae from an infected sowthistle plant collected in the field were put on 10 virus-free sowthistle seedlings, 1 aphid per plant. The apterae were allowed to larviposit for 2 days and then were transferred to a second virus-free plant, and 2 days later to a third plant. One aptera died during the first larviposition period. When the apterae were transferred, the larvae that had been born on the first 2 sets of plants were also transferred to a virus-free sowthistle seedling, 1 plant for the offspring of each aptera, and reared to maturity.

Transmission of virus by the maternal apterae to the first, second, and third sets of plants was 6/10, 8/9, and 9/9, respectively. During the first larviposition period, larvae were obtained from apterae Nos. 3, 5, 6, 7, and 10. None of the plants on which the larvae were reared developed symptoms. During the second larviposition period, larvae were obtained from all apterae except No. 2 which had died. The plant on which larvae from aptera No. 5 were reared developed symptoms of SYVV. Approximately 2 weeks later the larvae from each line were

transferred to a second set of virus-free seedlings, and again the plant fed upon by clone 5 developed symptoms. Clone 9 was used to establish a virus-free line of *H. lactucae* for future work; the rest were discarded.

The results suggested that SYVV might occasionally be transovarially passed, but further tests were put off for approximately a year. During this period the established clonal line (No. 9) was used in other experimental work, and substantial evidence was obtained as to its virus-free status (Sylvester and Richardson, 1969).

In 1968 another test for transovarial passage was made. Viviparae from clone 9 were put on SYVV-infected plants in a separate growth chamber to establish a viruliferous stock of aphids. Forty-nine apterae were taken from the viruliferous stock and put, 1 aphid per plant, on healthy sowthistle seedlings. After a larviposition period of 24 hours, the aphids were moved to a second set of virus-free seedlings and allowed to deposit larvae for 24 hours. The apterae were then discarded. After each larviposition period, the offspring from each aphid were counted and transferred to an individual test seedling and thereafter moved to new test seedlings at 48-hour intervals over a sequence of 5 or 6 test plants.

Thirty-six plants of the 49 of the first set of test seedlings fed upon by the maternal apterae developed symptoms of SYVV, while 46 of 48 (one aptera died) of the second set of test plants to which the apterae were transferred developed symptoms. Two apterae failed to transmit virus.

None of the 49 sets of larvae born during the first larviposition period transmitted virus, but of the 45 sets produced in the second larviposition period, 7 transmitted virus. Of these, 4 transmitted virus to at least 4 of the 5 successive test plants. Two of the sets of larvae transmitted virus only to the first member of the test plant series, and 1 transmitted only to the last member. Thus 6 sets of larvae transmitted SYVV to the first test plant fed upon, indicating that the incubation period of the virus was complete at the time of birth.

An experiment was done to compare transovarial passage of SYVV in larvae deposited by females that had their stylets amputated with larvae that were born on plants to normal females.

Thirty apterae, reared on a SYVV source, had the tip of the labium amputated. Twenty-four hours later the larvae produced by each female were caged on a healthy sowthistle seedling to test for virus transmission. The larvae were transferred to additional test seedlings at 48-hour intervals until each set had fed on 8 successive plants. Twenty-four of the 30 females produced an average of 2.8 larvae. Of the initial total of 68 larvae, 17 survived through the eighth transfer. No transmissions were obtained.

When the 30 apterae were removed for the operation, an additional 50 females were taken from the SYVV source plant and caged individually on healthy seedlings for larviposition. The females were moved to additional test plants the next day so that 2 successive sets of larvae from the 50 females were obtained for testing. The first 2 sets of larvae obtained from each aptera were tested for inoculativity by serially transferring them to healthy sowthistle seedlings at 48-hour intervals until they had fed on 8 successive sets of plants.

On day 3 of larviposition the 50 females were, at random, divided into 2 sets of 25 each. One set had the labium amputated and then were isolated for 24 hours of larviposition. The other set of 25 was again transferred to sowthistle seedlings for larviposition. The following day the larvae from each aphid in the 2 sets were transferred to healthy sowthistle plants, 1 plant for the offspring of each female. Again all sets of nymphs were tested for inoculativity by transferring them to a series of 8 test plants at 48-hour intervals.

The maternal apterae transmitted virus to 23 and 34 of the 50 test plants fed on during days 1 and 2 of transfer, respectively. Of the 25 normal apterae tested on day 3, 20 transmitted virus. No transmissions were obtained with the 50 sets of larvae produced by the apterae on day 1, or the 49 sets of larvae obtained on day 2. The average number of larvae in these 2 sets was 6.5 ± 2.1 and 4.5 ± 1.8, respectively. Two of the 25 sets of larvae obtained from the 25 normal apterae of the third day's transfer were inocula-

tive. Each set had 6 larvae in it. In one, the 6 larvae survived for the entire series of 8 transfers, and all 8 plants fed upon developed symptoms. In the other set, one larvae died during the third, and another during the eighth, test access period. The first 3 plants fed upon developed symptoms, the rest were negative, indicating that 1 of the 6 larvae was inoculative and that it died during the third test access period.

Seventeen sets of larvae, with a total of 46 individuals, were obtained from the 25 apterae that had the labium amputated, but no transmissions resulted. It was not possible to demonstrate transovarial passage of SYVV with a limited series of insects that produced larvae in the absence of plant feeding.

The experience with transovarial passage of SYVV in *H. lactucae* indicated that (1) it repeatedly occurred with a low frequency, (2) it apparently occurred after the maternal aphids had become inoculative, and (3) when it did occur, the larvae usually transmitted immediately—i.e., the incubation period of the virus was completed prior to birth.

Another experiment was done, to test this latter point, with a group of 63 larvae deposited on a SYVV source plant by previously virus-free adult *H. lactucae*. The larvae were born and reared to maturity on a virus source plant in a plant growth chamber with a 10-hour day at approximately 25° and a 14-hour night at approximately 18°. When the larvae had matured, or were in the last larval instar, they were transferred and caged, 1 per plant, on a set of healthy test seedlings. These aphids were the maternal series of vectors. Each day, until death, the maternal viviparae were transferred to a new test plant, and each day the larvae born by each aphid during the previous 24-hour test access period were removed, transferred, and caged as a group on a test seedling. These larvae had a test access period of 4 days at 25° and constant light; after this time the cage was removed and the survivors were counted. In this way the larvae produced each day from each female were tested for inoculativity during the entire reproductive period of the maternal aphids. One of the 63 maternal aphids failed to transmit virus, and 1 was lost. The results of the test on the

TABLE 1

LIFE TABLE AND TRANSMISSION STATISTICS OF MATERNAL *Hyperomyzus lactucae* VIVIPARAE ($n = 61$) AND TRANSMISSION BY THEIR OFFSPRING IN A TRANSOVARIAL PASSAGE EXPERIMENT OF SOWTHISTLE YELLOW VEIN VIRUS. THE TEST PLANT WAS *Sonchus oleraceus*

Age in days (x)	Survival[a] (l_x)	Natality[b] (n_x)	Reproductive[c] ($l_x n_x$)	Transmission[d] (daily transfers) (i_x)	Transmission rate[e] ($l_x i_x$)	Transovarial passage[f]
9	1.0	0.54	0.54	0.02	0.02	0/13
10	1.0	3.16	3.16	0.20	0.20	0/40
11	1.0	3.38	3.38	0.41	0.41	0/52
12	1.0	3.97	3.97	0.62	0.62	0/61
13	1.0	3.93	3.93	0.82	0.82	0/48
14	0.98	4.00	3.92	0.83	0.82	0/59
15	0.97	3.90	3.78	0.89	0.86	2/55
16	0.95	2.36	2.24	0.90	0.85	0/54
17	0.90	3.31	2.98	0.93	0.84	3/50
18	0.80	2.86	2.29	0.78	0.62	3/41
19	0.69	3.42	2.26	0.74	0.51	1/33
20	0.51	3.24	1.65	0.74	0.38	5/25
21	0.41	2.24	0.92	0.68	0.28	2/20
22	0.34	1.45	0.49	0.67	0.23	1/14
23	0.33	1.00	0.33	0.30	0.10	0/12
24	0.25	1.15	0.29	0.60	0.15	1/11
25	0.21	0.44	0.09	0.31	0.07	0/3
26	0.15	0.80	0.12	0.22	0.03	2/3
27	0.08	1.00	0.08	0.00	0.00	0/1
28	0.02	0.00	0.00	0.00	0.00	0/0

Net reproductive rate ($\sum l_x n_x$) = 36.4
Generation time ($\sum l_x n_x X \div \sum l_x n_x$) = 14.8
Net transmission rate ($\sum l_x i_x$) = 7.8
Mean weighted retention time ($\sum l_x i_x X \div \sum l_x i_x$) = 16.0

[a] Survival (l_x) is the probability of an aphid being alive at age X.

[b] Natality (n_x) is the average number of female offspring per female aphid at age X.

[c] Reproductive rate ($l_x n_x$) is the sample reproductive rate, the product of l_x and n_x.

[d] Transmission (i_x) is the age specific probability of transmission.

[e] Transmission rate ($l_x i_x$) is the sample transmission rate, the product of l_x and i_x.

[f] Ratio of lots of larvae transmitting to lots of larvae produced and tested.

remaining 61 inoculative aphids and their offspring are given in Table 1.

Beginning on day 7 of the reproductive period (when the incubation period was completed in approximately 95 % of the maternal viviparae, see Fig. 1, TOP test), SYVV was

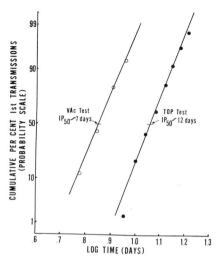

FIG. 1. Incubation period curves from a transovarial passage (TOP) and a 1st instar larval test (VAc) with the sowthistle yellow vein virus and the aphid *Hyperomyzus lactucae* (L.). In the TOP test the larvae were born and acquired virus during an 8-day period on virus source plants at a temperature cycle of a 10-hour day at 25° alternating with a 14-hour night at 18°. In the VAc test the temperature was a constant 25° and the larvae were born and acquired virus during a 24-hour period that maternal viviparae had access to a virus source plant. The test plants were *Sonchus oleraceus*.

transovarially passed to a low percentage of the larvae. It continued to be so until the end of the reproductive period. The data showed a tendency, after initiation, for the amount of transovarial passage to increase with age. This conclusion had some statistical support, as evidenced by a chi-square test for homogeniety of transmission in successive sets of larvae ($X^2 = 20.21$, with 10 d.f., $p < 0.05$).

Based upon a total of 484 sets of larvae produced and tested, with an average of 4.3 larvae per set, and a total of 20 sets inoculative, the probability of a larva being inoculative was estimated to be approximately 1 % (0.98). The number of maternal viviparae producing 0, 1, 2, 3, and 4 or more sets of inoculative larvae was 48, 7, 5, 1, 0, respectively. One of the 13 maternal aphids that produced a set of inoculative larvae was an alate, thus transovarial passage of SYVV can occur in both viviparous morphs of the vector.

Previous data (Sylvester and Richardson, 1969) had indicated that infection of adult *H. lactucae* with SYVV increased the mortality rate in comparison to noninoculative aphids. The number of larvae alive at the end of the 4-day test access period was recorded. During the period of transovarial passage, the sets of larvae that did not transmit virus involved 884 individuals, of which 800 (90.5%) survived the 4-day test access period. The 20 sets of larvae that did transmit involved 63 individuals, of which 50 survived, or 79.4%. A chi-square value of 6.61 with 1 d.f., and a $p < 0.02$, supports evidence for the conclusion that SYVV, when transovarially passed, lowers the survival potential of groups containing infected larvae.

The argument for transovarial passage involves an assumption that larvae produced on susceptible plants (sowthistle) were not acquiring and transmitting virus introduced by the maternal viviparae during the larviposition period of 24 hours.[2] Two lines of evidence support this assumption. One is that Duffus (1963) reported that aphids did not acquire SYVV from plants in less than 6 days following inoculation. This suggests that immediate acquisition of introduced virus would be a relatively rare event. The second line of evidence is the absence of a larval incubation period in the majority of the instances of transovarial passage. But this argument, in turn, depends upon the duration of the incubation period in 1st-instar larvae. A trial, done concurrently with

[2] A further assumption is that the results were not due to accidental contamination in the greenhouse. Absolute checks were not run, but nonrandom patterns in the results would support the assumption. Consecutive infections by specific lots of larvae, no transmission occurring during the vector incubation period, and a delay in the onset of transovarial passage until the inoculative potential of the maternal viviparae was almost fully established, all these suggest effects with assignable causes rather than random happenings.

the above transovarial passage experiment, was made to determine the incubation period in larvae that were born and acquired virus during a 24-hour period that maternal apterae had access to a virus source plant. Twenty-eight larvae were so tested, of which 24 lived for at least 7 days. These larvae were transferred, after removal from the virus source plant, at 24-hour intervals at 25° and constant light, to healthy sowthistle test plants until death. No transmissions occurred before the sixth set of test plants, although 16 out of the 24 insects were eventually demonstrated to be inoculative. The incubation period curve is given in Fig. 1 (VAc test). Thus there is evidence that SYVV undergoes an incubation period in 1st instar larvae of *H. lactucae*. The difference in the IP_{50} values for the VAc series (7 days) and the TOP series (12 days) presumably was due to the temperature at which the 2 sets of larvae were reared (Duffus, 1963). The VAc set was reared at a constant 25°, while the TOP set was reared at a 12-hour, 25° day and 14-hour, 18° night cycle for 8 days. The results with the VAc series support the assumption that the SYVV passed in the TOP experiment, even though a 4-day test access period was used, was not virus that had been acquired from the plants on which the inoculative maternal viviparae were fed and on which the larvae were born. Four days is less than the minimum incubation period found with 1st-instar larvae.

DISCUSSION

Aphid-borne circulative viruses usually are considered not to be transovarially passed. This is not surprising in view of the difficulty that has been met in attempting to demonstrate multiplication of any plant virus in an aphid vector. Stegwee and Ponsen (1958) presented evidence for the multiplication of PLRV in the aphid *Myzus persicae*, and Miyamoto and Miyamoto (1966) recently reported a low percentage of transovarial passage of PLRV during tests made in winter months.

The present work provides some evidence for the transovarial passage of SYVV in the aphid *H. lactucae*, and as such gives additional support for the hypothesis of multiplication of this virus in this vector

(Duffus, 1963; Richardson and Sylvester, 1968; Sylvester and Richardson, 1969). Perhaps transovarial passage was to be expected since SYVV was found in nuclei of cells of the salivary gland of viruliferous insects (Richardson and Sylvester, 1968), although it might be unexpected to find it to be transovarially passed so infrequently. This, however, might be associated with the particular aphid clone being used in our laboratory.

Most of the leafhopper/planthopper-borne viruses, e.g., rice dwarf (Fukushi, 1933, 1935), clover club leaf (Black, 1950), rugose leaf curl (Grylls, 1954), rice stripe (Yamada and Yamamoto, 1955), European wheat striate mosaic (Watson and Sinha, 1959), and oat dwarf tillering (Lindsten, 1961) are transovarially passed to a relatively high proportion of the offspring of viruliferous females. Wound-tumor virus (WTV) and potato yellow dwarf virus were originally reported to be transovarially passed at a very low frequency (Black, 1953), although later the efficiency of passage of WTV was found to vary with the race of the vector (Nagaraj and Black, 1962).

In most leafhopper-borne viruses that are transovarially passed, as with SYVV, the larvae are viruliferous at hatching if the incubation period of the virus has been completed in the maternal females at the time of oviposition. However, in the case of WTV an additional posthatching incubation period of 6–9 days was reported to be needed (Sinha and Shelley, 1965). The amount of transovarial passage of European wheat striate mosaic virus was dependent upon the age of the maternal females at the time of virus acquisition (Sinha, 1960).

None of the viruses are transmitted by sperm, and it would be of interest to know in the case of such a virus as SYVV, which is found in nuclei, whether or not transmission through sperm would occur. The lack of sperm transmission may be related to the mechanism by which eggs are infected. Nasu (1965) presented electron micrographs that indicated that rice dwarf virus entered the egg on the membrane surface of one type (L-symbiote) of the bacterium-like symbiotes of the mycetome of the green rice leafhopper vector, *Nephotettix cincticeps*.

Both aphids and leafhoppers, as well as many other arthropods, have intracellular bacterium-like and/or yeast-like symbiotes associated with specialized cells (mycetocytes). These cells may or may not be aggregated into an organ, the mycetome. The symbiotes, while present in both sexes, apparently are passed from generation to generation only via the egg. Current data indicate that they are nutritionally or metabolically involved in the life processes of their hosts.

Aposymbiotic individuals occur, both under natural and experimental conditions, but apparently no one has attempted to determine whether or not transovarial passage of viruses takes place when the symbiotes are absent from the mycetocytes.

The symbiotes are incorporated into the egg after the maturation divisions. In the parthenogenic phase of the reproductive cycle of aphids there is a single maturation division of the oogonia, without reduction, and parthenogenesis is of the diploid type. In the sexual phase, as in the case of leafhoppers, oogensis involves two maturation divisions, one reduction and one equational. Female aphids have two X chromosomes, while males, due to the extrusion of an extra X chromosome during the single maturation division, have but one X chromosome. In spermatogenesis therefore, two types of gametes are produced, with and without an X chromosome. Only those with the X chromosome mature, and consequently fertilization always restores the XX female condition.

Be this as it may, after the maturation divisions, and during cleavage of the nuclei that eventually develop into the cells of the blastoderm, the surface of the cytoplasm that surrounds the yolk becomes a syncytium. Some of the daughter nuclei migrate internally and posteriorly into the yolk mass and form mycetoblasts that later develop into mycetocytes. At the posterior end of the egg the syncytium is incomplete and the periplasm thin, and here develops a blastopore-like region of contact between the egg and the cushion of follicular cells of the maternal ovarian follicle. Associated with these follicular cells are maternal mycetocytes with their symbiotes. It is in this area that the maternal symbiotes invade the egg. Invasion can be by "migrant forms" of the symbiotes, liberated from maternal mycetocytes, which actively move through or between the follicular cells and into the egg. In other cases specialized maternal mycetocytes enter the blastopore-like area, fuse with the cells and then pour their contents into the egg. In any event, symbiotes of maternal origin are transferred and become incorporated in the developing mycetocytes of the egg.

Given this mechanism of transovarial perpetuation of intracellular symbiotes, it would appear that transovarial passage of viruses would only necessitate association of the virus with a migrant or invasive form of either a symbiote or a fusing maternal mycetocyte. The single example investigated to date (Nasu, 1965) apparently is of the former type.

Reliable evidence for virus multiplication in leafhopper vectors has been gained bv demonstrating continuous passage through a series of successive generations (Fukushi, 1935; Black, 1950). The extremely low per centage of transovarial passage of SYVV found in our work, along with the tendency for the longevity of infected insects to be reduced, would mitigate the feasibility of this experimental approach to the problem of multiplication of SYVV in *H. lactucae*.

ACKNOWLEDGMENTS

The author expresses his appreciation of Jean Richardson and Geoffrey M. Behncken for their technical assistance.

REFERENCES

BLACK, L. M. (1950). A plant virus that multiplies in its insect vector. *Nature* 166, 852–853.

BLACK, L. M. (1953). Occasional transmission of some plant viruses through the eggs of their insect vectors. *Phytopathology* 43, 9–10.

BRADLEY, R. H. E. (1960). Effect of amputating stylets of mature apterous viviparae of *Myzus persicae*. *Nature* 188, 337–338.

DUFFUS, J. E. (1963). Possible multiplication in the aphid vector of sowthistle yellow vein virus, a virus with an extremely long insect latent period. *Virology* 21, 194–202.

FUKUSHI, T. (1933). Transmission of the virus through the eggs of an insect vector. *Proc. Imp. Acad. (Tokyo)* 9, 457–460.

FUKUSHI, T. (1935). Multiplication of virus in its vector. *Proc. Imp. Acad. (Tokyo)* 11, 301–303.

GRYLLS, N. E. (1954). Rugose leaf curl—a new virus disease transovarially transmitted by the leafhopper *Austroagallia torrida*. *Australian J. Biol. Sci.* 7, 47–58.

LINDSTEN, K. (1961). Studies on virus diseases of cereals in Sweden. II. On virus diseases transmitted by the leafhopper *Calligypona pellucida* (F.). *Kgl. Lantbruks-Högskol. Ann.* 27, 199–271.

MIYAMOTO, S., and MIYAMOTO, Y. (1966). Notes on aphid-transmission of potato leafroll virus. *Sci. Rept. Hyogo Univ. Agr.* 7, 51–56.

NAGARAJ, A. N., and BLACK, L. M. (1962). Hereditary variation in the ability of a leafhopper to transmit two unrelated plant viruses. *Virology* 16, 152–162.

NASU, S. (1965). Electron microscopic studies on transovarial passage of rice dwarf virus. *Japan. J. Appl. Entomol. Zool.* 9, 225–237.

RICHARDSON, J., and SYLVESTER, E. S. (1968). Further evidence of multiplication of sowthistle yellow vein virus in its aphid vector, *Hyperomyzus lactucae*. *Virology* 35, 347–355.

SINHA, R. C. (1960). Comparison of the ability of nymph and adult *Delphacodes pellucida* Fabricius, to transmit European wheat striate mosaic virus. *Virology* 10, 344–352.

SINHA, R. C., and SHELLEY, S. (1965). Studies on the transovarial transmission of wound-tumor virus. *Phytopathology* 55, 324–327.

STEGWEE, D., and PONSEN, M. B. (1958). Multiplication of potato leaf roll virus in the aphid *Myzus persicae* (Sulz.). *Entomol. Exptl. Appl.* 1, 291–300.

SYLVESTER, E. S., and RICHARDSON, J. (1969). Additional evidence of multiplication of the sowthistle yellow vein virus in an aphid vector—serial passage. *Virology* 37, 26–31.

WATSON, M. A., and SINHA, R. C. (1959). Studies on the transmission of European wheat striate mosaic virus by *Delphacodes pellucida* Fabricius. *Virology* 8, 130–163.

YAMADA, M., and YAMAMOTO, H. (1955). Studies on the stripe disease of rice plant. I. On the virus transmission by an insect, *Delphacodes striatella* Fallen. *Okayama Agr. Expt. Stat. Spec. Bull.* 52, 93–112.

A Plant Virus Lethal to Its Insect Vector

D. D. JENSEN

INTRODUCTION

The evidence that certain plant viruses multiply also in their insect vectors is now so convincing that the idea is no longer resisted. In this category are the viruses of rice stunt (Fukushi, 1939), aster yellows (Kunkel, 1937; Black, 1941; Maramorosch, 1952), clover club-leaf (Black, 1950), and wound-tumor virus (Black and Brakke, 1952).

The fact that these now appear to be viruses of animals as well as of plants has resulted in the extension by Maramorosch (1954) and Andrewes (1957) of the organismal theory of virus origin to suggest

VIROLOGY, 1959, Vol. 8, pp. 164-175.

that plant viruses, and viruses commonly considered to be vertebrate viruses, were originally arthropod viruses.

Green (1935), Laidlaw (1938), Burnet (1945), Andrewes (1952), and others have speculated that viruses originated by retrograde evolution from parasitic microorganisms. The basis for this belief has been the generalization in biology that the more recent the relationship of parasite and host, the more likely is it to be characterized by damage to the host. In contrast, hosts which accommodate their parasites with little if any apparent harm are assumed to have had a long enough association with the parasite for the evolution of a compatible relationship.

Host injury caused by plant viruses has, until very recently, been recognized only in the plants. The insect vectors of some plant viruses appeared to be symptomless but true hosts, and therefore may have harbored these viruses longer than have the known plant hosts.

The first evidence that a plant virus could alter the tissue of its insect vector was provided by Littau and Maramorosch (1956). They reported that aster yellows virus caused the cells of the fat body of *Macrosteles fascifrons* (Stål) to have more stellate nuclei than occurred in virus-free leafhoppers. However, there is no evidence as yet that this virus is harmful to the leafhopper vector. Kunkel (1926) and Severin (1947) compared the longevity of infective aster leafhoppers with that of virus-free leafhoppers and found no difference. Kunkel (1926) and Dobroscky (1929, 1931) also failed to find any cytological difference between infective and virus-free aster leafhoppers.

In Japan, Yoshii and Kiso (1957) reported that, in some but not all respects, the virus causing dwarf disease of orange has a metabolic effect on the plant hopper vector, *Geisha distinctissima* Wal., similar to that found in infected orange leaves. Both oxygen consumption and total phosphorus were reduced in a similar manner in host plant and vector. The authors do not indicate whether or not viruliferous insects have reduced longevity or other evidence of adverse effects due to the virus. However, the decreased utilization of oxygen would suggest that infective vectors are more likely to be suffering than benefiting from the presence of this virus in their bodies.

The present paper reports experimental evidence that Western X-disease virus of stone fruits causes the premature death of viruliferous *Colladonus montanus* (Van Duzee), one of the leafhopper vectors of the virus (Jensen, 1958, 1959).

Although this virus has been found in the field only in stone fruits, it has been transmitted experimentally to celery, *Apiu graveolens* L., (Jensen, 1956) and to periwinkle, *Vinca major* L., by the writer.

Colladonus montanus only rarely succeeds in acquiring virus from peach trees or in transmitting virus to peach, *Prunus persica* (L.) Batsch. However, it is a fairly efficient vector of the virus from and to celery (Jensen, 1957).

MATERIALS AND METHODS

Western X-disease virus of stone fruits occurs as different strains in various areas of western North America. Four of these occur in northern California, with the most severe strain known as peach yellow leaf roll virus. The present experiments were conducted with this virulent strain. It was obtained from peach near Marysville, California, and has been maintained for several years in the greenhouse in peach, celery, and periwinkle.

Celery, var. Golden Self Blanching and var. Green Jumbo, grown from seed in the greenhouse, was used for test plants and virus source plants. The test plants were growing in 4-inch pots and varied in height from 2–5 inches when fed upon by insects. At the completion of the test feedings, some of the experimental plants were sprayed with malathion before being returned to the greenhouse; others were left unsprayed in order that, after symptoms developed, they could be used as virus sources for leafhoppers.

All virus transmission during these experiments was accomplished by means of leafhoppers. *Colladonus montanus* was used almost exclusively, with *Colladonus geminatus* (Van Duzee) being involved in a few tests. The test insects were reared on celery in the greenhouse. The leafhopper stock colonies were shown to remain noninfective by periodically testing 30 to 50 leafhoppers from a stock cage on a series of healthy celery plants.

The leafhopper longevity figures given are based on the length of survival on the test plants, in days, after an incubation period of the virus in the insects of approximately 30 days.

Experimental procedures will be described in the appropriate sections.

EXPERIMENTS AND RESULTS

Longevity of Insects with and without Access to Diseased Plants

In order to determine the effect of the virus on the longevity of a large number of insects from the same stock colony, most of them were tested in groups of ten rather than singly. Young nymphs, most of them in the second or third instar, were divided into two groups each of approximately 225–250 individuals. This was done by collecting the nymphs from the stock cage by means of an aspirator and transferring them into two separate cages. The selection was a random one and the two transfer cages were used alternately in receiving the nymphs. One group was then caged on an infected celery plant and the other group was placed on a healthy celery plant. After an acquisition feeding period of 21 days on diseased plants, the infective group was transferred to a healthy celery plant and held for 9 more days before being transferred to test celery plants. The healthy control group of leafhoppers was transferred to a new celery plant each time the infective group was transferred.

Five males and ten females from each of the two main groups were caged singly on celery plants and checked daily for longevity and virus transmission. This was done to determine the approximate percentage of viruliferous leafhoppers present in the infective group. The remaining insects in each main group were tested in lots of ten. These were transferred to new celery plants twice weekly and counted by catching them individually in an aspirator.

Although the infective group had started with approximately the same number of nymphs (225–250) as the noninfective group, 30 days later, when tests were begun, only 110 were alive compared to 221 leafhoppers in the noninfective control group. At this time all insects had reached the adult stage.

Table 1 and Figs. 1 and 2 summarize the results. Of the 15 insects tested singly from the infective group, 12 transmitted virus and had a mean longevity of 38 days on the test plants. One of the 3 nontransmitters died in 3 days, which was too short a time to determine whether or not it had acquired virus, and the 2 obviously nonviruliferous leafhoppers lived for 54 and 94 days, respectively. From these single tests it is evident that at least 2 of the 15 insects failed to acquire virus during the 21 days on the inoculum plant. It may therefore be assumed that an undetermined number of leafhoppers in the infective groups also failed to acquire virus.

Longevity of the 15 insects tested singly from the noninfective group ranged from 17 to 142 days, with a mean of 82 days.

It is of some interest that the 5 males in each of the two groups of 15 leafhoppers tested singly had a longer average life than did the 10

TABLE 1

EFFECT OF WESTERN X-DISEASE VIRUS ON LONGEVITY OF *Colladonus montanus*

Test type	Total insects	Insects or groups transmitting	Longevity in days	
			Range	Mean
Single insects				
Infective	15	12	24–59	38
Noninfective	15	0	17–142	82
Groups of 10				
Infective	110	11	3–132	24
Noninfective	221	0	3–154	51

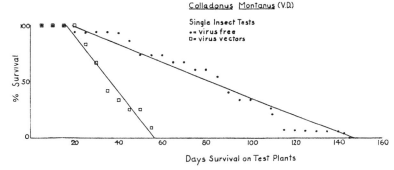

FIG. 1. Survival of twelve *Colladonus montanus* leafhoppers which transmitted Western X-disease virus compared with that of fifteen nonviruliferous leafhoppers, of the same age and from the same colony, which had fed only on healthy plants.

females. In the noninfective group, the longevity of the 5 males ranged from 87 to 114 days with an average of 106 days. Longevity of the 10 females ranged from 17 to 142 days with an average of 71 days. In the infective group, 4 of 5 males transmitted virus to an average of 1.75 plants. They had a longevity of 25, 52, 55 and 59 days, with an average of 48 days. Nine of 10 females transmitted virus. One of these lived only 3 days and transmitted virus to 1 plant. The other 8 females lived from 24 to 45 days for an average of 30 days. They transmitted virus to from 2 to 5 plants for an average of 3.7 per insect.

The mean longevity of the 110 leafhoppers from the infective group, tested in lots of 10, was 24 days compared to 51 days for 221 individuals in the noninfective control groups.

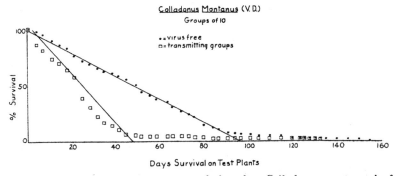

Fig. 2. Survival of twenty-two groups of virus-free *Colladonus montanus* leaf-hoppers compared with that of eleven groups which transmitted Western X-disease virus. Not all individuals in the transmitting groups were viruliferous.

The virus transmission records for the eleven infective groups indicate that practically all of the individuals which were transmitting virus died within the first 40 days on the test plants. Only two of eleven infective groups transmitted virus after 35 days. One group transmitted after 41 days and there was no transmission after 45 days. In one group, 9 of the 10 leafhoppers died in 11 days. The single survivor, apparently having failed to acquire virus, lived for 104 days without transmitting virus to any of the plants fed upon during the time it was being tested alone.

There was no apparent difference in the range of longevity between the infective groups (3–132 days) and the noninfective groups (3–154 days). This is because an undetermined percentage of the individuals in the transmitting groups apparently failed to acquire virus during the acquisition feeding period on the diseased plants. These nonviruliferous leafhoppers appeared to live as long as did control leafhoppers which had fed only on healthy plants.

The greater mean longevity of insects tested singly over that of comparable insects tested in groups is believed to be due primarily to the fact that the latter were caught individually in an aspirator twice weekly for counting. This type of handling inevitably results in injuries to some insects.

Longevity of Transmitting and Nontransmitting Leafhoppers Given Identical Feeding Times on Virus-infected Plants

In each of the experiments reported in this section, all of the leafhoppers involved had identical treatment and were tested singly instead of in groups. In a given experiment, nymphs were transferred from a single stock colony to a diseased celery plant. Acquisition feeding periods in excess of 4–7 days required use of more than one inoculum plant because diseased celery plants do not live long after symptoms develop (Jensen, 1956). Following the acquisition feeding period, the insects were transferred from the diseased celery plants to a healthy celery plant and held for the completion of the latent period of the virus in the leafhoppers. The time allowed for this was usually 30 to 40 days from the first day on the virus source.

The insects were then caged singly on celery plants to determine the longevity and virus transmission record of each. Survival was checked daily in all experiments. The test insects were transferred to new plants either daily, twice weekly, or weekly. Table 2 summarizes the results of experiments of this type conducted during 1957 and 1958.

The percentage of individual leafhoppers acquiring virus during the acquisition feeding period is a function of the time on the diseased plant, and there was no evidence that some individuals are unable to acquire or to transmit virus. For example, in experiments 7, 8, and 9 all leafhoppers came from the same stock colony and were placed on the source plant together. They were then removed to healthy plants after 3, 7, or 16 days on inoculum. After 3 days on the source plant, only 3 of 11 later transmitted virus, whereas after 16 days, only 1 of 10 failed to transmit virus.

In each experiment the mean longevity of the leafhoppers which failed to transmit virus was markedly greater than that of those which transmitted virus. Survival on the test plants averaged 50.6 days per insect for 64 nontransmitters and only 20.2 days for 116 leafhoppers which transmitted virus.

The mean longevity figures for the nontransmitting insects are considered to be very conservative. Some of the very short-lived insects, whose survival data were averaged in with the nontransmitters, probably died early because they carried virus, but failed to transmit it before death. Viruliferous leafhoppers usually do not transmit an infective charge of this virus to every plant upon which they feed. Thus there were examples of vectors which transmitted virus to only the first test plant fed upon, whereas others transmitted only to plants at or near the end of the test series. Had the first examples started the test series a day later and had the second examples died a day or two earlier than they did, their longevity records would have been averaged with those listed as nontransmitters.

TABLE 2

REDUCED LONGEVITY OF *Colladonus montanus* DUE TO
WESTERN X-DISEASE VIRUS[a]

Experiment	Days on source plant	Trans-mission record	No. of insects	Longevity in days	
				Range	Mean
1	7	+	15	6–28	13
		−	4	6–42	26
2	46	+	8	5–38	17
		−	7	5–118	26
3	46	+	16	1–32	13
4	26	+	14	5–25	16
		−	1	75	75
5	17	+	8	14–44	24
		−	2	22–132	77
6	17	+	8	21–79	34
		−	2	97–129	113
7	3	+	3	9–42	24
		−	8	8–68	49
8	7	+	7	7–19	12
		−	3	11–68	40
9	16	+	9	6–28	17
		−	1	68	68
10	11	+	4	17–28	23
		−	4	14–46	38
11	21	+	12	3–59	38
		−	2	54–94	74
12	7	+	4	26–47	34
		−	6	47–117	78
13	7	+	6	4–25	16
		−	10	4–94	46
14	4	+	2	15–21	18
		−	14	3–95	49

[a] Longevity is measured from first day on test plant and follows completion of the incubation period of the virus in the leafhopper. Transmitting and non-transmitting insects had the same feeding time on diseased and healthy plants. Mean longevity for 116 transmitters = 20.2 days. Mean longevity for 64 non-transmitters = 50.6 days.

In experiments 2 and 3 the test insects had exceptionally long feeding periods of 46 days on inoculum. All 16 insects in experiment 3 transmitted virus. In experiment 2, 7 of 15 were listed as nontransmitters. However, it is probable that 6 of these 7 actually had acquired virus because they lived only 3, 6, 13, 13, 15, and 21 days, respectively. The seventh individual, apparently lacking virus, lived 118 days.

Although the total number of virus-transmitting insects was almost twice that of the nontransmitters in these tests, in no experiment did the maximum longevity of a vector exceed the maximum longevity of the nonvectors. In one test, experiment 7, the maxima were equal. In all other tests the maximum longevity for the nonvectors was considerably greater than that of the vectors. A mean of the maxima proved to be 85.4 days and 36.6 days, respectively.

Tests with Colladonus geminatus

Preliminary experiments with *Colladonus geminatus* indicate that the longevity of this species also is reduced by Western X-disease virus. In the few tests conducted, the differences in longevity between transmitting and nontransmitting insects were consistent, but not as great as occurred with *Colladonus montanus*. For many years large colonies of *Colladonus geminatus* could be reared successfully in the greenhouse throughout the year. However, during the last few years we have been unable to maintain this species in the greenhouse in sufficient numbers for extensive tests.

DISCUSSION

There are over 200 insect viruses known that kill their hosts, but plant viruses and vertebrate viruses transmitted by insects have usually been considered harmless to their vectors. Examples are known of some disease-causing agents that injure the insects by which they are transmitted. Thus, the body louse, vector of the rickettsia causing typhus fever, suffers high mortality from this cause (Zinsser, 1935). Although at one time grouped with virus diseases, typhus fever is known to be caused by a rickettsia. Indications that viruses also may be deleterious to their insect vectors have appeared only very recently.

The report by Littau and Maramorosch (1956) suggests that the role played by aster yellows virus in the body of the aster leafhopper is more than passive multiplication and transmission. However, extensive tests by Kunkel (1926) and Severin (1947) demonstrate that this virus is not harmful to the vector in terms of longevity. Thus it is still not known if the cytological effects reported are in any sense deleterious to the leafhopper.

In the present study of the effect of Western X-disease virus on its leafhopper vector, *Colladonus montanus*, it seems evident that the reduction in the longevity of virus-transmitting individuals is caused by the virus per se and does not result from some indirect effect such as impaired nutrition provided by infected host plants.

It is true that a virus can alter the effectiveness of a plant as a host of insects. However, it is of special interest that in all published cases known to the writer, the virus is considered to render the host plant more suitable rather than less suitable for the insects involved.

Kennedy (1951) stated that *Aphis fabae* Scop. was more productive of offspring on sugar beet, *Beta vulgaris* L., leaves infected with beet mosaic virus than on healthy leaves of comparable age. Severin (1946) reported that nine species of leafhoppers completed their nymphal development on celery or asters, *Callistephus chinensis* Nees., infected with aster yellows virus, but the adults died within a few days after transfer to healthy celery and asters. Maramorosch (1958) found that *Dalbulus maidis* Del. and W., a leafhopper incapable of transmitting aster yellows virus, dies within 4 days on healthy asters, but lives as long on asters carrying aster yellows virus as it does on corn, its normal host. After 5 weeks on infected asters, the leafhopper could even live on healthy asters.

If, in the experiments with *Colladonus montanus*, the longevity of insects which had fed on diseased celery plants had been compared only with that of insects which had never fed on a virus source plant, one might infer that the premature death of the former was due to an impairment of the physiological qualities of a diseased plant. However, even in these tests the longevity of the individuals which did not transmit virus was approximately equal to that of leafhoppers maintained only on healthy celery.

In most of the work (Table 2) the only evident variable was the presence or absence of the plant virus in the insect vector. In a given experiment all insects came from the same colony, all fed the same period of time on the diseased plant, and each insect was tested separately for virus transmission and longevity. Since the test plants require 30 days or more for symptom development, the identity of the individual leafhoppers which transmitted virus could not be determined, in many instances, until after the insects had already died.

The difference between the mean longevity of transmitting and nontransmitting leafhoppers is highly significant statistically. Moreover, the absolute difference is probably even greater than indicated, because there can be little doubt that some of the insects which died very early without transmitting virus (and therefore were averaged with the nonvectors) actually carried virus.

An alternative explanation cannot be found in the possibility that there are genetic differences among the leafhoppers involving correlation between greater longevity and failure to acquire virus. All individuals appear to be potential vectors if given sufficient time on the inoculum plant.

Analysis of the maximum longevity figures for transmitting and nontransmitting leafhoppers also indicates that the virus itself shortens the life of the insect. If the virus had no effect on the leafhopper, the maximum longevity among transmitting insects should, on a chance basis, exceed the maximum of nontransmitting individuals some of the time. However, this does not happen, despite the fact that there were approximately twice as many transmitting insects as nontransmitters.

The knowledge that a plant virus, such as that of Western X-disease, can be lethal to its insect vector as well as to some of its plant hosts, makes the organismal theory of virus origin more tenable. The hypothetical evolution of plant viruses from arthropod-inhabiting viruses, which in turn may have been derived from parasitic organisms, becomes more plausible as evidence for some of the stages in this postulated transition are actually found to exist in nature. Western X-disease virus appears to provide an example of a virus which has not yet evolved to the point that it has ceased to injure its insect vector.

REFERENCES

ANDREWES, C. H. (1952). The place of viruses in nature. *Proc. Roy. Soc.* B139, 313–326.

ANDREWES, C. H. (1957). Factors in virus evolution. *Advances in Virus Research* 4, 1–24.

BLACK, L. M. (1941). Further evidence for multiplication of the aster-yellows virus in the aster leafhopper. *Phytopathology* 31, 120–135.

BLACK, L. M. (1950). A plant virus that multiplies in its insect vector. *Nature* 166, 852–853.

BLACK, L. M., and BRAKKE, M. K. (1952). Multiplication of wound-tumor virus in an insect vector. *Phytopathology* 42, 269–273.

BURNET, F. M. (1945). *Virus as Organism.* Harvard Univ. Press, Cambridge, Massachusetts.

DOBROSCKY, I. D. (1929). Is the aster-yellows virus detectable in its insect vector? *Phytopathology* 19, 1009–1015.

DOBROSCKY, I. D. (1931). Morphological and cytological studies on the salivary glands and alimentary tract of *Cicadula sexnotata* (Fallen), the carrier of aster-yellows virus. *Contrib. Boyce Thompson Inst.* 3, 39–58.

FUKUSHI, T. (1939). Retention of virus by its insect vectors through several generations. *Proc. Imp. Acad. (Tokyo)* **15**, 142–145.

GREEN, R. G. (1935). On the nature of filtrable viruses. *Science* **82**, 443–445.

JENSEN, D. D. (1956). Insect transmission of virus between tree and herbaceous plants. *Virology* **2**, 249–260.

JENSEN, D. D. (1957). Differential transmission of peach yellow leaf roll virus to peach and celery by the leafhopper, *Colladonus montanus*. *Phytopathology* **47**, 575–578.

JENSEN, D. D. (1958). Reduction in longevity of leafhoppers carrying peach yellow leaf roll virus. *Phytopathology* **48**, 394. (Abstract.)

JENSEN, D. D. (1959). Insects, both hosts and vectors of plant viruses. *Pan-Pacific Entomologist* **35**, 65–82.

KENNEDY, J. S. (1951). Benefits to aphids from feeding on galled and virus-infected leaves. *Nature* **168**, 825.

KUNKEL, L. O. (1926). Studies on aster yellows. *Am. J. Botany* **13**, 646–705.

KUNKEL, L. O. (1937). Effect of heat on ability of *Cicadula sexnotata* (Fall.) to transmit aster yellows. *Am. J. Botany* **24**, 316–327.

LAIDLAW, P. M. (1938). *Virus Diseases and Viruses*. Cambridge Univ. Press, London and New York.

LITTAU, V. C., and MARAMOROSCH, K. (1956). Cytological effects of aster-yellows virus on its insect vector. *Virology* **2**, 128–130.

MARAMOROSCH, K. (1952). Direct evidence for the multiplication of aster-yellows virus in its insect vector. *Phytopathology* **42**, 59–64.

MARAMOROSCH, K. (1954). Biological transmission of plant viruses by animal vectors. *Trans. N. Y. Acad. Sci.* [2] **16**, 189–195.

MARAMOROSCH, K. (1958). Healthy and yellows asters as food plants for corn leafhoppers. *Intern. Congr. Microbiol. 7th Congr.* p. 260. Stockholm, Aug. 3–9, 1958.

SEVERIN, H. H. P. (1946). Longevity, or life histories, of leafhopper species on virus-infected and on healthy plants. *Hilgardia* **17**, 121–137.

SEVERIN, H. H. P. (1947). Longevity of noninfective and infective leafhoppers on a plant nonsusceptible to a virus. *Hilgardia* **17**, 541–543.

YOSHII, H., and KISO, A. (1957). Studies on the nature of insect-transmission in plant viruses (II). Some researches on the unhealthy metabolism in the viruliferous plant hopper, *Geisha distinctissima* Wal., which is the insect vector of the dwarf disease of Satsuma orange. *Virus (Osaka)* **7**, 315–320.

ZINSSER, H. (1935). *Rats, Lice, and History*. Little, Brown, Boston, Massachusetts.

365

DIRECT EVIDENCE FOR THE MULTIPLICATION OF ASTER-YELLOWS VIRUS IN ITS INSECT VECTOR*

By KARL MARAMOROSCH

(From the Laboratories of The Rockefeller Institute for Medical Research)

Although transovarial passages (5, 6, 10, 11) of two plant viruses through the eggs of their vectors provided evidence of virus multiplication in these vectors, the evidence was considered inadequate by some workers (1). This stimulated a return to the problem. It seemed that the question of whether or not any given plant virus multiplied in its insect vector could easily be settled if the virus were carried in serial passages from insect to insect, with the inoculum adequately diluted at each passage. Such a test was made for the animal virus of equine encephalomyelitis by Merrill and TenBroeck (25), but no similar evidence was available for any plant virus. The discovery by Black (3) that aster-yellows virus could be transmitted by needle inoculations to its insect vector, the aster leafhopper *Macrosteles divisus* Uhler, made it possible to obtain such evidence for aster-yellows virus in its carrier insect. A preliminary report of work on the problem has already been presented (20). This paper describes in detail ten consecutive passages through the leafhopper in experiments started in March 1950, and carried out over a period of 13 months.

MATERIALS.—All experiments were carried out under controlled conditions of temperature, light, humidity, and wind velocity. Figure 1 represents a diagram of one of the temperature control chambers used. The inside dimensions were 65 × 75 × 75 cm. A removable ceiling made of 0.020-in. (0.5-mm.) transparent cellulose acetate was found to reduce the light intensity by only 2 per cent and at the same time to insulate the working part of the box sufficiently. Six holes, 0.5 cm. in diameter, were made in the celluloid to avoid excessive water vapor condensation on the ceiling. Two inner walls were perforated by 13 rows of holes, 0.5 cm. in diameter, 4 cm. apart. These holes served primarily for air flow, but were also used for the insertion of metal blocks which supported the platform at desired levels. Behind one of the perforated walls a heater of high-resistance wire was placed and covered by a metal box with a blower. The speed of this blower was regulated by a rheostat. The air flow was directed through the space below the proper inside box and back into it

* Awarded an A. Cressy Morrison Prize in Natural Science in 1951 by the New York Academy of Sciences.

PHYTOPATHOLOGY, 1952, Vol. 42, pp. 59-64.

through the opposite wall, as indicated in the diagram. It proved desirable to cover the holes below the platform by pieces of cardboard. A gas bulb type thermostat (Minneapolis Honeywell) was placed behind the wall opposite to the heater. The boxes were kept in an air-conditioned room at 10° C. and the inside temperature maintained at 25° ± 0.5° C. Cool air from the room entered each box through holes in the outer walls and mixed continuously with the warm air inside. Fluorescent lamps were chosen as the source of light because of their low temperature, in spite of some disadvantages like low intensity and excessive weight of electric resistance (ballast) equipment, which could be partially or completely overcome. Each box was lighted by 19 fluorescent tubes, mounted on a panel as close together as their widths made practical. The ballasts were placed outside the room so that their heat was not dissipated in the refrigerated area. By means of separate switches, each fluores-

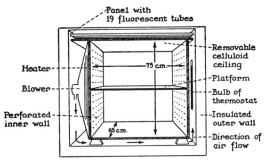

FIG. 1. Diagram of a temperature control chamber, with fluorescent lights (door removed).

cent tube could be connected with either one or two ballasts. By the use of double ballasts for single lights, the intensity was increased by approximately 60 per cent. With new tubes at a distance of 44 cm. (19 in.) from the plastic ceiling, the maximum intensity of light was 4000 foot-candles, whereas with single ballasts at the same distance it was 2500 foot-candles. The ballast arrangements were suggested by Went's description of the Earhart Plant Research Laboratory in Pasadena (31). The lights were turned on for 16 hr. a day by a standard automatic electric clock.

China asters (*Callistephus chinensis* Nees), used as test plants, were grown from commercial seed in flats and transplanted to 2½-in. pots.

A stock colony of virus-free *Macrosteles divisus* Uhler was kept in an insectary (Fig. 2) on rye plants, which are immune from aster yellows.

A specially constructed microsyringe, calibrated to 1/8000 cc., described by McMaster and Hogeboom (24), permitted an accurate measurement of the volume of inoculum introduced into each insect. Ordinary metal hypodermic needles of 23 to 26 gauge and Pyrex micropipettes cemented to them with a paste of litharge and glycerine were used (21) (Fig. 3). When a colony of insects was employed, the insects were macerated in a commercially available TenBroeck tissue grinder (29). Single insects were ground in a similar micromortar of small dimensions (8).

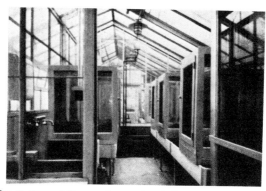

FIG. 2. View of the insectary. (Photograph by J. A. Carlile.)

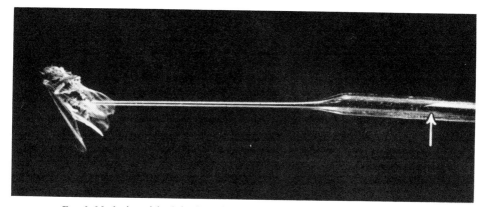

FIG. 3. Method used for injecting a leafhopper. Arrow points to the end of a hypodermic needle that was cemented into a Pyrex capillary pipette. (Photograph by J. A. Carlile.)

METHODS.—The viruliferous insects, which served as virus source, were obtained by feeding 100 virus-free leafhoppers from stock cultures containing approximately equal numbers of males and females on diseased aster plants for 2 weeks at 25° C. When tested individually for 2 days on asters, 83 of them proved infective. The 100 insects, weighing approximately 140 mgm., were crushed in the tissue grinder and 999.860 cc. of neutral buffered saline added at the time of maceration, to make approximately a 1:7000 dilution of the insect pulp. In subsequent passages the weight of the survivors was taken as the basis for making a 1:1000 dilution. Single insects weigh at least 10 times as much as the inoculum used for their injection (1.2 to 1.4 mg., as compared to the weight of 1/8000 cc. = 0.12 mg., approximately). Therefore the actual dilution of the original inoculum in each consecutive passage increased by a factor of 10^{-4}.

The diluted pulp was centrifuged at 3000 r.p.m. for 10 min. at 0° C. and the supernatant fluid was used for injections. The injections were performed under a fluorescent light and a magnifying glass in a coldroom at 0° C., which immobilized the insects. An attempt was made to insert the needle between the third and fourth segment of the abdomen, thus introducing the measured

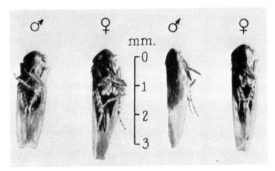

FIG. 4. Male and female *Macrosteles divisus* Uhler. Note larger size of females. (Photograph by J. A. Carlile.)

amount of 1/8000 cc. into the abdominal cavity. This procedure was a modification of leafhopper inoculations developed by Storey (27) and Black (3). The essential difference consisted of the introduction of a very small but accurately measured volume of inoculum. Figure 3 shows an insect during injection. The insects were pushed off the needle by means of an insect pin sealed in a glass rod; they were then slowly warmed to room temperature. Subsequently they were caged on rye plants (*Secale cereale* L.), and placed in chambers at 25° C. Females were employed for the injections because they were somewhat larger and therefore more easily injected. The size of the leafhoppers is illustrated in figure 4. Injected insects were transferred every 10 days to fresh rye plants and after 30 days the survivors were tested individually for 48 hr. on young aster plants. They were then macerated, diluted, and used for the next passage. The aster plants were kept under observation in a greenhouse for 6 weeks after the removal of the insects. Noninjected control insects from the same stock culture were caged on aster plants and transferred on the same days as the injected leafhoppers.

EXPERIMENTS AND RESULTS.—*Serial passage.*—The results of infectivity tests of the first six passages were not known at the time of maceration of the survivors. These passages are summarized in Table 1, A. One hundred viruliferous insects were used as a source of virus in the first transfer. The leafhopper pulp (140 mg.) was diluted 1:7000, so that the dilution of the virus in the insect juices actually was greater than stated. Parts of these diluted juices were injected into 200 virus-free leafhoppers which were maintained for the suc-

TABLE 1

Serial Passage of Aster-Yellows Virus through the Aster Leafhopper

Passage[a]	No. of injected insects	Days after injection on:		Survivors[c]	Calculated dilution
		Rye	Asters[b]		
A.					
1	200	30	2	36 (8)	$10^{-3.8}$
2	300	30	2	16 (3)	10^{-8}
3	150	30	2	2 (0)	10^{-12}
4	300	30	2	34 (5)	10^{-16}
5	100	30	2	5 (0)	10^{-20}
6	200	30	2	22 (5)	10^{-24}
B.					
7	100	6	54*	8 (2)	10^{-28}
8	240	40	25**	12 (4)	10^{-32}
9	50	19	13*	16 (6)	10^{-36}
10	50	30	20	4 (1)	10^{-40}

[a] The diluted insect juice in the fourth passage was filtered through sintered glass. Penicillin was added in the fourth, fifth, sixth, and seventh passages.

[b] Individual insects were transferred to individual aster plants: *three times weekly; **every 5 days.

[c] Number of infective survivors in parentheses. In series A, all 100 control insects for each passage survived, and in series B all 20 control insects for each passage survived.

ceeding 30 days on rye plants at 25° C. The 36 insects that survived were tested individually for 48 hr. on young aster plants. After 3 weeks this test showed that eight hoppers were infective. In the meantime the 36 insects were used as a source of virus for the next passage. Three hundred insects were injected; 16 survived 30 days and were used for the third passage. Three of them were later found to have been infective. In the third passage, 150 insects were injected and only two survived. These two survivors were macerated and, in an attempt to reduce the high mortality rate, penicillin was added and the supernatant filtered through a coarse glass filter. Of 300 injected insects in this passage, 34 survived and five proved infective. Thus the virus was not lost in the third passage in spite of the negative infectivity test. Penicillin was also added in the next three passages. In the fifth passage five insects survived but none of these proved infective; in the sixth passage, five of 22 survivors transmitted the virus.

The following four passages (Table 1, B) were made with some modifications of the previously used method. The 22 survivors of the sixth passage were macerated with the addition of penicillin, and 100 virus-free insects were injected. Eight survived a period of 60 days and two of them were infective. The eight survivors served as a source for the injection of 240 insects, of which 12 survived 65 days and four were infective. The insects of these two passages were not kept on rye continuously, but after a 6-day and a 40-day period, respectively, they were caged on asters and transferred three times weekly or every 5 days. Only the four infective survivors of the eighth passage were used for the inoculum of the ninth group. The injected insects were transferred three times weekly to fresh asters after an initial period of 19 days on rye. After 32 days, 16 of the 50 injected leafhoppers survived and four of them proved infective. The tenth and last passage, with 50 injected leafhoppers, was kept 30 days on rye, then tested on aster plants, and of four survivors one proved to be infective. The estimated dilution used to inoculate the insects of the tenth passage in the series, if no multiplication had occurred, would be at least 10^{-40} but aster-yellows virus in insect juices has been found infective at dilutions of 10^{-3} but not 10^{-4} or higher.

In experiments which will be discussed in more detail elsewhere (23), the concentration of virus in the first and ninth passages was measured by the use of a new method. The tests showed no decrease in virus concentration of the inoculum used in the ninth passage over that used in the first, and provided further direct evidence for multiplication of aster-yellows virus in the insect host.

Transfers of virus from "noninfective" viruliferous insects.—It was found, in two instances, that virus was carried over to the next group of insects although infectivity tests of the source insects proved negative. This occurred in the third and fifth passages. It is possible that some insects that did not transmit virus during the 48-hr. test feeding period were nevertheless infective, or that the incubation period of the virus in some insects was not completed by the time of their maceration. An attempt was therefore made to find whether or not very long incubation periods may account for the negative infectivity tests. The insects of the seventh passage were kept for 54 days on test plants, and not, as in the first six passages, for but 2 days. They were transferred to fresh plants three times weekly. The survivors were macerated individually and diluted to 10^{-3} and groups of 30 insects injected with each dilution. Insects No. 5 and No. 30 were infective in the seventh passage. The virus from No. 30 passed to two injected insects, whereas none of the insects injected with juice of No. 5 became infective. But the noninfective No. 21 of the seventh passage also contained enough virus to render two insects of the eighth passage infective. This may mean that in insect No. 21 the incubation period of the virus was not completed in the long span of 60 days which had elapsed since it was injected. This appears likely because in insect No. 5 of the seventh group the required incubation period was shown to be 52 days. It should be mentioned that in other tests of insects that acquired the virus by feeding, the average incubation period at 25° C. was 12 days. It was shown by Black (4) that aster-yellows virus can be recovered and transferred from viruliferous insects a number of days before the incubation is completed.[1]

Control experiments.—The control insects, amounting to 100 for each of the first six passages, came from the same stock as the injected ones and all proved virus-free. During winter months, when the last four passages were made, and outside contamination was unlikely to occur, the number of control insects was reduced to 20 for each passage. This was considered as a sufficient number because the stock of leafhoppers lived and bred entirely on rye plants, and the possibility of contamination of the stock culture in the insectary was therefore practically eliminated. In the seventh, eighth, and ninth passages insects were transferred to aster plants three times weekly by means of "leaf cages" (22). Individual hoppers were confined to single cages that were fastened to leaves. From five to ten control plants were inoculated at each transfer and all remained healthy.

To confirm the immunity of rye from aster-yellows, established long ago by Kunkel in early experiments with the disease (12), 50 viruliferous females were caged on rye and kept on it until some nymphs of the next generation reached the third instar stage. The 100 largest nymphs were caged individually on asters at 25° C. for 4 weeks. None of them transmitted aster yellows.

In a preliminary test it was found that at 25° C. approximately 47 per cent of insects acquired aster-yellows virus in a one-day infection feeding. It seemed desirable to define more accurately the length of time during which insects could be kept, without acquiring the virus, on inoculated test plants in which the incubation period was not completed. Forty aster plants were inoculated by means of infective insects, five feeding on each plant. Together with these infective adult insects, single virus-free nymphs were caged on the plants. After 24 hr. the infective adults and the test nymphs were removed, the adults discarded, and the nymphs caged on rye. Forty virus-free female leafhoppers were caged on the plants for 24 hr., then removed to rye and replaced by another group of 40 virus-free females. This was repeated until, on the 9th day, the first plant in the group showed symptoms of disease. The 40 insects

[1] Transfer from such insects can be described as "blind." This term is used in experimental transmission of animal viruses for the method whereby transfer to a healthy animal is made from an inoculated one at a time when no signs of infection can be noted.

which were removed on each day and kept at 25° C. on rye for 21 following days, were then tested on asters for one week. Of 312 survivors, one picked up virus on the 7th day, that is, 2 days before the first disease symptoms were observed. On the 8th day an additional nine insects acquired aster-yellows virus. Of the 40 inoculated plants all but three eventually became diseased. Ninety control insects, tested on asters, proved virus-free. The test showed that at 25° C. under the conditions of the experiment none of the tested insects were able to acquire the virus during the first 6 days of the incubation period of the virus in the plant. Therefore it was also concluded that the 2-day test feeding after each of the first six passages, as well as the transfers on asters in the later passages which were made every 2 to 5 days, could not have accounted for any increase of the virus in the tested insects.

Mortality of injected insects.—The high mortality of injected insects during the second and subsequent transfers presented a serious problem to the continuation of the serial passage experiment. It actually may have accounted for Black's failure to succeed with similar experiments in 1939–1942.[2] It was known from earlier tests by Black that the mortality could be decreased by filtration, but filtration also reduced the amount of virus in the inoculum.[3] Aster-yellows virus is presumably large and can be filtered only with difficulty. A preliminary test was made to find whether or not the mortality was due to an increase in pathogenicity of the virus towards the vector. This hypothesis could not be excluded in view of the fact that the serial passage eliminated the alternating plant host entirely from the life cycle of the virus. Ordinarily, when the virus alternates between plant and insect vector, no deleterious effect on the vector can be observed, although it would be difficult to detect any small disturbances or even small differences in the percentage that died. An alternative hypothesis could explain the increased mortality as due to bacterial and fungus contamination in injected insects. Undoubtedly many injected insects die of septicemia, and the mechanical injury even without infection may be responsible for some deaths.

An attempt was made to compare the mortality rate of insects injected with virus-containing and virus-free insect juices. Fifty virus-free females were injected with a 1:100 dilution of juices from infective leafhoppers, and another group of 50 virus-free females of the same age injected with a 1:100 dilution of juices from virus-free hoppers. Both groups of injected insects were transferred five times during 30 days to fresh rye plants and kept continuously at 25° C. under identical controlled conditions. The death rate in the two groups was almost exactly the same. On the 31st day the 10 and 12 survivors, respectively, of the viruliferous and virus-free leafhoppers were macerated and diluted 1:100, and two groups of 50 virus-free females were injected with

[2] Personal communication.
[3] Personal communication.

373

the dilutions. The injections were carried out with a single needle, the virus-free dilution being injected first. Utmost care was exercised to prevent excessive wounding. The 1/8000 cc. of inoculum was measured in the same way as in the serial passages. A pronounced decrease in the survival of the virus-carrying insects was observed during the first 3 days following injection (from 50 to 24, as compared to 50/42 in the virus-free group), and after 9 days the number decreased to 13, as compared to 32 in the second group. But on the 23rd day the number of survivors in both groups reached the same level (12 and 13, respectively). Noninjected insects decreased very slightly in number, due to death, and of 50 control insects in the two tests survivors numbered 40 and 37, respectively, by the 30th day of the experiments.

Dilution end-point.—It seemed desirable to find the dilution end-point of aster-yellows virus from insect juice in view of the fact that evidence for multiplication was derived from the calculated "dilution" in the serial passage. From earlier experiments by Black (4) it was known that a dilution of 10^{-3}, but not 10^{-4}, will render injected insects infective.

Several tests were made and a more detailed account will be given elsewhere in a study of virus concentration as related to the length of incubation periods in inoculated insects. Only one of the experiments will be briefly mentioned. Groups of 30, 45, 50, and 40 insects, respectively, were injected with dilutions of 10^{-1}, 10^{-2}, 10^{-3}, and 10^{-4} of juices from virus-containing leafhoppers. The injected insects were transferred on every day to individual fresh aster plants in colonies of not more than three, for 48 days, and afterwards three times weekly until the 64th day, when the last insect died. Transmission was obtained in the groups injected with 10^{-1}, 10^{-2}, and 10^{-3} dilutions. No transmission occurred with a 10^{-4} dilution. In two other tests negative results with 10^{-4} dilutions and transmission with 10^{-3} also confirmed Black's finding.

The positive infectivity test in the first transfer of the serial passage experiment occurred within 32 days, as shown by the eight insects that were rendered infective (Table 1). It seems very likely that the dilution of the inoculum used, $10^{-3.8}$, was near the dilution end-point. It is still possible, however, that occasionally an insect would become infective following an injection of a somewhat higher dilution.

DISCUSSION.—Earlier evidence indicated that several viruses multiply in both plants and insects. Experimental evidence was presented for the multiplication of rice stunt (10, 11), aster-yellows (4, 13, 14, 15, 19), club-leaf (5, 6), and wound-tumor virus (7, 18). These viruses have three characteristic features in common: the high specificity of vectors, the retention of the virus, and the incubation period. These features had led long ago to the assumption that such plant viruses might possibly multiply in their vectors. The opposite view was expressed in the past 15 years by a few workers (1, 2, 9, 26, 28, 30).

The aster-yellows virus was carried in 10 serial passages in the aster leafhopper. If the virus had been diluted without multiplication, the final dilution used to inoculate the tenth group of the series would have been 10^{-40}. This, of course, is inconceivable for a number of reasons. The virus of aster-yellows derived from viruliferous insects was shown to have a dilution end-point below 10^{-4}. No virus is known to have a dilution end-point[4] above 10^{-10}. In a recent paper Black pointed out that a mass of hydrogen weighing the same as a female leafhopper (1.7 mgm.) contains only about 5.1×10^{20} molecules (6). Therefore, the serial passage provided adequate direct evidence for multiplication of the aster-yellows virus in the aster leafhopper. Further evidence was provided when the concentrations of virus in the first and ninth transfers were compared and it was found that no decrease occurred in the virus concentration during the nine passages.

It should be pointed out that leafhoppers are sucking insects and do not take up living plant cells. Since viruses multiply only inside of living cells, the multiplication must have occurred in cells of the insect.

A few of the implications of plant virus multiplication in insects have recently been pointed out by Black (6). The virus of aster-yellows can no longer be considered as solely a plant virus. It is really both a plant and an animal virus and may therefore serve as a connecting link between the two groups. This will have to be considered in any future classification of viruses, heretofore separated into animal, plant, and bacterial groups. It allows also some speculation as to the origin of the yellows group of plant viruses. They could have originated as insect or animal viruses. Some of them have the capacity of passing through the egg of the vector to the progeny and are thus maintained indefinitely in insects without the necessity of alternating plant hosts (6, 11). An adaptation permitting them to multiply in plants may possibly have come about as a further step in evolution, and the passage through the egg may then have been gradually lost.

The ability of some viruses to multiply in such diversified hosts as plants and animals suggests strongly that they are living organisms. The early hypothesis of a precursor responsible for virus multiplication, which even in recent years received some support, can hardly account for aster-yellows multiplication. It seems unlikely that a large molecule-precursor would occur in two hosts that are so unrelated.

The high specificity of yellows viruses in relation to their insect vectors can easily be explained on the basis of multiplication. The specificity also supports

[4] The highest dilution end-points of 10^{-10}, of viruses derived from tissues, without concentration, were found for Russian Far East Encephalitis, Venezuelan Equine Encephalitis, Western Equine Encephalitis, and Eastern Equine Encephalitis (Olitsky, Peter K., personal communication), also for St. Louis Encephalitis (16) and yellow fever (17). Tobacco-mosaic virus in tobacco plant juices has a dilution end-point of 10^{-7} (Kunkel, L. O., personal communication).

the hypothesis of the origin of these viruses in insects. The aster-yellows virus is certainly better adapted to its vector, in which it causes no visible harm, than to plant hosts in which it invariably causes disease symptoms and sometimes death.

The possible harmful influence of the virus on the vector after it was passed from insect to insect has been pointed out. Although preliminary results had first suggested such deleterious effect, closer analysis does not permit such a conclusion at present.

The "blind" passage of virus was most likely due to a very long incubation period in some injected insects. On the other hand, it is possible that some injected insects harbored virus but never became infective because the virus did not reach the saliva. It is hoped that further investigations will elucidate this possibility.

The finding that the incubation period varied markedly in the vector, in relation to the dose, may indicate an essential difference between the mechanism of infection of plants and animals. Wounding may be a necessary condition for the infection of plants but not of animals.

The basic study of yellows viruses promises to be of importance to animal workers as well as plant workers.

SUMMARY

The virus of aster yellows was carried in the vector *Macrosteles divisus* through 10 serial passages. The transfer from insect to insect was made by means of injections, of measured volumes of 1/8000 cc. per insect, into the abdominal cavity. The insect pulp was diluted with neutral buffered saline to 10^{-3} of the weight of the surviving leafhoppers. In the first six passages each group of injected hoppers was kept for 30 days, following injection, on rye plants immune from aster yellows, then tested 48 hr. on aster plants and used for the next transfer. In the later passages insects were tested on asters and transferred three times weekly to a fresh set of plants for periods up to 60 days. Direct evidence was provided for the multiplication of the virus in the insect vector, as some insects of all but the third and fifth groups were found infective. The estimated dilution used to inoculate the tenth group of the series, if no multiplication had occurred, would have been 10^{-40}, but the dilution end-point of the virus from macerated insects was found to be below 10^{-4}. A comparison of virus concentration in the inoculum of the first and ninth passages showed no decrease in concentration. It is concluded that the aster-yellows virus, multiplying in both its plant and insect hosts, can be considered an animal as well as a plant virus.

LITERATURE CITED

1. BAWDEN, F. C. Plant viruses and virus diseases. 3rd ed., revised. 335 pp. Chronica Botanica Co., Waltham, Mass. 1950.

2. BENNETT, C. W., and HUGH E. WALLACE. Relation of the curly top virus to the vector, Eutettix tenellus. Jour. Agr. Res. [U. S.] **56**: 31–52. 1938.

3. BLACK, L. M. Mechanical transmission of aster-yellows virus to leafhoppers. (Abstr.) Phytopath. **30**: 2. 1940.

4. ————. Further evidence for multiplication of the aster-yellows virus in the aster leaf hopper. Phytopath. **31**: 120–135. 1941.

5. ————. Multiplication of clover club-leaf virus (Aureogenus clavifolium) in its vector. (Abstr.) Phytopath. **39**: 2. 1949.

6. ————. A plant virus that multiplies in its insect vector. Nature **166**: 852–853. 1950.

7. ————, and M. K. BRAKKE. Serial passage of the wound-tumor virus through its leafhopper vector. (Manuscript in preparation.)

8. BUGHER, JOHN C. A micromortar especially adapted to virus studies in insects. Proc. Soc. Exp. Biol. and Med. **43**: 422–424. 1940.

9. FREITAG, J. H. Negative evidence on multiplication of curly top virus in the beet leafhopper, Eutettix tenellus. Hilgardia **10**: 305–342. 1936.

10. FUKUSHI, T. Multiplication of virus in its vector. Proc. Imp. Acad. Japan **11**: 301–303. 1935.

11. ————. Retention of virus by its vectors through several generations. Proc. Imp. Acad. Japan **15**: 142–145. 1939.

12. KUNKEL, L. O. Studies on aster yellows. Amer. Jour. Bot. **13**: 646–705. 1926.

13. ————. Effect of heat on ability of Cicadula sexnotata (Fall.) to transmit aster yellows. Amer. Jour. Bot. **24**: 312–327. 1937.

14. ————. Insects in relation to diseases of fruit trees and small fruits. Jour. Econ. Entom. **31**: 20–22. 1938.

15. ————. Heat cure of aster yellows in periwinkles. Amer. Jour. Bot. **28**: 761–769. 1941.

16. LENNETTE, EDWIN H., and HILARY KOPROWSKI. Neutralization tests with certain neurotropic viruses. Jour. Immunol. **49**: 375–385. 1944.

17. ————, and ————. Influence of age on the susceptibility of mice to infection with certain neurotropic viruses. Jour. Immunol. **49**: 175–191. 1944.

18. MARAMOROSCH, KARL. Influence of temperature on incubation and transmission of the wound-tumor virus. Phytopath. **40**: 1071–1093. 1950.

19. ————. Effect of dosage on length of incubation period of aster-yellows virus in its vector. Proc. Soc. Exp. Biol. and Med. **75**: 744. 1950.

20. ————. Serial passage of aster-yellows virus through the aster leafhopper. (Abstr.) Phytopath. **41**: 25. 1951.

21. ————. A simple needle for micro-injections. Nature **167**: 734. 1951.

22. ————. Handy insect-vector cage. Jour. N. Y. Entomol. Soc. **59**: 49–50. 1951.

23. ————. New evidence for multiplication of aster-yellows virus in its vector. Nature (in press).

24. McMASTER, P. D., and G. H. HOGEBOOM. Formal Progress Report No. 683. Off. Sci. Res. and Dev. 1942.

25. MERRILL, MALCOLM H., and CARL TENBROECK. Multiplication of equine encephalomyelitis virus in mosquitoes. Proc. Soc. Exp. Biol. and Med. **32**: 421–423. 1934.

26. SMITH, KENNETH M. Viruses and virus diseases. I. Jour. Roy. Hort. Soc. **74:** 482–491. 1949.
27. STOREY, H. H. Investigations of the mechanism of the transmission of plant viruses by insect vectors. I. Proc. Roy. Soc. London, B, **113:** 463–485. 1933.
28. ————. Transmission of plant viruses. Bot. Rev. **5:** 240–272. 1939.
29. TENBROECK, CARL. A simple grinder for soft tissues. Science **74:** 98–99. 1931.
30. WATSON, M. Λ., and F. M. ROBERTS. A comparative study of the transmission of Hyoscyamus virus 3, potato virus Y and cucumber virus 1 by the vectors Myzus persicae (Sulz), M. circumflexus (Buckton), and Macrosiphum gei (Koch). Proc. Roy. Soc. London, B, **127:** 543–576. 1939.
31. WENT, F. W. The Earhart Plant Research Laboratory. Chronica Botanica **12:** 89–108. 1950.

STRUCTURES RESEMBLING MYCOPLASMA IN DISEASED PLANTS AND IN INSECT VECTORS

Karl Maramorosch, Eishiro Shikata and Robert R. Granados

INTRODUCTION

Fungi, bacteria, and viruses have been recognized for many years as infectious agents of disease in plants. Since diseased plants often manifest conspicuous yellowing, many names of diseases contain the word "yellow," irrespective of the causative disease agent. The so-called yellows-type diseases have been of special interest for many years as they cause serious economic losses to cultivated plants. In addition, intriguing biologic interactions have been discovered between the disease agents, the infected plants, and the insects that carry the agents to susceptible hosts. The insect vectors, so far as known, are limited to species belonging to a few families of leafhoppers and planthoppers (*Cicadellidae*). Yellows-type diseases are characterized by the growth of slender, adventitious shoots; chlorosis without spotting; clearing of veins; growth stimulation of normally dormant buds; malformation; stunting; virescence of flowers; sterility; and an abnormally erect, upright growth habit.

Filterable, graft-transmissible agents of yellows-type diseases of plants have been customarily considered as viruses because no bacteria, rickettsiae, fungi, or protozoa have been implicated as possible etiologic agents in diseased plants or in insect vectors. In several instances, leafhopper vectors were found to act as alternate hosts and reservoirs of the disease agents. Attempts to purify the causative agents and characterize them by electron microscopy have met with formidable difficulties.

The demonstration of leafhopper-borne plant-pathogenic viruses *in situ* in cells of diseased plants and in insect carriers (Fukushi *et al.*, 1960; Shikata *et al.*, 1964) suggested that the same techniques could be used for the localization and characterization of yellows-type disease agents. From 1963 to 1965, Dr. Eishiro Shikata, while on leave from Hokkaido University, studied thin sections of plants infected with aster yellows at the Boyce Thompson Institute. None of the thin sections revealed virus-like particles. The findings, reported in an abstract (Maramorosch *et al.*, 1968), are discussed in detail for the first time in this paper.

In 1967, Doi *et al.* in Japan described structures resembling mycoplasma or psittacosis-lymphogranuloma-trachoma (PLT) bodies in the phloem elements of plants naturally infected with mulberry dwarf, potato witches' broom, Japanese aster yellows, and paulownia witches' broom. Morphologically the structures were similar to those observed by us in American aster yellows-

TRANSACTIONS OF THE NEW YORK ACADEMY OF SCIENCES, 1968, Vol. 30, pp. 841-855.

infected plants. Doi and coworkers made a careful study of the fine structure of the bodies and suggested that these mycoplasma-like organisms were probably the causal agents of the respective diseases. No attempts were made to detect similar bodies in the respective insect vectors. Ishiie *et al.* (1967), working in the same laboratory as Doi, applied antibiotics to mulberry dwarf-diseased plants and observed that the mycoplasma or PLT-like structures were partly eliminated by the application of chlortetracycline hydrochloride (Aureomycin ® *) or tetracycline hydrochloride (Achromycin ® *), but not of kanamycin. The successful treatment consisted of root dipping or foliage spraying with 100 ppm of the tetracycline antibiotics. The plants were not permanently cured, and the disease reappeared several weeks after the treatment was stopped.

The reports of Doi *et al.* and Ishiie *et al.* prompted further work in our laboratory with aster yellows and corn stunt, as well as collaborative work with Drs. E. Shikata, T. Matsumoto, and K. C. Ling, in studying a sugarcane disease in Taiwan and a rice disease in the Philippines. The present paper will summarize earlier, pertinent findings with aster yellows and corn stunt that seemed to support the viral etiology and describe recent findings and a reevaluation of the conclusions, indicating the possible mycoplasma etiology of these, as well as of several other, leafhopper-borne diseases.

ASTER YELLOWS

The aster yellows disease is prevalent throughout the Nearctic zone of North America. A detailed description of the disease was made by Smith (1902), who was unable to find any parasitic organism and suggested at the time that aster yellows might be a virus disease. The pioneering work of L. O. Kunkel at the Boyce Thompson Institute established that the disease agent of aster yellows is transmitted from plant to plant in the eastern United States by the aster leafhopper, known today as *Macrosteles fascifrons* Stål (*Cicadula sexnotata* Fall.) (Kunkel, 1926). Mechanical transmission by rubbing or by needle puncture has never been successful in transmitting the disease agent to plants. An incubation period of at least nine days is required before the signs of disease appear. Production of chlorophyll is inhibited and general chlorosis sets in. In different plant species the disease causes widely different degrees of yellowing and malformation. Many economically important plants, such as carrots, lettuce, spinach, celery, onions, and others, succumb to the disease.

Kunkel (1926) found that aster leafhoppers confined to diseased plants required at least nine days before they were able to transmit the disease agent acquired by feeding. This protracted incubation period corresponds in length to the incubation period in the plant, and Kunkel suggested that the etiologic agent multiplies in both plants and leafhopper vectors.

The infectious agent of aster yellows can be inactivated by comparatively low temperatures that do not kill the insect vectors, and permit the heat cure of woody plants, such as *Vinca rosea*, infected with aster yellows (Kunkel, 1937b, 1938, 1941). Approximately 32° C was found as the critical temperature above which transmission by insects ceased. *Vinca* plants maintained for

*Product of Lederle Laboratories, a Division of American Cyanamid Co., Pearl River, N.Y.

several days at 44°C became permanently cured of aster yellows, while infective leafhoppers, subjected for eight days to 36°C, lost infectivity permanently. Such insects could be reinfected by repeated confinement to diseased plants. The etiologic agent of aster yellows was not attenuated by passage through different hosts, but an attenuated strain was obtained by heat treatment (Kunkel, 1937a). Aster yellows in middle and southern Europe (Richter, 1936; Heinze & Kunze, 1955; Valenta *et al.*, 1962; Książek, 1960; Sukhov & Vovk, 1945; Rischkov, 1943) and in Japan (Fukushi, 1930) is very similar to the American disease.

In 1940 Black succeeded in mechanically transmitting the disease agent to leafhoppers by needle inoculation. This technique provided the first bioassay and permitted a new approach to the study of the etiologic agent. Black attempted filtration experiments which were designed to demonstrate the "filterability" of the disease agent. Passage through Berkefeld N and V filters was difficult and usually accompanied by the passage of unidentified bacteria, considered an apparently normal contaminant of the preparation (Black, 1943). Infectivity was associated with a large size agent, labile, and presumed to form aggregates.

Mechanical transmission to insects was used by Black (1941) to demonstrate the multiplication of the agent in leafhoppers. The same technique was also used by Maramorosch (1952) for a serial passage through ten groups of insects, demonstrating the proliferation of aster yellows in leafhopper vectors. The length of incubation varied with the dosage of the inoculum (Maramorosch, 1950). In 1955 Kunkel found interference between two strains of aster yellows, not only in inoculated plants, but also in leafhopper vectors. Interactions among three strains in plants and insects have been reported by Freitag (1958, 1964, 1968). Interactions between European and American strains have been tested by Valenta (1959). Cytopathic changes have been described in leafhoppers carrying the aster yellows agent (Littau & Maramorosch, 1956, 1960).

Most of the accumulated experimental evidence seemed to favor the virus etiology of aster yellows, paralleling findings made with other, proven virus diseases of plants. Yet, attempts to purify the etiologic agent and to characterize it morphologically and chemically have met with remarkable difficulties. Dr. R. L. Steere (personal communication) has tried since 1950 to purify aster yellows, first by differential centrifugation, then by using butanol, and finally by agar gel filtration (Steere, 1967). In the latter, infectivity seemed distributed throughout the column. All tests indicated that the agent was fairly large, confirming the conclusion reached by Black in 1943. Lee and Chiykowski (1963) tried differential centrifugation but were unable to determine the size or to concentrate the infectious agent. Infectivity appeared not only in the low speed, but also in the high speed supernatant fractions. The only electron micrographs that were published (Protsenko, 1958, 1959) showed a highly heterogenous, unpurified accumulation of particles of various sizes; so-called "virus particles" of 30 millimicrons in diameter and of cubical symmetry were suspected as the infectious agent, but no attempts were made to link them experimentally (by insect injection) with infectivity.

ELECTRON MICROSCOPY OF THIN SECTIONS

In 1964 Dr. Eishiro Shikata began the study of thin sections of aster yellows diseased plants in an effort to localize the infectious agent. To preserve the cell structure, plant tissues were excised from diseased *Nicotiana rustica* L. or *Callistephus chinensis* Nees plants and fixed in 6% glutaraldehyde in 0.1 M phosphate buffer solution with 0.2 M sucrose for 90 minutes, then postfixed in 1% osmium tetroxide for 60 minutes. After dehydration in graded ethanol or acetone, the materials were embedded in epoxy resin. Thin sections of up to 50 millimicrons in thickness were cut with diamond knives on a MT-1 Porter-Blum microtome, and stained with a 6% uranyl acetate aqueous solution for 60 minutes, and with lead citrate for 15 minutes. Details of the procedure have been described (Shikata *et al.*, 1966; Hirumi *et al.*, 1967); observations were made with a Siemens Elmiskop I, or with a JEM electron microscope. Controls consisting of plant material from healthy specimens were prepared and examined in the same manner as the diseased material.

Since it was generally accepted that the disease agent was a virus, attempts were concentrated on finding virus-like particles. However, no rod-shaped or spherical particles were detected in thin sections of aster yellows diseased plants. Since the same techniques have been successfully employed in our laboratory for the localization of the leafhopper-borne wound tumor virus (Shikata *et al.*, 1964; Shikata & Maramorosch, 1965a & b, 1966a, 1967a & b; Granados *et al.*, 1967, 1968c; Hirumi *et al.*, 1967) and the aphid-borne pea enation mosaic virus (Shikata et al., 1966; Shikata & Maramorosch, 1966b), the inability to find virus particles in aster yellows diseased plants was at first interpreted as due to either very low concentration or the absence of virus in the cells.

Unexpectedly, in phloem cells of chlorotic adventitious shoots from diseased China aster plants, there consistently appeared accumulations of pleomorphic bodies, ranging in size from 80 to 800 millimicrons, spherical to irregularly elongated in shape, as shown in FIGURE 1. All structures were bounded by a single unit membrane, about 75 to 90 angstroms thick, and devoid of a cell wall. Although some small bodies in the range of 80 to 100 millimicrons (elementary bodies?) were observed, larger forms were more prevalent. Typical structures contained what seemed to be a central nuclear area, with strands of presumed DNA and a peripheral cytoplasmic area containing ribosome-like granules. Very few of the bodies had vacuoles. *N. rustica* plants, infected with aster yellows, contained bodies similar to those just described (Maramorosch *et al.*, 1968). No similar bodies were observed in healthy material from both plant species prepared in the same manner.

CORN STUNT

The corn stunt disease affects only two species of plants: *Zea mays* L., the cultivated maize or corn, and *Euchlena mexicana* Schrad., a wild grass believed to be related to maize. Several species of leafhoppers are now known to transmit the infectious agent of the disease. The first insect vector, *Dalbulus maidis* DeL. & W., was discovered by Kunkel (1946), who also identified the disease, named it, and studied its transmission (1948). Kunkel reported that the incubation period of the etiologic agent in the plant and in the leafhopper was 14 days or more. In 1950 Niederhauser and Cervantes found that the related species, *D. elimatus* DeL. & W., acted as a vector on the high plateau of Mexico where the disease is of economic importance. Granados *et al.* (1966) discovered the third vector, *Graminella nigrifrons* (Forbes), and

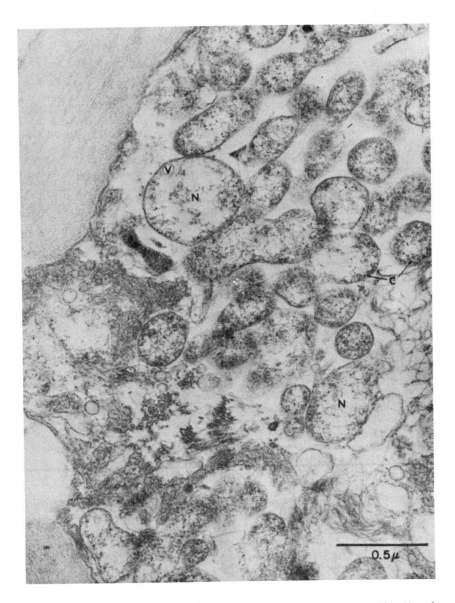

FIGURE 1. Mycoplasma-like bodies in a phloem cell of a young chlorotic, adventitious shoot from a China aster plant infected with aster yellows. A central nuclear-like area (N) with net-like strands, the peripheral cytoplasmic area (C) with ribosome-like granules, and a vacuole (V) are indicated. Mag. x48,500.

recently the fourth species, able to transmit corn stunt (Granados *et al.*, 1968a, b). Several strains of the disease agent occur in nature, and interference of strains has been described in plants and in insect vectors (Maramorosch, 1958). Leafhoppers can be infected mechanically, by needle inoculation, with extracts from diseased plants or insects (Maramorosch, 1951), but all attempts to infect plants mechanically and to purify the causative agent have failed.

Following Shikata's work with aster yellows virus, which came to a temporary close with his return to Japan in 1965, Dr. Robert R. Granados began to study thin sections of corn leafhoppers, *D. elimatus*, prepared in the same manner as sections from aster yellows diseased material.

In infective leafhoppers, mycoplasma-like bodies, 80 to 800 millimicrons in diameter, were observed in the ventral ganglia cells (FIGURE 2) and in the filter chamber region of the intestine (FIGURE 3). All bodies were bounded by a single unit membrane about 70 to 85 angstroms thick. Bodies with cell walls were never observed, although several hundred sections have been examined. The mycoplasma-like bodies possessed two main types of internal structures. One type, found mainly in the ventral ganglia cells (FIGURE 2), contained ribosome-like granules about 10 to 15 millimicrons in size in a ground substance of intermediate to high density. In these bodies, nuclear areas with net-like strands were not very prominent. A second type, found in the intestinal cells (FIGURE 3), had large zones of net-like strands, presumed to be nuclear areas. The cytoplasm in this type consisted of ribosome-like granules in a ground substance of light density. Elementary-like bodies, 80 to 95 millimicrons in diameter, were common in many of the infected cells (FIGURE 2). Mycoplasma-like structures have not been found in controls from stock colonies of *D. elimatus* raised on healthy plants.

Young, chlorotic, adventitious shoots of diseased corn plants, fixed and embedded in epoxy resin, were prepared by Mrs. Lorraine S. Ward in the same manner as described for aster yellows, and shipped to Dr. Shikata at Hokkaido University for examination. Mycoplasma-like bodies, similar to those found by Dr. Granados in the insect vectors, were present in the phloem cells of diseased corn plants (FIGURE 4). In addition, small spherical bodies and elongated filamentous structures were also found. They resembled bodies described for human mycoplasma species (Anderson & Barile, 1965). The filamentous bodies detected in corn cells did not clearly reveal the presence of unit membranes.

The finding of mycoplasma-like bodies in corn stunt diseased plants, as well as in leafhopper vectors carrying the disease agent, and their absence in healthy plants and in stock insects, is of particular significance because it is the first reported instance of mycoplasma-like bodies in insect vectors of a plant disease.

Preliminary results of tetracycline treatment of corn stunt inoculated plants indicated that the disease can be arrested by antibiotic treatment. These studies are being continued and expanded to treatments of infective insect vectors. It now appears that transmission can be impaired temporarily by the injection of tetracycline into leafhopper vectors.

OTHER YELLOWS-TYPE DISEASES

In Taiwan Shikata *et al.* (1968) found mycoplasma-like bodies in phloem elements of sugarcane plants infected with the white leaf disease agent, but

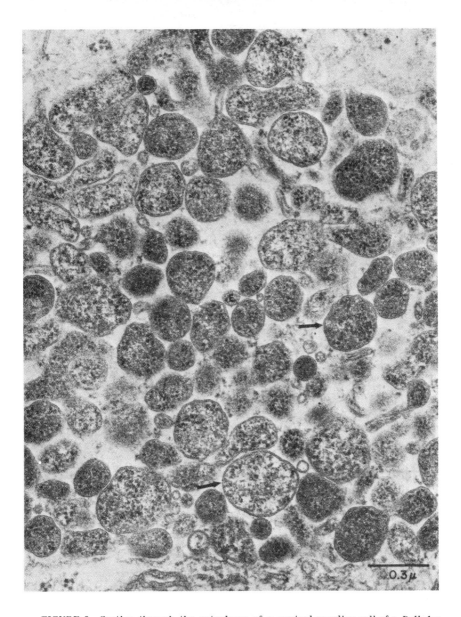

FIGURE 2. Section through the cytoplasm of a ventral ganglion cell of a *Dalbulus elimatus* leafhopper infected with corn stunt. Mycoplasma-like bodies bounded by a single unit membrane (arrows) contain ribosome-like granules in a ground substance of intermediate to high density. Note elementary-like bodies (E) which range in size from 80-90 m μ. Mag. x52,500.

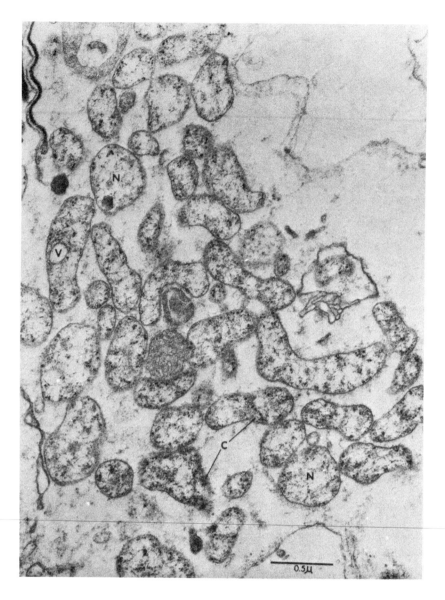

FIGURE 3. Mycoplasma-like bodies in an intestinal cell of a *Dalbulus elimatus* leaf-hopper infected with corn stunt. These bodies show the same internal structures described in FIGURE 1. N = central nuclear-like area; C = peripheral cytoplasmic area with ribosome-like granules; V = vacuole. Mag. x34,500.

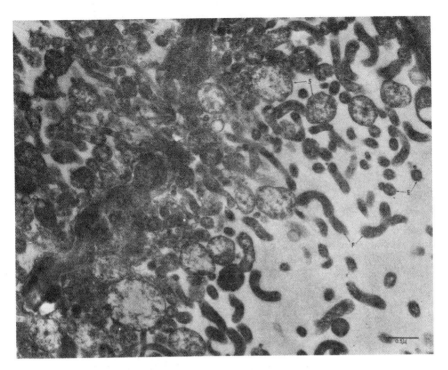

FIGURE 4. Section through a phloem cell of a corn plant infected with corn stunt. Note spherical (S) and filamentous (F) mycoplasma-like bodies. Compare with FIGURES 2 and 3. Numerous elementary-like bodies (E) are probably cross sections through filaments. Mag. x18,500.

no virus-like particles could be detected in such plants. The phloem of healthy sugarcane plants was free from mycoplasma-like bodies. In addition, a rice disease in the Philippines, known as yellow dwarf, has also been examined and similar mycoplasma-like bodies have been detected (Shikata *et al.*, 1968). Recently Dr. Petru Ploaie, on leave from the Institute of Biology "Traian Savulescu" in Bucharest, has been working at the Boyce Thompson Institute under the U.S. National Academy and Rumanian Academy of Sciences exchange program. While at the Boyce Thompson Institute, Dr. Ploaie examined thin sections from plants infected with Crimean yellows from the USSR, stolbur from Rumania, and para-stolbur and clover dwarf from Czechoslovakia. In all four diseases, mycoplasma-like bodies have been observed, while healthy plants were devoid of such bodies. No virus-like particles were found in any of the infected plants.

Maniloff (1967) demonstrated that the fine structure of different species of mycoplasma can be distinguished by electron microscopy. If the bodies detected in yellows-diseased plants should indeed prove to be species of mycoplasma, it will be of interest to study possible differences in their fine structure. Attempts are under way in several laboratories to isolate and culture these bodies, in order to establish whether they are the etiologic agents of the respective diseases. Until now, no successful cultivation has been achieved.

Antibiotic treatments seem to provide a useful approach to the control of several yellows-type diseases. The work in Japan with mulberry dwarf by Ishiie *et al.* (1967) has been called by us to the attention of colleagues at the Pioneering Virus Laboratory of the U. S. Department of Agriculture in Beltsville, Md. Recently Davis *et al.* (1968) of that laboratory confirmed Ishiie's findings, using aster yellows inoculated plants, as well as aster leaf-hoppers carrying the disease agent. They found that chlortetracycline at 100 ppm suppressed the development of disease signs in treated plants, and injection of the antibiotic into leafhoppers at 1000 ppm, simultaneously with extracts containing the disease agent, prevented subsequent transmission.

OTHER STRUCTURES RESEMBLING MYCOPLASMA-LIKE BODIES

Electron microscopy, in itself, is not adequate to positively identify mycoplasmas. Cell walls are sometimes not seen well in electron micrographs, and it may be that in some stages of the life cycle a cell wall is not visible in the Chlamydozoaceae (trachoma, lymphogranuloma venereum, ornithosis, etc.). Similarly, bacterial L forms have no cell wall and are pleomorphic. Nevertheless, the bodies found in infected plants and insects are quite typical for mycoplasma (Drs. K. Hummeler, D. Armstrong, D. R. Anderson, and L. Dienes, personal communication).

An electron microscopy study by Hirumi *et al.* (1967) of the nervous system of *Agallia constricta* revealed not only the invasion of the central nervous system by the plant-pathogenic wound-tumor virus, but also uncovered the presence of bodies that superficially resembled mycoplasma of yellows-diseased plants. Hemocytes of *A. constricta*, studied by Dr. Granados, were found to contain similar structures (FIGURE 5). However, the bodies, present in virus-carrying as well as in virus-free individuals, were characterized by a rippled cell wall, indicating that they were rickettsiae, probably symbiotic species known to occur in leafhoppers (Nasu, 1965).

Normal animal and plant cells may contain mitochondria that, in some stages of development or degeneration, bear a superficial resemblance to the mycoplasma-like bodies described in yellows-diseased plants. However, the internal structure of the mycoplasma-like bodies differed from such mitochondria, and they did not contain cristae. In addition, the bodies that were found only in diseased plants and in infective insects, but not in controls, were accompanied by elementary-like bodies.

DISCUSSION

The presence of filterable, mycoplasma-like forms in nature is apparently fairly common, and the filterable organisms described in 1936 by Laidlaw and Elford are now considered to belong to the mycoplasma group. Diseases of birds and of higher animals, including man, are known to be caused by various mycoplasma species. Yet the existence of mycoplasma-infecting plants or insects has not been considered in the past. One might wonder how such mycoplasma would differ from those of higher animals, what their characteristics would be, and whether their host range would be limited to a few species of invertebrates and to plants, or whether they could also infect mammals.

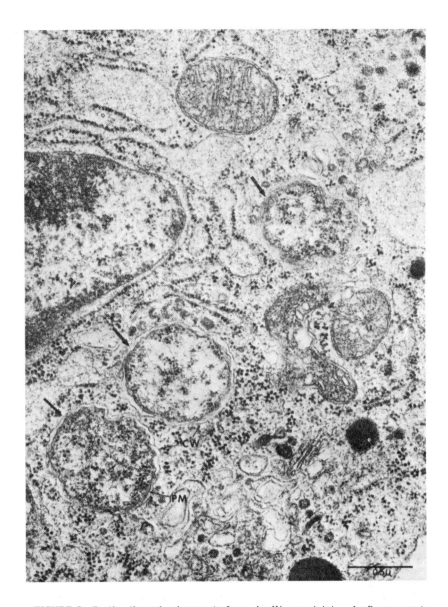

FIGURE 5. Section through a hemocyte from *Agallia constricta*, a leafhopper vector of the plant pathogenic wound tumor virus. Three rickettsia-like structures (arrows) can be seen in the cell cytoplasm. The characteristic rippled cell well (CW) is obvious and the underlying plasma membrane (PM) can be seen in several places. Note the similarity of the internal structures when compared with mycoplasma-like bodies in FIGURES 1-4. Mag. x37,500.

Most of the data reported in the past for the infectious agents of aster yellows or corn stunt can apply equally well to viruses as to mycoplasma, PLT, or L-forms of bacteria. Small size, interference of strains, filterability, resistance to most antibiotics and even cytopathic effects in vitro are features common to both viruses and PPLO. Sensitivity to 32°C has not, of course, been associated with mycoplasma species infecting warm-blooded animals, but it is conceivable that species found in plants or in insects could be affected by such comparatively low temperatures. In this connection it might be worthwhile to point out the similarity between the infectious agent of aster yellows and the *Drosophila* sterility factor (Ehrman, 1967). Both react to heat administered to the carriers. Since aster yellows does not pass through the egg to the progeny of vectors, its presence in leafhoppers can only be ascertained by testing their transmitting ability. Kunkel (1938) demonstrated complete "cure" of vectors by exposing them to 36°C for eight days. While the eastern yellows strain proved heat labile, exposure of other strains to 32°C was not effective (Chapman, 1949; Granados, 1965). In *Drosophila*, heat shocks interfere with the transovarial infection of successive generations, although heat does not cure the carriers entirely (Ehrman, 1967). It now appears that the cytoplasmic, inherited factor of *Drosophila* sterility may also belong to the mycoplasma group (Ehrman, personal communication).

CONCLUSIONS

In conclusion, it now appears that the so-called yellows-type diseases of plants, until now considered to be caused by leafhopper-borne viruses that were believed to multiply in infected plants as well as in insect vectors, might be caused by various species of mycoplasma-like organisms. Attempts are under way in several laboratories to isolate and culture these etiologic agents, but until now cultivation has not been achieved. The Koch postulates have not yet been satisfied in the case of aster yellows, corn stunt, or other yellows-type diseases in which mycoplasma-like bodies have been demonstrated by electron microscopy. These diseases had been arbitrarily classified as virus diseases merely on the basis of their transmission by leafhoppers and the type of disease syndrome. Now the combined results of electron microscopy observations and chemotherapy experiments strongly suggest that they might be caused by mycoplasma-like organisms, and not by viruses.

The practical implications of the findings are seen in the feasibility of applying antibiotic therapy for the cure of yellows-type diseases of plants. It can be expected that several diseases of uncertain etiology, including economically important diseases of the coconut palm (Maramorosch, 1964), will be reinvestigated in the light of present findings. If such diseases should prove to be caused by mycoplasma-like organisms, their chemotherapy might become economically sound.

Several other insect-transmitted plant pathogens may be found to be mycoplasma-like agents. It will be interesting to review their beneficial and harmful effects (Maramorosch & Jensen, 1963) in this new perspective.

REFERENCES

ANDERSON, D. R. & M. F. BARILE. 1965. Ultrastructure of *Mycoplasma orale* isolated from patients with leukemia. J. Natl. Cancer Inst. 36: 161-167.

BLACK, L. M. 1940. Mechanical transmission of aster-yellows virus to leaf hoppers. Phytopathology 30: 2.

BLACK, L. M. 1941. Further evidence for multiplication of the aster-yellows virus in the aster leaf hopper. Phytopathology 31: 120-135.

BLACK, L. M. 1943. Some properties of aster-yellows virus. Phytopathology 33: 2.

CHAPMAN, R. K. 1949. Some factors affecting the transmission of aster-yellows virus by the six-spotted leafhopper, *Macrosteles divisus* (Uhl.). Ph.D. Thesis. Univ. of Wisconsin, Madison, Wis.

DAVIS, R. E., R. F. WHITCOMB & R. L. STEERE. 1968. Chemotherapy of aster yellows disease. Phytopathology 58: In press.

DOI, Y., M. TERENAKA, K. YORA & H. ASUYAMA. 1967. Mycoplasma- or PLT group-like microorganisms found in the phloem elements of plants infected with mulberry dwarf, potato witches' broom, aster yellows, or paulownia witches' broom. (In Japanese, English summary.) Ann. Phytopath. Soc. Japan 33: 259-266.

EHRMAN, L. 1967. A study of infectious hybrid sterility in *Drosophila paulistorum*. Proc. Natl. Acad. Sci. USA 58: 195-198.

FREITAG, J. H. 1958. Cross-protection tests with 3 strains of the aster yellows virus in host plants and in the aster leafhopper. Phytopathology 48: 393.

FREITAG, J. H. 1964. Interaction and mutual suppression among three strains of aster yellows virus. Virology 24: 401-413.

FREITAG, J. H. 1968. Interactions of plant viruses and strains in their insect vectors. *In* Viruses, Vectors, and Vegetation. K. Maramorosch, ed. Interscience Publishers, New York, N.Y. In press.

FUKUSHI, T. 1930. Aster yellows in Japan. (In Japanese). Agriculture & Gardening 5: 557-584.

FUKUSHI, T., E. SHIKATA, I. KIMURA & M. NEMOTO. 1960. Electron microscopic studies on the rice dwarf virus. Proc. Japan Acad. 36: 352-357.

GRANADOS, R. R. 1965. Strains of aster-yellows virus and their transmission by the six-spotted leafhopper, *Macrosteles fascifrons* (Stål). Ph.D. Thesis. Univ. of Wisconsin, Madison, Wis.

GRANADOS, R. R., J. S. GRANADOS, K. MARAMOROSCH & J. REINITZ. 1968a. Corn stunt virus: Transmission by three cicadellid vectors. J. Econ. Entomol. 61: in press.

GRANADOS, R. R., R. D. GUSTIN, K. MARAMOROSCH & W. N. STONER. 1968b. Transmission of corn stunt virus by the leafhopper, *Deltocephalus sonorus* Ball. Contrib. Boyce Thompson Inst. (In press.)

GRANADOS, R. R., H. HIRUMI & K. MARAMOROSCH. 1967. Electron microscopic evidence for wound-tumor virus accumulation in various organs of an inefficient leafhopper vector, *Agalliopsis novella*. J. Invertebrate Pathol. 9: 147-159.

GRANADOS, R. R., K. MARAMOROSCH, T. EVERETT & T. P. PIRONE. 1966. Transmission of corn stunt virus by a new leafhopper vector, *Graminella nigrifrons* (Forbes). Contrib. Boyce Thompson Inst. 23: 275-280.

GRANADOS, R. R., L. S. WARD & K. MARAMOROSCH. 1968c. Insect viremia caused by a plant-pathogenic virus: Electron microscopy of vector hemocytes. Virology 34: 790-796.

HEINZE, K. & L. KUNZE. 1955. Die europäische Asterngelbsucht und ihre Übertragung durch Zwergzikaden. Nachrbl. Deut. Pflanzenschutzdienstes (Brunswick) 7: 161-164.

HIRUMI, H., R. R. GRANADOS & K. MARAMOROSCH. 1967. Electron microscopy of a plant-pathogenic virus in the nervous system of its insect vector. J. Virol. 1: 430-444.

ISHIIE, T., Y. DOI, K. YORA & H. ASUYAMA. 1967. Suppressive effects of antibiotics of tetracycline group on symptom development of mulberry dwarf disease. (In Japanese, English summary.) Ann. Phytopath. Soc. Japan 33: 267-275.

KSIAZEK, D. 1960. Experiments with mechanical transmission of yellow-dwarf virus (*Allium virus* 1 Melhus) and aster yellows virus (*Callistephus virus* 1 A Smith) on some species of *Allium* by sap inoculation method. (In Polish, English summary.) Acta Agrobotan. (Warsaw) 9: 75-87.

KUNKEL, L. O. 1926. Studies on aster yellows. Am. J. Botany 13: 646-705.

KUNKEL, L. O. 1937a. Isolation of mild strains of aster yellows from heat-treated leafhoppers. J. Bacteriol. 34: 132.

KUNKEL, L. O. 1937b. Effect of heat on ability of *Cicadula sexnotata* (Fall.) to transmit aster yellows. Am. J. Botany 24: 316-327.

KUNKEL, L. O. 1938. Insects in relation to diseases of fruit trees and small fruits. J. Econ. Entomol. 31: 20-22.

KUNKEL, L. O. 1941. Heat cure of aster yellows in periwinkles. Am. J. Botany 28: 761-769.

KUNKEL, L. O. 1946. Leafhopper transmission of corn stunt. Proc. Natl. Acad. Sci. USA 32: 246-247.

KUNKEL, L. O. 1948. Studies on a new corn virus disease. Arch. Ges. Virusforsch. 4: 24-46.

KUNKEL, L. O. 1955. Cross protection between strains of yellows-type viruses. Advances in Virus Research 3: 251-273.

LAIDLAW, P. P. & W. J. ELFORD. 1936. A new group of filterable organisms. Proc. Roy. Soc. (London) Ser. B. 120: 292-303.

LEE, P. E. & L. N. CHIYKOWSKI. 1963. Infectivity of aster-yellows virus preparations after differential centrifugations of extracts from viruliferous leafhoppers. Virology 21: 667-669.

LITTAU, V. C. & K. MARAMOROSCH. 1956. Cytological effects of aster-yellows virus on its insect vector. Virology 2: 128-130.

LITTAU, V. C. & K. MARAMOROSCH. 1960. A study of the cytological effects of aster yellows virus on its insect vector. Virology 10: 483-500.

MANILOFF, J. 1967. Organization of small cells: The pleuropneumonia-like organisms. J. Cell Biol. 35(2, pt.2): 87A.

MARAMOROSCH, K. 1950. Effect of dosage on length of incubation period of aster-yellows virus in its vector. Proc. Soc. Exptl. Biol. Med. 75: 744.

MARAMOROSCH, K. 1951. Mechanical transmission of corn stunt virus to an insect vector. Phytopathology 41: 833-838.

MARAMOROSCH, K. 1952. Direct evidence for the multiplication of aster-yellows virus in its insect vector. Phytopathology 42: 59-64.

MARAMOROSCH, K. 1958. Cross protection between two strains of corn stunt virus in an insect vector. Virology 6: 448-459.

MARAMOROSCH, K. 1964. A survey of coconut diseases of unknown etiology. Food and Agriculture Organization, Rome.

MARAMOROSCH, K. & D. D. JENSEN, 1963. Harmful and beneficial effects of plant viruses in insects. Ann. Rev. Microbiol. 17: 495-530.

MARAMOROSCH, K., E. SHIKATA & R. R. GRANADOS. 1968. Mycoplasma-like bodies in leafhoppers and diseased plants. Phytopathology 58: In press.

NASU, S. 1965. Electron microscopic studies on transovarial passage of rice dwarf virus. Jap. Jour. Appl. Entomol. Zool. 9: 225-237.

NIEDERHAUSER, J. S. & J. CERVANTES. 1950. Transmission of corn stunt in Mexico by a new insect vector, *Baldulus elimatus*. Phytopathology 40: 20-21.

PROTSENKO, A. E. 1958. Elektronoskopiya fitopatogennykh virusov. I. Virus zheltukhi astr. [Electron micrography of phytopathogenic viruses I. Aster yellows virus.] Mikrobiologiya 27: 131-132.

PROTSENKO, A. E. 1959. Electron microscopy of the aster yellows virus (*Leptomotropus callistephi* Ryzhkov). Biol. Plant. Acad. Sci. Bohemoslav. 1: 187-191.

RICHTER, H. 1936. Die Gelbsucht der Sommerastern. Nachrbl. Deut. Pflanzenschutsd. 16: 66-67.

RISCHKOV, V. L. 1943. Kok-saghyz yellows. Compt. Rend. Acad. Sci. URSS, N.S. 41: 90-92.

SHIKATA, E. & K. MARAMOROSCH. 1965a. Electron microscopic evidence for the systemic invasion of an insect host by a plant pathogenic virus. Virology 27: 461-475.

SHIKATA, E. & K. MARAMOROSCH. 1965b. Plant tumour virus in arthropod host: Microcrystal formation. Nature 208: 507-508.

SHIKATA, E. & K. MARAMOROSCH. 1966a. An electron microscope study of plant neoplasia induced by wound tumor virus. J. Natl. Cancer Inst. 36: 97-116.

SHIKATA, E. & K. MARAMOROSCH. 1966b. Electron microscopy of pea enation mosaic virus in plant cell nuclei. Virology 30: 439-454.

SHIKATA, E. & K. MARAMOROSCH. 1967a. Electron microscopy of wound tumor virus assembly sites in insect vectors and plants. Virology 32: 363-377.

SHIKATA, E. & K. MARAMOROSCH. 1967b. Electron microscopy of the formation of wound tumor virus in abdominally inoculated insect vectors. J. Virol. 1: 1052-1073.

SHIKATA, E., K. MARAMOROSCH & R. R. GRANADOS. 1966. Electron microscopy of pea enation mosaic virus in plants and aphid vectors. Virology 29: 426-436.

SHIKATA, E., K. MARAMOROSCH, K. C. LING & T. MATSUMOTO. 1968. On the mycoplasma-like structures encountered in the phloem cells of American aster yellows, corn stunt, Philippine rice yellow dwarf and Taiwan sugar cane white leaf diseased plants. Ann. Phytopath. Soc. Japan 34(2): In press.

SHIKATA, E., S. W. ORENSKI, H. HIRUMI, J. MITSUHASHI & K. MARAMOROSCH. 1964. Electron micrographs of wound-tumor virus in an animal host and in a plant tumor. Virology 23: 441-444.

SMITH, R. E. 1902. Growing China asters. Hatch Expt. Sta. Mass. Agr. Coll. Bull. 79.

STEERE, R. L. 1967. Gel filtration of aster yellows virus. Phytopathology 57: 832.

SUKHOV, K. S. & A. M. VOVK. 1945. On the identity between yellow of kok-saghyz and yellow of aster and its possible relation to big bud in tomato. Compt. Rend. Acad. Sci. URSS, N.S. 48: 365-368.

VALENTA, V. 1959. Interference studies with yellows-type plant viruses. I. Cross protection tests with European viruses. II. Cross protection tests with European and American viruses. Acta Virol. (Prague) 3: 145-152.

VALENTA, V., M. MUSIL & S. MIŠIGA. 1961. Investigations on European yellows-type viruses. I. The stolbur virus. Phytopathol. Z. 42: 1-38.

ACERIA TULIPAE KEIFER (ACARINA: ERIOPHYIDAE) IN RELATION TO THE SPREAD OF WHEAT STREAK MOSAIC [1]

John T. Slykhuis [2]

The discovery of an eriophyid mite on wheat and the demonstration of its ability to transmit wheat streak mosaic virus (*Marmor virgatum* McK.) were reported earlier (13). Workers in Nebraska, Kansas, and Oklahoma have since found the same species of mite and have verified its function as a vector of wheat streak mosaic in their areas[3]. Eriophyid mites collected from wheat in various areas where wheat streak mosaic occurs have been identified as *Aceria tulipae* Keifer.

Amos et al (1) and Massee (5, 6) reported that *Eriophyes ribis* (Westw.) Nal. transmitted "Reversion," a destructive disease of black currants. There is evidence that "Reversion" is caused by a virus and if so this is the only previous instance recorded in which a mite has been implicated in the transmission of a virus disease of plants.

This paper includes a discussion of *A. tulipae* in relation to wheat streak mosaic and other chlorotic symptoms on wheat, and a report on experiments with factors that influence the dispersal, perpetuation, and control of the mite in conjunction with the virus disease it carries.

[1] Contribution No. 1406 from the Botany and Plant Pathology Division, Science Service, Canada Department of Agriculture, Ottawa, Ontario.

[2] Plant Pathologist, Plant Pathology Laboratory, Lethbridge, Alberta, Canada.

The writer is indebted to Dr. H. H. Keifer, California Department of Agriculture, Sacramento, California, for identifying mites collected on wheat and wild grasses. He is also indebted to J. E. Moffatt for technical assistance in designing cages for the mites, and to Dr. M. W. Cormack for many helpful suggestions during the preparation of the manuscript.

[3] Wheat mosaic project review, held at Kansas State College, June 2-3, 1953.

ADVANCES IN VIRUS RESEARCH, 1965, Vol. 11, pp. 97-137.

MATERIALS AND METHODS.—The eriophyid mites are so small that a 30- to 40-power stereoscopic microscope was a valuable aid when working with them. Since leaves infested with *A. tulipae* are usually tightly rolled, metal hair clips were utilized to hold the leaves flat on a gass slide to facilitate observation of the mites. Individual mites or eggs were readily transferred with a single squirrel hair of suitable flexibility glued to a wooden handle about the size of a pencil. Sometimes the mites were transferred by placing short pieces of infested leaves against the leaves of plants to be infested. In other experiments it was convenient to use an electric fan to blow mites from a few mite-infested plants to a large number of plants to be infested.

The methods of caging infested plants varied with the nature of the experiment. Sometimes it was necessary to ascertain that only 1 mite fed on an individual plant. In such cases mites or eggs were placed singly on wheat seedlings grown from surface-sterilized seeds sown in sterilized soil in 2.3 cm × 20 cm test tubes tightly plugged with cotton. Sometimes infested plants growing in pots or flats were caged under cylindrical celluloid cages with open bases pressed into the soil around the plants (Fig. 1, A and C). The cages varied in size from 2.5 cm × 20 cm for individual plants to 10 cm × 25 cm for several plants. The ends of the larger cages were reinforced with metal rings cemented to the celluloid. White nylon taffeta cloth was cemented over the top and over the 2 ventilator openings in the sides. This cloth allowed diffusion of air but prevented the passage of mites.

A cage large enough to contain several pots of plants was desirable for maintaining stock colonies of mites. A suitable large cage consisted of a celluloid cylinder approximately 2 ft. high and 2 ft. in diameter, the base of which was cemented securely in a groove in a weatherproof plywood disc. The celluloid was supported by an inside framework of heavy wire welded at the joints. White nylon taffeta cloth was cemented over 2 large ventilator holes on opposite sides of the cylinder. The top was also covered with nylon taffeta in the form of a sleeve, which could be tied to close the cage. A stoppered glass or copper tube tied in the sleeve facilitated watering the pots without opening the cage (Fig. 1, B).

Non-infective mites were acquired by transferring eggs to healthy wheat seedlings in large test tubes where the eggs hatched and the mites multiplied rapidly. The mites were transferred to healthy wheat seedlings in 6-in. pots placed in large celluloid cages.

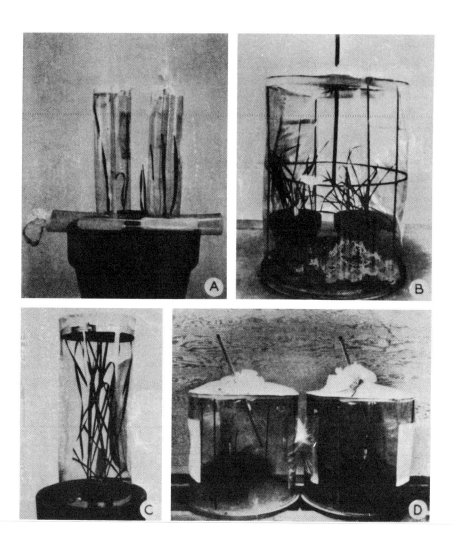

Fig. 1. Celluloid cages used in transmission experiments and for rearing eriophyid mites on wheat. A) Cages, 2.5 × 20 cm, for individual plants. B) Large cage into which several pots can be placed. Note the tube to facilitate watering without opening the cage. C) Cages, 10 × 25 cm, with ends reinforced with metal rings cemented to the celluloid. D) Double cage made by connecting 2 large cages with nylon taffeta cloth forming an opening between the 2 chambers.

Under these conditions the mites multiplied prolifically on the wheat.

SYMPTOMS ASSOCIATED WITH A. TULIPAE ON WHEAT.— Wheat plants naturally infested with *A. tulipae* show various symptoms including a marginal leaf roll, varying degrees of leaf chlorosis and necrosis, stunting, and, in extreme cases, death of the plants. The mites, wheat streak mosaic virus, and apparently a hitherto-unrecognized factor operate either singly or in combination to produce these symptoms.

Mite damage.—All collections of *A. tulipae* from wheat, including mites reared from eggs on healthy plants, cause a longitudinal leaf roll that is sometimes so extreme that the leaves resemble garlic (Fig. 2, A). This symptom is more extreme on plants infested during or before stooling. On field or older greenhouse-grown plants with tougher foliage the rolling is usually confined to the leaf margins. Mites reared from up to 10 eggs hatched on 82 individual healthy plants caused no apparent chlorosis until they became numerous, i.e. several hundred mites per plant. They then caused a chlorotic leaf spotting and eventually necrosis.

Wheat streak mosaic virus.—This virus, transmitted by artificial sap inoculation or by mites that acquired it from artifically infected plants, causes light green to yellow dashes and streaks (Fig. 3, A). In more advanced stages of the disease, a more general chlorosis and stunting result. Varying degrees of necrosis may develop, sometimes leading to death of the plant.

Non-manually transmitted factor carried by A. tulipae.—Observations and experiments have indicated that *A. tulipae* often carries a non-manually transmitted factor causing chlorosis, necrosis, and stunting. This factor apparently induces 2 types of symptoms on Kharkov 22 M.C. winter wheat. One type (Fig. 3, B) appears first as light green spots about 0.5 mm × 1 mm in size. These spots intensify to yellow and may become necrotic. They enlarge and coalesce to form chlorotic or necrotic areas and may render the entire leaf chlorotic or necrotic. The other type of chlorosis is evident first as a light green mottle, but develops into a yellowing that may include the entire leaf (Fig. 3, C). Either type of chlorosis results in loss of functional leaves, stunting, and often death of plants.

The additional factor was suspected when it was observed that wheat naturally infected with wheat streak mosaic in the field usually developed more severe chlorosis, necrosis, and stunting than wheat infected by manual methods. It was also found that mites from naturally diseased wheat usually induced more severe symptoms on wheat than mites from non-infective

397

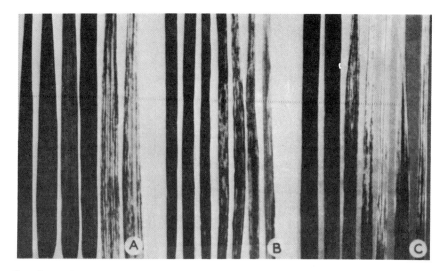

FIG. 3. Leaves of Kharkov 22 M.C. wheat showing 3 types of chlorotic symptoms induced by mites from naturally diseased wheat: A) wheat streak mosaic; B) a chlorotic and necrotic spotting; C) a blotchy type of chlorosis.

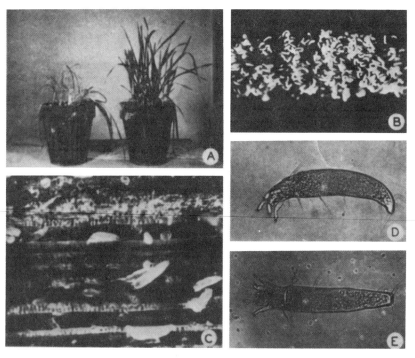

FIG. 2. *A. tulipae* reared on Kharkov 22 M.C. winter wheat. A) mite-infested plants with tightly rolled leaves (left), normal plants (right); B) an extremely heavy population of mites on the outside surface of a tightly rolled leaf; C) eggs and various stages of mites on the upper surface of a wheat leaf; D) lateral view of an adult mite about 250μ long; E) ventral view of adult mite.

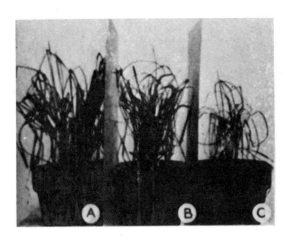

Fig. 4. Kharkov 22 M.C. winter wheat infested with A) non-infective mites, B) mites that acquired wheat streak mosaic virus from manually inoculated wheat, C) mites collected from naturally diseased wheat. The rolling and looping of leaves was caused by the severe infestation of mites. Note the slight stunting and chlorosis in B as compared with the severe stunting, chlorosis and necrosis in C.

colonies that acquired the streak mosaic virus by feeding on manually infected plants (Fig. 4).

The effects of the non-manually transmitted factor were distinguished from wheat streak mosaic in 2 different experiments. When mites from naturally diseased wheat were tested individually for infectiousness on 263 individual wheat plants, severe cholorosis developed on 149 of the latter plants. Wheat streak mosaic could be transmitted artificially from 83 of these chlorotic plants but not from the remaining 66. In another experiment, 10 severely chlorotic and stunted plants were selected from a field of diseased winter wheat. Wheat streak mosaic was transmitted both manually and by mites from only 5 of the plants. Although streak mosaic could not be transmitted from the other 5 plants, mites from them induced severe chlorotic symptoms. As mentioned above, mites originating from eggs hatched on 83 healthy wheat plants caused no severe chlorosis. These results indicate that the chlorosis was caused by an undefined factor, probably virus in nature, that was carried by mites from the naturally diseased plants but was not transmitted manually.

EXPERIMENTS ON THE TRANSMISSION OF WHEAT STREAK MOSAIC WITH A. TULIPAE. —*Transmission of various isolates.*—After non-infective colonies of *A. tulipae* had been established from eggs hatched on healthy plants, it was possible to test the ability of the mites to transmit various isolates of wheat streak mosaic. The isolates included several from various locations in Alberta, a mild and a moderately severe isolate from South Dakota, and the type collection of yellow streak mosaic from Salina, Kansas[4]. Young Kharkov 22 M.C. wheat plants were inoculated manually with the isolates. As soon as symptoms were evident on the inoculated plants, non-infective mites were transferred to them and to healthy check plants. After 10 days on the source plants, about 10 mites were transferred to each of 8 to 24 test plants. Wheat streak mosaic symptoms developed on all the plants colonized with mites that had fed on wheat manually inoculated with any of the isolates, whereas the 18 controls, colonized with the mites that had not fed on diseased wheat, remained healthy. The identity of each isolate was checked by manual transmission to other wheat plants. It was thereby demonstrated that *A. tulipae* from wheat could transmit all the isolates of wheat streak mosaic tested from Alberta, South Dakota and Kansas.

Infective stages of the vector.—Like some other eriophyids (2, 3), *A. tulipae* has 3 instars. Measurements of *A. tulipae* from wheat showed the following size variations in the various stages: eggs $35 \times 42\mu$ to $46 \times 65\mu$, first-instar nymphs $33 \times 80\mu$ to $47 \times 150\mu$, second-instar nymphs $38 \times 140\mu$ to $57 \times 206\mu$, adults $38 \times 173\mu$ to $63 \times 285\mu$. All these stages, including nymphs in the first and second molts, can usually be found on infested wheat. The shortest life cycle observed at about 25°C was 7 days from egg to egg. Males have not been recognized in this species (4).

Tests were made on the infectiveness of all stages of *A. tulipae* reared on streak-mosaic-infected wheat. Two individuals of a stage were transferred to a single wheat seedling growing in a large test tube. Ten plants were infested in this way for each stage of the mite. After 2 weeks in a greenhouse at 20°–25°C. the plants were tested for streak mosaic by manual transmission to healthy plants. The results of 2 experiments showed that all stages of *A. tulipae* except the eggs may be infective. The combined results of the 2 experiments

[4] The isolate was supplied by H. H. McKinney, Senior Pathologist, Division of Cereal Crops and Diseases, Bureau of Plant Industry, United States Department of Agriculture.

show the percentage of plants infected by mites transferred in various stages of development as follows: egg 0, first-instar nymph 30, first molt 55, second-instar nymph 55, second molt 70, adult 35.

Acquisition of the virus.—Experiments described above showed that when *A. tulipae* was reared on diseased wheat all stages except the eggs could be infective. It was therefore evident that first-instar nymphs could acquire wheat streak mosaic virus from diseased plants. However, it was still necessary to determine whether second nymphs and adults could acquire the virus. About 200 eggs, first-instar nymphs, second-instar nymphs and adults respectively from a non-infective colony of mites were placed on separate groups of mite-free plants that had been artificially infected with wheat streak mosaic virus. On each of the following 3 days mites were removed from the various groups and 2 or 3 mites were placed on each of 5 to 7 test plants. The results of this type of experiment repeated on 3 occasions showed that mites that had access to diseased plants only when in the first nymphal instar, including those placed on diseased plants when in the egg stage or first nymphal instar, infected 42 of the 86 plants on which they were tested. Mites that had fed on diseased plants only in the second nymphal instar infected 14 of 49 test plants. However, mites that had fed on diseased plants only after they had become adults old enough to be distinguished with certainty from second nymphs by their larger size and darker color, did not infect any of 63 test plants. Experiments of a preliminary nature showed that nymphs can become infective during a period of 30 minutes on diseased plants, but the actual feeding time was not determined.

Persistence of the virus in the vector.—The persistence of wheat streak mosaic virus in *A. tulipae* was tested by utilizing a *Triticum* $\times$ *Agropyron* hybrid that was a favorable host for the mites but immune from the virus. About 200 nymphs and adult mites were placed on each of 10 of the hybrid plants, and each day for 10 days 3 mites were transferred from each hybrid plant to each of 3 wheat test plants. The development of streak mosaic symptoms on the wheat indicated whether or not the mites were still infective. Two weeks after the mites had been applied to the hybrid plants the latter were all tested by artificial inoculation of wheat to ascertain that they had remained free from virus infection despite the feeding of the infective mites on them. It was found that even though the *Triticum* $\times$ *Agropyron* plants on which the infective mites were colonized remained virus-free, some of the

401

mites remained infective up to 6 days on these immune plants. The life span of the infective mites could not be determined because of the rapid development and overlapping of stages of the new generation of mites; therefore the evidence to date is not sufficient to ascertain whether the infective mites lost infectivity before death.

DISPERSAL OF MITES AND VIRUS.—The incidence of streak mosaic in various parts of infected wheat fields often bore an obvious relationship to the distance and direction from the apparent source of infection. The proportion of infected plants was greatest near the source. Frequently, the incidence was high for a much greater distance eastward than westward from the source, indicating an influence of the prevailing west winds. Since the mites are wingless, the influence of wind could be either direct by blowing the mites from infested plants, or indirect by affecting the direction of flight of insects, such as thrips or aphids, that could conceivably carry the mites.

The direct effect of wind on the spread of mites and wheat streak mosaic was tested by using 10-in. electric fans as sources of wind. A soil bed 12 ft. long, 15 in. wide, and 4 in. deep was prepared in each of 4 separated greenhouse compartments. Wheat was seeded in each bed. After the wheat emerged, potted wheat plants infested with mites and infected with mosaic were placed, with or without a fan, at one end of the respective beds in the following arrangements: 1) the source plants were heavily infested with mites and infected with streak mosaic, but a fan was not used, 2) a fan was placed behind source plants that were heavily infested with mites and infected with streak mosaic, 3) a fan was placed behind source plants that were infested with mites but not infected with streak mosaic, 4) a fan was placed behind source plants that were infected with streak mosaic but free from mites. The fans were operated for approximately 2 hours each day for 1 week. Since the experiment was conducted during early spring, there was little difficulty from insect infestations. However, there were several very windy days during the course of the experiment and absolute control was not maintained over movement of air in the greenhouses. Nevertheless, as shown in Table 1, the influence of the fans on the dispersal of mites from mosaic-infected or mosaic-free plants was striking. There was little spread of mites from mite-infested diseased plants when a fan was not used. When the mites were absent the fan did not spread mosaic from the diseased plants.

A further check on the movement of mites by air

TABLE 1.—*Dispersal of A. tulipae and wheat streak mosaic virus by wind from electric fans*

Source	Symptoms	Percentage of plants developing symptoms at various distances from the source plants						
		1st foot	2nd foot	4th foot	6th foot	8th foot	10th foot	12th foot
Mosaic & mites (no fan)	Leaf roll	48.9	2.0	1.9	1.6	3.9	3.9	2.0
	Mosaic	38.2	2.0	1.9	1.6	5.9	2.0	2.0
Mosaic & mites (fan)	Leaf roll	100.0	100.0	100.0	100.0	100.0	100.0	100.0
	Mosaic	100.0	100.0	100.0	97.0	98.5	95.1	75.0
Mites only (fan)	Leaf roll	100.0	100.0	100.0	100.0	100.0	100.0	100.0
	Mosaic	0.0	0.0	0.0	0.0	0.0	0.0	0.0
Mosaic only (fan)	Leaf roll	0.0	0.0	0.0	0.0	0.0	0.0	0.0
	Mosaic	0.0	0.0	0.0	0.0	0.0	0.0	0.0

was obtained by placing vaseline-coated microscope slides in the path of air blowing past mite-infested wheat in the greenhouse. Mites were caught in the vaseline and could be identified readily with a microscope. Mites have also been caught on vaseline-coated slides exposed on windy days near naturally diseased wheat crops.

Thrips and aphids were frequently present on wheat plants infested with *A. tulipae*, and occasionally mites have been seen clinging to these insects. Experiments were therefore conducted to determine whether thrips or aphids could play a part in spreading the mites and hence streak mosaic. Four double cages were prepared by connecting 2 large cylindrical cages with a 6-in. sleeve of nylon taffeta cloth (Fig. 1, D). Two pots of mite-infested, mosaic-diseased wheat were placed in one side of each of the double cages and 2 pots of young, healthy test plants were placed in the other side. The infested plants were at least 2 ft. from the test plants in the opposite compartment of each cage. The nylon taffeta cloth covering the ventilators and forming the connections between the compartments was of such a close weave that air currents were negligible and hence would not disturb the mites on the plants in the cages. In 2 experiments, about 200 thrips were introduced on the infested plants in 2 of the cages, whereas the other 2 cages were kept thrips-free for controls. Within 3 or 4 days an estimated $\frac{1}{3}$ of the thrips that had been applied to the mite-infested plants had migrated to the 16 test plants in the other compartment of each of the cages, but observations up to 6 weeks later showed no evidence that they had carried mites to the test plants. Similarly attempts to transmit wheat streak mosaic virus from the test plants to other wheat plants failed.

Natural infestations of unidentified species of aphids on diseased mite-infested wheat were employed in 2 experiments on the spread of mites by aphids. Winged aphids flew from the diseased plants to test plants in the opposite compartment of the cages, but subsequent examination and transmission tests for the presence of mosaic virus did not indicate that any mites had been carried to the test plants by the aphids.

Although the above tests gave negative results on the spread of *A. tulipae* by unidentified species of wheat-infesting thrips or aphids, more comprehensive experiments under various environmental conditions and with other species of insects may reveal a relation between insects and the spread of *A. tulipae*.

HOSTS OF MITES AND VIRUS.—Earlier work (8, 9, 11, 12) demonstrated that a number of wild and cultivated grasses can be infected with wheat streak mosaic by manual inoculation. Grass plants other than wheat that have been found naturally infected include the following annuals: *Aegilops cylindrica* Host., *Bromus japonicus* Thunb., *B. tectorum* L., *Cenchrus pauciflorus* Benth., *Echinochloa crusgalli* (L.) Beauv., *Eragrostis cilianensis* (All.) Lutati, *Panicum capillare* L., *P. dichotomiflorum* Michx., and *Setaria viridis* (L.) Beauv. Perennials on which the disease has been found naturally include *Elymus virginicus* L. and *Sitanion hystrix* (Nutt.). More recently the author has found wheat streak mosaic on wild oats (*Avena fatua* L.) and on commercial varieties of barley (*Hordeum vulgare* L.) and oats (*Avena sativa* L.) in Alberta.

The susceptibility of a number of grasses to wheat streak mosaic was compared in the greenhouse by mite transmission as well as by manual inoculation. The series tested by mite transmission was infested by dispersing the mites from the diseased plants with a fan. After a sufficient incubation period, all plants were tested for virus infection by manual transmission to wheat. Non-inoculated plants of each grass were held as controls.

The results of tests on cultivated and wild annual grasses (Table 2) showed that all grasses that were readily infected with the virus by manual inoculation were also readily infected by mites. Among the plants that were more difficult to infect, the cultivated and wild millets and the 2 corn varieties appeared to be more susceptible to infection from mite than from manual inoculation. The mites reproduced and maintained sparse to moderate populations on several grasses including barley, rye, and several species of wild and cultivated millet. The wheat varieties were the only hosts highly susceptible to infestation by the mites.

A number of perennial grasses[5] were also tested for susceptibility to wheat streak mosaic and to the mites. The following grasses did not become infected with the virus by either manual inoculation or mite transmission, and the mites did not become established on them: *Agropyron cristatum* (L.) Gaertn., *A. elongatum* (Host.) Beauv., *A. intermedium* (Host.) Beauv., *A. repens* (L.) Beauv., *A. smithii* Rydb., *A. trachycaulum* (Link) Malte, *Agrostis alba* L., *Bromus inermis* Leyss., *Festuca elatior* L., *F. rubra* L., *Hordeum jubatum* L., *Phleum pratense* L., and *Poa pratensis* L.

[5] Seed obtained from R. W. Peake, Canada Department of Agriculture, Experimental Farms Service, Lethbridge, Alberta.

Table 2.—Susceptibility of annual grasses to wheat streak mosaic and A. tulipae

Species	Variety	Reaction to virus		Susceptibility to mites
		Manual inoculation	Mite inoculation	
CULTIVATED GRASSES				
Avena sativa L.	Victory	M*	M	0
Echinochloa crusgalli L. Beauv.	Japanese millet	M (F)	M	+
Hordeum vulgare L.	Trebi	M	M	+
	Vantage	M	M	+
	O.A.C. 21	M	M	+
Panicum miliaceum L.	Proso millet	M	M	0
Secale cereale L. (winter type)	Dakold	M (F)	M (F)	+
Setaria italica (L.) Beauv.	Hungarian millet	M (F)	M (F)	+
Triticum dicoccum Schrank	Vernal	M (F)	L	++
Triticum durum Desf.	Mindum	M	M	+++
Triticum timopheevi Zhukov.		M	M	++
Triticum aestivum L. (spring types)	Lee	M	M	++++
	Marquis	M	M	+++
	Rescue	M	M	+++++
	Thatcher	M	M	+++++
Triticum aestivum L. (winter types)	Jones' Fife	M	M	+++++
	Kharkov 22 M.C.	M	M	+++++
	Minter	M	M	+++++
	Pawnee	M	M	+++++
	Yogo	M	M	+++
Zea mays L.	Northern Cross	O	L M	+
	Golden Rush	O	L M	0
WILD GRASSES				
Avena fatua L.	Wild oats	M (F)	M (F)	0
Bromus japonicus Thunb.	Japanese chess	M (F)	M (F)	0
Bromus secalinus L.	Cheat	M	M (F)	0
Bromus tectorum L.	Downy brome	M	M (F)	0
Digitaria sanguinalis (L.) Scop.	Crab grass	M (F)	M	0
Echinochloa crusgalli (L.) Beauv.	Barnyard grass	M (F)	M	+
Eragrostis cilianensis (All) Lutati	Stink grass	M (F)	M	+
Panicum capillare L.	Witch grass	M (F)	M (F)	0
Setaria lutescens (Weigel) Hubb.	Yellow foxtail	O	O	0
Setaria verticillata (L.) Beauv.	Bristly foxtail	M (F)	M	+
Setaria viridis (L.) Beauv.	Green foxtail	M (F)	M	+

*M = mosaic symptoms; F = few plants showing symptoms; L = local chlorotic spots; O = no mosaic, or no mites; + = few mites; ++ = moderate survival of mites; +++ = abundance of mites.

Although mites from wheat transmitted the virus to *Elymus canadensis* L., attempts to rear the mites on this grass were not successful. Moderate populations of mites were reared on young plants of *Poa compressa* L. and *Oryzopsis hymenoides* (Roem. & Schult.) Ricker. Both these grasses can be infected with the virus. Mosaic symptoms may develop on *P. compressa*, but *O. hymenoides* is a symptomless carrier (8).

A comparison was made of the susceptibility of 45 *Triticum* × *Agropyron* hybrids[6] to wheat streak mosaic by manual and mite inoculation. All hybrids readily infected by manual inoculation were also readily infected by mite inoculation. The mosaic-susceptible plants were readily colonized by the mites. Several hybrids that did not develop systemic symptoms of streak mosaic developed local lesions, which on the mite-infested plants appeared as a chlorotic speckling. Other hybrids were symptomless carriers. Some of the symptomless carriers of the virus were readily colonized by the mites.

Mites identified as *Aceria tulipae* were found on *Hordeum jubatum, Elymus canadensis,* and *Agropyron smithii* collected in southern Alberta. These grasses occur in spring wheat areas far removed from winter wheat production. *H. jubatum* is especially widespread and common throughout the Canadian spring wheat belt, and mites were found on it in widely scattered locations in Alberta and Saskatchewan. *Elymus canadensis* has occasionally been infected with wheat streak mosaic (8). There was therefore a particular interest in determining whether or not *A. tulipae* from these perennial grasses could be reared on wheat and whether or not *A. tulipae* from wheat could be reared on any of these grasses. Results to date have not shown that these host exchanges can be made, thus indicating that there are different strains of *A. tulipae* and that these 3 grasses are not perennial hosts of the strain found on wheat.

In both South Dakota, U. S. A., and in southern Alberta, Canada, the author has found wheat streak mosaic on spring wheat only in or near districts where winter wheat was grown. This indicates that winter wheat is an important host of the virus and vector. The importance of perennial grasses as harboring hosts in either winter or spring wheat areas has not as yet been determined.

FACTORS INFLUENCING THE SURVIVAL OF MITES AND

---

[6] Tested in co-operation with J. E. Andrews, Canada Department of Agriculture, Experimental Farms Service, Lethbridge, Alberta.

VIRUS.—*Temperature tolerance.*—When *A. tulipae* was first discovered, nothing was known about its means of overwintering nor of the low temperature tolerance of the various stages. The condition of the mites was observed on naturally infested plants collected from fields after major changes in the weather throughout the winters of 1952–53 and 1953–54. The plants were searched for mites within 1 hour after bringing them into the laboratory from out-of-doors. On every date, all stages of the mites, including eggs, could be found in apparently good condition. The majority of the eggs hatched when placed in 100 per cent relative humidity at 25°C.

Mites and eggs were subjected to rapid cooling tests to determine their freezing temperature[7]. When the mites or eggs were placed on the cooling stage and insulated from the surrounding atmosphere by 2 sheets of glass sealed over the stage, they could be observed continuously with a binocular microscope. The temperature was recorded with a thermocouple. Mites were cooled to sub-freezing temperatures in 10–15 minutes, and they could be held as low as −26.0°C for several minutes without freezing. But mites in the nymphal and adult stages, whether reared in the greenhouse or removed directly from field plants in mid-winter, froze at temperatures between −26.5°C and −28.0°C. The eggs did not appear to freeze until the temperature was lowered to about −31.0° or −32.0°C. Some eggs held at −30.7°C for 2.5 minutes without freezing hatched when incubated at room temperature.

The effect of longer periods of sub-freezing temperatures on the survival of mites on winter wheat plants was tested in temperature-controlled rooms. Yogo wheat in 6-in. pots was infested with mites and was hardened by exposure to 5°C for 2 nights, 0°C for 7 nights, and −5°C for 21 nights. During the day, the plants were kept in a greenhouse. After the hardening period, 5 pots of the mite-infested wheat were placed at each of the following temperatures: −5°, −10°, −15°, −20°, and −25°C. Pots of infested plants were subjected to these temperatures for a period of 1, 2, 4, 8, or 16 days. Immediately after removal from the cold rooms, the plants were searched for living mites. Eggs were also removed and tested for hatchability. The wheat plants were placed in the greenhouse and later checked for survival after the cold treatment. Under these conditions the mites and eggs appeared to be considerably more tolerant to low temperatures than

[7] The cooling apparatus was developed by Dr. R. W. Salt, Science Service Laboratory, Lethbridge, Alberta.

TABLE 3.—*Survival of Yogo winter wheat and A. tulipae after exposure to sub-freezing temperatures for various periods of time*

		Time at sub-zero temperatures				
		1 day	2 days	4 days	8 days	16 days
−5° C	Wheat	33ᵃ	20	O	O	O
	Mites	H	H	H	M	M
	Eggs	80	80	65	20	30
−10° C	Wheat	20	O	O	O	O
	Mites	H	H	H	L	O
	Eggs	80	33	82	9	O
−15° C	Wheat	O	O	O	O	O
	Mites	H	M	O	O	O
	Eggs	60	87	25	27	O
−20° C	Wheat	O	O	O	O	O
	Mites	M	O	O	O	O
	Eggs	53	20	18	O	O
−25° C	Wheat	O	O	O	O	O
	Mites	O	O	O	O	O
	Eggs	O	O	O	O	O

ᵃ Numerals indicate percentage of survival of wheat or hatchability of eggs; H = high survival of mites; M = medium survival of mites; L = low survival of mites, i.e., only an occasional living mite; O = no survival of wheat or mites, or no eggs hatchable.

TABLE 4.—*Survival of A. tulipae on detached wheat leaves placed in various humidities at 3 temperatures*

Temp.	R.H. (%)	Days at each temperature and humidity											
		1	2	3	4	5	6	7	8	9	10	11	12
25° C.	0	O*											
	25	O											
	50	L	O										
	75	L	O										
	100	H	H	H	H	H	H	M	M	M	L	L	O
15° C.	0	M	O										
	25	M	O										
	50	M	O										
	75	H	O										
	100	H	H	H	H	H	H	H	M	M	L	L	L
5° C.	0	M	O										
	25	M	L	L	O								
	50	H	H	M	L	O							
	75	H	H	M	M	L	L	L	L	L	O		
	100	H	H	H	H	H	H	H	H	H	H	H	H

* H = high survival, mites appeared normal; M = medium survival; L = low survival; O = no living mites found, all desiccated or overgrown by saprophytic fungi.

the wheat (Table 3). In other experiments[8], healthy Yogo winter wheat showed considerably more tolerance to low temperatures under similar experimental conditions than the mite-infested mosaic-diseased Yogo showed in the above experiment. It is also probable that winter wheat can tolerate lower temperatures under field conditions than under the conditions of these experiments. Nevertheless, it appears likely that the mites or their eggs can survive the lowest temperatures that the varieties of winter wheat grown in Alberta can survive.

Although controlled experiments have not been performed on high temperature tolerance, mites have been reared satisfactoriiy in celluloid cages in the greenhouse during the summer, when the temperature in the cages occasionally approached 50°C.

Humidity tolerance. — The influence of various humidities on the survival of mites on detached leaves placed at 5°, 15°, and 25°C was tested (Table 4). The mites perished sooner at the lower humidities and higher temperatures. Rapid mortality appeared to be directly related to the rapidity with which the mites were desiccated. The mites appeared normal at humidities near 100 per cent at all temperatures until

[8] Unpublished data from experiments performed by Dr. D. W. A. Roberts, Science Service Laboratory, Lethbridge, Alberta.

TABLE 5.—*Hatchability of eggs of A. tulipae held at various humidities and temperatures for different periods of time before incubation at 100 per cent R.H. and 25° C.*

Temp.	R.H. (%)	No. of eggs out of 10 that hatched after exposure to specified humidities and temperatures for							
		1 day	2 days	3 days	4 days	5 days	6 days	7 days	8 days
25° C.	0	0	0	0	0	0	0	----	----
	25	0	0	0	0	0	0	----	----
	50	2	0	0	0	0	0	----	----
	75	10	10	4	0	1	0	----	----
15° C.	0	2	0	0	0	0	0	0	0
	25	2	0	0	0	0	0	0	0
	50	8	0	2	0	0	0	0	0
	75	10	6	7	2	5	0	0	0
	100	10	10	10	10	10	10	10	10
5° C.	0	4	2	0	0	0	0	0	0
	25	5	2	3	7	0	0	0	0
	50	5	3	2	2	2	0	0	0
	75	10	6	10	3	3	3	3	0
	100	10	10	10	10	10	10	10	10

the leaves became chlorotic and began to decompose. Decomposition began more quickly at 25°C than at the lower temperatures, and consequently the mites perished more quickly. The survival of mites appeared to be directly related to the micro-environment supplied by the leaves, and this was determined by the condition of the leaves.

The effect of various humidities on the hatchability of eggs stored on glass slides at 5°, 15°, and 25°C was tested. The eggs were selected from vigorous, young wheat plants infested with a thriving colony of mites. Ten eggs were placed on each of a number of glass slides, which were immediately placed in chambers at the desired humidities and temperatures. Each day a slide was removed from each chamber, examined to note the condition of the eggs, and then placed at 100 per cent R.H. at 25°C. Under these conditions undamaged eggs hatched within 4 days.

Although the eggs hatched readily at 25°C when the relative humidity was near 100 per cent, hatching was almost completely arrested at 15° and 5°C. Similarly, very few eggs hatched even at 25°C when the relative humidity was lowered to about 75 per cent, and none hatched at relative humidities of 50 per cent or lower. The storage of eggs at 100 per cent R.H. for 8 days at 15° or 5°C before removal to 25°C at 100 per cent R.H. was not detrimental to hatchability (Table 5). However, storage at 75 per cent R.H. or lower soon reduced hatchability. Shrivelling and loss of hatchability was most rapid at the lower humidities and higher temperatures.

Age and condition of host plant.—In attempts to rear *A. tulipae* on wheat at various stages of development it was found that the plants were infested very readily up to and during the stooling stage. Infective mites usually caused excessive damage to plants infested in the 1- to 3-leaf stage. Plants not infested until near the heading stage did not support vigorous colonies. It was also apparent in the field that the mites were frequently abundant on immature plants but scarce or absent on plants nearing maturity. A preference was shown for young, succulent tissues of the plant.

A comparison was made of immature and mature wheat plants as natural carriers of *A. tulipae* and wheat streak mosaic. Shortly after harvest, ripe, diseased plants and stubble were collected from a winter wheat crop that had been severely infected with wheat streak mosaic and infested with mites. Volunteer plants in the stooling stage were collected from the edge of the same field. The plants were transplanted into pots. Wheat was seeded in the same pots, which were then placed in separate mite-proof cages. The 21 young plants that grew from seed sown in the 2 pots with the immature wheat became infested with mites and developed wheat streak mosaic. None of the 42 plants that grew from seed in 4 pots with mature, diseased wheat, or the 28 plants in 3 pots with stubble from diseased plants, showed any evidence of mites or wheat streak mosaic.

An additional comparison was made of stubble and young plants as carriers of mites and wheat streak mosaic. Pots of Kharkov 22 M.C. wheat grown to the 1-leaf stage in the greenhouse were placed in various positions in a field. Some pots were placed beside spring-planted winter wheat that had remained vegetative until late fall and had become infested with *A. tulipae* and infected with wheat streak mosaic. Other pots were placed in various positions in a strip of clean summerfallow 53 yd. wide located east of the immature wheat. Two other pots were placed in a plot of stubble left from a mosaic-infected winter wheat crop that had been harvested in mid-August. After a set of pots had been in the field for 1 week it was replaced by a new set. Plants taken from the field were put in the greenhouse where they were fumigated with nico-fume to reduce the danger of mites spreading from plant to plant. Observations were made periodically for about 3 weeks, and the development of streak mosaic symptoms was recorded as an indication of the spread of mites with the virus in the field.

The infections resulting among the 12 plants in each of 1–3 pots exposed for 1 week at each location in the field are shown in Table 6. Since the results from plants exposed on successive weeks were often very similar, the data for several of the alternating weeks are omitted from the table to save space. The data show that when the pots of test plants were placed near the immature, diseased wheat a high percentage of plants became infected. The farther the pots were from the immature wheat, the fewer the plants that became infected. There was no evidence that the stubble of a diseased crop acted as a source of virus or mites. The rate of virus spread also varied considerably with the date. From 70 per cent to 100 per cent of the test plants became infected in pots exposed near the immature, diseased wheat for a week at any time from early August to mid-October, but after the latter date the percentage of infection dropped off rapidly to nil by the end of November. This reduced rate of spread late in the fall season was probably related to the effects of cool weather on the mites.

Earlier experiments with streak mosaic showed that the virus could not be recovered by manual transmission from mature wheat plants (10, 12). Mature plants are also not suitable hosts for *A. tulipae*. It therefore appears safe to conclude that stubble or mature plants are not a source of mosaic or mite infestation in the field. On the other hand, volunteer or other immature wheat at the edge of fields or in summerfallows may become infested with mites carrying the virus, and such infected plants are the real danger to the new crops of winter wheat.

Destruction of the host by cultivation.—Frequently the summerfallow land on which winter wheat is to be planted is infested with volunteer wheat that is diseased and infested with mites. Occasionally a field of winter wheat appears so severely damaged with wheat streak mosaic by late spring that it is advisable to destroy it and plant a spring crop. In both of the above situations the diseased, mite-infested plants are a menace to wheat that may be planted in the same field; hence the diseased plants must be destroyed. However, it has been noticed that wheat emerging soon after diseased plants were destroyed by cultivation often develop the disease. Earlier work showed that wheat streak mosaic virus loses infectivity rapidly in plant tissues that have begun to decompose (12). On the other hand, the virus can remain infectious for a

TABLE 6.—Spread of streak mosaic to young greenhouse-grown wheat exposed in pots near fields of diseased wheat for weekly periods from early August to late November

Position of pots of wheat in the field	Percentage plants infected when exposed for week starting						
	Aug. 24	Sept. 11	Sept. 26	Oct. 9	Oct. 16	Oct. 30	Nov. 13
1. Edge of patch of spring seeded winter wheat naturally infected with streak mosaic	88.8	100.0	70.0	97.3	48.6	28.2	3.7
2. In summerfallow strip, 8 yards east of #1	75.0	85.0	11.7	23.8	4.1	0.0	0.0
3. In summerfallow strip, 18 yards east of #1	70.8	63.6	4.1	15.0	12.5	9.0	0.0
4. At edge of winter wheat stubble, 50 yards east of #1	0.0	20.0	0.0	0.0	0.0	0.0	0.0
5. 35 yards within winter wheat stubble 90 yards east of #1	4.1	14.2	0.0	0.0	7.6	0.0	0.0

considerable time in plant tissues that have dried rapidly (7, 10). However, the loss or retention of infectivity of the virus in plant tissues is of little consequence unless the vector can survive to infest a subsequent crop of wheat.

Experiments in the greenhouse showed that mites could survive long enough on diseased wheat plants severed from their roots and mixed with the surface soil to infest wheat plants emerging from seed sown in the soil several days later. The proportion of young plants infested in this manner was influenced by the depth to which the infested leaves were buried, the temperature and the moisture of the soil, and the date of seeding.

The significant influence of covering infested leaves with soil on the degree of infestation of wheat sown in the soil was strikingly illustrated in experiments in the greenhouse. Twenty-five wheat seeds were sown 2 in. deep the same day that infested wheat leaves were added at various levels to the soil in 8 in. pots. There were 4 replicates of each treatment. The pots were watered and held in a greenhouse at a temperature of about 20°C. After the wheat had emerged, a high percentage of plants became infested with mites and developed wheat streak mosaic in the pots in which the infested leaves had been left on the surface of the soil (Table 7). Infestation and disease were strikingly reduced when the leaves were buried under as little as 1 in. of soil, and only a trace of mite-infestation occurred when the leaves were buried to greater depths.

The influence of various temperatures and moistures on the survival of mites on infested plants left on the surface or covered with soil was compared. A loam soil was used in the experiment. The soil for the dry series was thoroughly air-dried and for the wet series liberally watered for several days before the beginning of the experiment. About 10 g. of mite-infested mosaic-diseased wheat leaves were added to each 6-in. pot of soil.

TABLE 7.—*A. tulipae infestation and streak mosaic infection in wheat sown 2 in. deep in soil to which mite-infested, diseased wheat leaves were added on the surface and at various depths below the surface*

Position of infested trash in the soil	Percentage mite infestation	Percentage streak mosaic
On surface	100.0	100.0
1″ below surface	19.4	43.5
2″ below surface	19.0	34.5
3″ below surface	3.8	9.0
4″ below surface	3.7	7.5

TABLE 8.—*Survival of A. tulipae on infested leaves added to the surface or incorporated in wet and dry soil at various above-freezing temperatures*

Temp.	Days after placing infested leaves on the soil											
	0	1	2	4	6	8	10	12	14	16	18	20
A. Infested leaves covered by about 1 in. of soil												
Soil wet												
25° C.	H[a]	H	H	M	O							
20° C.	H	H	H	H	H	H	M	O				
15° C.	H	H	H	H	H	H	H	L	O			
10° C.	H	H	H	H	H	H	H	H	H	M	M	
Soil dry												
25° C.	H	H	H	H	M	L	O					
20° C.	H	H	H	H	M	L	O					
15° C.	H	H	H	H	H	H	M	L	O			
10° C.	H	H	H	H	H	H	H	M	M	L	O	
B. Infested leaves placed on the surface of the soil												
Soil wet												
25° C.	H	H	H	M	M	M	L	O				
20° C.	H	H	H	H	M	M	M	L	O			
15° C.	H	H	H	H	H	H	M	M	L	L	O	O
10° C.	H	H	H	H	H	H	H	H	M	L	O	O
Soil dry												
25° C.	H	L	L	O								
20° C.	H	M	M	L	O							
15° C.	H	H	H	M	L	O						
10° C.	H	H	H	H	M	M	L	O				

[a] H = high survival of mites; M = medium survival; L = low survival; O = no living mites found, all desiccated or overgrown by saprophytic fungi.

The leaves were covered with 1 in. of soil in one experiment and left on the surface of the soil in the other. Pots of each treatment were kept in rooms with temperatures of 10°, 15°, 20°, and 25°C. The leaves in each treatment were examined periodically until there were no longer any living mites. It was found that the mites survived a few days longer at the lower than at the higher temperatures (Table 8). They survived longer on leaves under moist than under dry conditions at the lower temperatures. At the higher temperatures the mites survived longer in dry than in moist soil when the leaves were buried, but when they were left on the surface of the soil the mites survived longer under moist conditions. These results are in accordance with earlier experiments, which indicated that the rate of destruction of mites on infested leaves is related to the rate of desiccation or decomposition of the host leaves.

Tests were made on the carry-over of infestations to wheat seeded in 2 pots of each treatment at intervals of 1 or 2 days up to 20 days after infested leaves were added to the soil under the conditions of the preceding experiment. The least carry-over of infestation occurred when the leaves were buried in moist soil kept at 25°C. A high degree of carry-over of infestation occurred at all temperatures from 10°–25°C when the leaves were added near the surface of soil that was kept dry until the date of seeding. Under these conditions the rate of infestation was high on wheat seeded the same day on which the infested leaves were added to the soil, but it dropped off rapidly on wheat seeded 1 or more days later. No infection occurred on wheat seeded more than 6 days after the infested leaves had been added to the soil.

As yet, controlled experiments on the elimination of the mites by cultivation have not been performed in the field. Obviously weather conditions will influence the results of various methods of cultivation. However, the experiments in the greenhouse have indicated some hazards in seeding wheat without taking adequate precautions for eliminating volunteer or other infested wheat long enough before seeding to ensure complete elimination of the mites. Under field conditions this may necessitate the keeping of land free from green growth for more than a week before seeding. Field experiments may show the relative merits of various methods of cultivation.

DISCUSSION.—The study of the spread of wheat streak mosaic and its vector *Aceria tulipae* in southern Alberta has indicated the paramount importance of wheat, and especially winter wheat, in the perpetuation of the disease. Although a number of wild grasses and cultivated plants can be infected with the virus, both manually and by the vector, wheat is the host most susceptible to the virus and it is the most suitable host known for the rapid multiplication of the strain of *A. tulipae* associated with the disease on wheat. As wheat streak mosaic has not been found on spring wheat in areas where winter wheat is not grown, it appears that winter wheat is important for the overwintering and propagation of the vector and the disease. Some perennial grasses may be of some importance in the perpetuation of both the virus and the vector.

The important phases in the annual cycle of wheat streak mosaic appear to be associated with living wheat plants. Winter wheat that becomes infested with

417

the mites and thus infected with the disease in the fall carries the vector and the virus over winter. Next spring and summer the mites continue to multiply on infested wheat and carry the disease to any susceptible host nearby, such as spring wheat, volunteer wheat of any type, and some annual grass weeds. Infestations may build up during the summer on volunteer wheat growing in summerfallow land adjacent to diseased crops. Even when the summerfallow is cultivated, young plants emerging within a few days can become infested with mites that have not yet perished on the infested plants uprooted by the cultivation. In addition, a few plants often survive the cultivation and so perpetuate the vector and the disease. If the summerfallow is not kept free from infested volunteer wheat for a sufficient period before a new winter wheat crop is planted on the same land, a serious infestation of mites and the disease may result.

The dates for seeding winter wheat appear to be of considerable importance, in that the earlier seedings are more subject to severe infection. This may be attributed to a greater abundance of mite-infested, diseased plants, including spring wheat, in the summer and early fall, more favorable conditions for dispersal of mites, and a longer period during which the mites can infect new plants before the onset of winter.

Effective control measures for wheat streak mosaic in southern Alberta are both simple in principle and compatible with recommended agronomic practices. Fields in or near which winter wheat is to be seeded should be kept free from volunteer wheat long enough before seeding the new crop to ensure complete elimination of the mites that carry the virus. It is important to avoid seeding winter wheat before spring wheat is mature in adjacent fields. A helpful precaution is to avoid seeding winter wheat before early September in areas where wheat streak mosaic is a threat.

If the disease is controlled satisfactorily in winter wheat it will not be a problem in spring wheat. Spring wheat should not be planted adjacent to severely diseased winter wheat. It is possible to replace a severely diseased winter wheat crop with spring wheat if it can be efficiently destroyed soon enough to ensure elimination of the mites before the spring wheat is seeded.

SUMMARY

The eriophyid mite *Aceria tulipae* Keifer was proved an efficient vector of wheat streak mosaic virus (*Marmor virgatum* McK.). Evidence was obtained that this mite often carries an additional factor possibly a virus that also causes severe chlorosis, necrosis, and stunting of wheat. Unlike wheat streak mosaic virus, this factor has not been transmitted manually. The mites themselves caused a longitudinal rolling of wheat leaves but they did not cause chlorosis unless they became numerous.

When *A. tulipae* was reared on diseased wheat, all stages except the eggs carried wheat streak mosaic virus. Nymphs could acquire the virus, but the older adults could not. The virus persisted in the vector for at least 6 days.

Wind was shown to be a major factor in the dispersal of *A. tulipae* and hence of wheat streak mosaic virus.

A. tulipae transmitted wheat streak mosaic virus to the species of wild and cultivated grasses that were readily infected by manual inoculation. Corn and several species of wild millets were more readily infected with the virus by mite transmission than by manual inoculation. Although the mites could be reared on barley, rye, and several wild annual grasses, wheat was the most favorable host tested. The mites were also reared on the perennial grasses *Poa compressa* L. and *Oryzopsis hymenoides* (Roem. & Schult.) Ricker, both of which can be infected with the virus. Although *A. tulipae* was found in nature on *Hordeum jubatum* L., *Agropyron smithii* Rydb., and *Elymus canadensis* L., attempts to rear mites from these grasses on wheat were unsuccessful. Similarly, attempts to rear mites from wheat on these grasses failed.

All stages of *A. tulipae* survived the winter on winter wheat. The mites survived lower temperatures than hardy varieties of winter wheat artificially hardened and exposed to various subfreezing temperatures in temperature-controlled rooms.

Experiments and observations have indicated that mite infestations, and hence the danger of streak mosaic infection, can be eliminated by destroying infested living wheat plants by cultivation. However, mites survived long enough on infested leaves buried in or placed on the surface of soil to infest wheat seeded 6 days later. Since the mites soon perished on leaves that became desiccated or partially decomposed, the rate at which the mites were eliminated was influenced by temperature and moisture conditions in the soil.

1. Amos, J., R. G. Hatton, R. C. Knight, and A. M. Massee. 1927. Experiments in the transmission of "Reversion" in black currants. Ann. Rept. East Malling Res. Stat. 1925, II Supplement, 126-150.
2. Bailey, S. F., and H. H. Keifer. 1943. The tomato russet mite, Phyllocoptes destructor Keifer: its present status. Jour. Econ. Entom. **36**: 706-712.
3. Hassan, A. S. 1928. The biology of the Eriophyidae, with special reference to Eriophyes tristriatus (Nalepa). U. of Cal. Publ. in Ent. **4**: 341-394.
4. Keifer, H. H. 1938. Eriophyid studies. Bul. Dept. Agr., State of Calif. **27**: 181-206.
5. Massee, A. M. 1925. Entomology.—Programme of research with brief progress reports. Ann. Rept. East Malling Res. Stat., 1924: 139-142.
6. Massee, A. M. 1927. Entomology.—Ann. Rept. East Malling Res. Stat. 1926: 63-65.
7. McKinney, H. H. 1947. Stability of labile viruses in desiccated tissue. Phytopathology **37**: 139-142.
8. McKinney, H. H. and H. Fellows. 1951. Wild and forage grasses found to be susceptible to the wheat streak-mosaic virus. U. S. Dept. Agr. Pl. Dis. Reptr. **35**: 441-442.
9. McKinney, H. H., and W. J. Sando. 1951. Susceptibility and resistance to the wheat streak-mosaic virus in the genera Triticum, Agropyron, Secale and certain hybrids. U. S. Dept. Agr. Pl. Dis. Reptr. **35**: 476-479.
10. Sill, W. H., Jr. 1953. Some characteristics of the wheat streak-mosaic virus and disease. Trans. Kans. Acad. Sci. **56**: 418-424.
11. Sill, W. H., Jr., and R. V. Connin. 1953. Summary of the known host range of the wheat streak mosaic virus. Trans. Kans. Acad. Sci. **56**: 411-417.
12. Slykhuis, J. T. 1952. Virus diseases of cereal crops in South Dakota. South Dakota Ag. Exp. Sta. Tech. Bul. 11.
13. Slykhuis, J. T. 1953. Wheat streak mosaic in Alberta and factors related to its spread. Can. Jour. Agr. Sci. **33**: 195-197.